NETTER'S ATLAS OF HUMAN EMBRYOLOGY

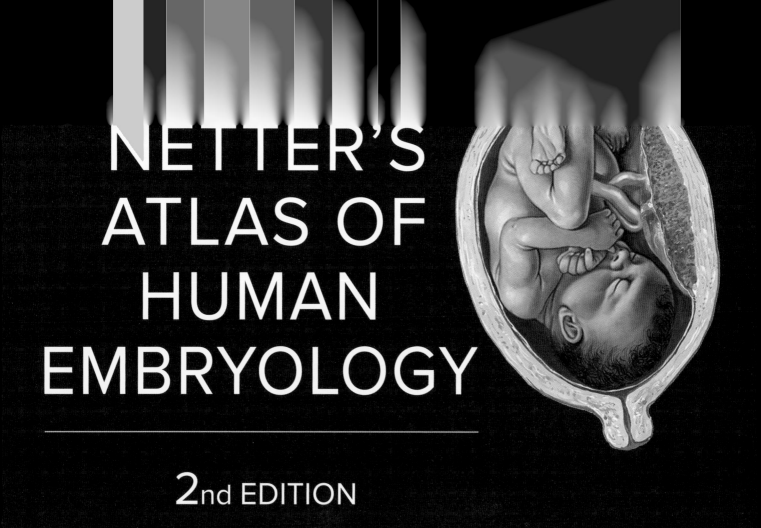

NETTER'S ATLAS OF HUMAN EMBRYOLOGY

2nd EDITION

Larry R. Cochard, PhD

Associate Professor (Retired), Medical Education

Feinberg School of Medicine, Northwestern University

Chicago, Illinois

Angelique N. Dueñas, PhD

Assistant Professor, Medical Education

Feinberg School of Medicine, Northwestern University

Chicago, Illinois

Illustrations by

Frank H. Netter, MD

Contributing Illustrators

Carlos A. G. Machado, MD

John A. Craig, MD

Tiffany S. DaVanzo, MA, CMI

Paul Kim, MS, CMI

DragonFly Media

Kristen W. Marzejon, CMI

James A. Perkins, MS, MFA

ELSEVIER

Elsevier
1600 John F. Kennedy Blvd.
Ste 1800
Philadelphia, PA 19103-2899

NETTER'S ATLAS OF HUMAN EMBRYOLOGY, SECOND EDITION   ISBN: 978-0-443-11761-9

Copyright © 2025 by Elsevier Inc. All rights reserved.

Notice

Previous edition copyrighted 2012.

Publisher: Elyse O'Grady
Senior Content Strategist: Marybeth Thiel
Publishing Services Manager: Shereen Jameel
Senior Project Manager: Mani Chandrasekaran
Design Direction: Patrick Ferguson

Printed in India

Last digit is the print number: 9   8   7   6   5   4   3   2   1

Working together
to grow libraries in
developing countries

www.elsevier.com • www.bookaid.org

To **Dr. David Langebartel**

As my teacher and mentor at the University of Wisconsin—Madison, he stressed the relationship between embryology and adult anatomy, and he did so with energy, authority, and a considerable amount of humor.

And to the memory of
Dr. Leslie B. Arey

He was a colleague at the beginning of my career at Northwestern. It was a privilege and a very humbling experience for a young, green anatomist to teach with the 20th-century master of embryology, anatomy, and histology.

-Larry R. Cochard, PhD

To **Dr. Lisa M.J. Lee**

As my teacher and mentor at the University of Colorado Anschutz Medical Campus, she introduced me to not just the wonders of embryology, but also encouraged me on my path to becoming an anatomy educator. I will always remember your words of "trust your gut(tube)!"

-Angelique N. Dueñas, PhD

PREFACE

The goals of the first edition remain. This book is intended for first-year medical students, dental students, and other beginning students of embryology. As an atlas, it is a showcase for the incomparable artwork of Dr. Frank H. Netter. The theme throughout this book is an emphasis on morphological patterns in the embryo and how they relate to the organization and function of structures in the adult. Another important focus is the embryological basis of congenital birth defects. Descriptive embryology can be an educational goal, but the study of embryology is more effective, rewarding, and relevant when it is placed in a biological or clinical context that goes beyond the embryo itself. The focus on morphological themes in prenatal development makes it easier to learn adult anatomy and to understand an abnormality in a patient. In keeping with this idea, this *Atlas* contains some Netter plates of adult anatomy. These include parts of the body where complex anatomy has embryonic relevance. They also provide context to help show the relationships between primordia and derivatives.

Like anatomy, embryology is a very visual subject that lends itself to an atlas format. Embryological pictures can also be difficult and frustrating for students because of the three-dimensional complexity of the embryo and the unfamiliar structures, terminology, and relationships. To address this problem, the book consists of more than just labeled images. It contains tables, schematics, concepts, descriptive captions, summaries, chapter glossaries, and concise text at the bottom of each page that address the major events and processes of normal and abnormal development. Histological principles are briefly covered to help the uninitiated understand the many references to embryonic tissues in this book.

Little was known about the genetic and molecular basis of development when Dr. Netter drew most of his illustrations, and an atlas is not the ideal medium to convey this type of information. We believe it is important, though, to introduce the subject and include examples of the control of development. Illustrations from the *Atlas* are used to introduce cellular, molecular, and genetic concepts such as induction, apoptosis, growth factors, and genetic patterning and determination. These are, by necessity, selective and include major events (e.g., limb development, segmentation of the head) or processes that have broad significance in development (e.g., the interactions between epithelia and connective tissue in organ development).

The terminology tables at the end of each chapter include major structures, potentially confusing structures, and histological or anatomical terms that provide context. The glossary is also an opportunity to include terms that did not make it into a chapter or to elaborate on important ones. Another effective learning tool is an appendix at the end of the book that summarizes all of the major congenital anomalies and their embryonic basis.

Chapter 1 is an overview of the major developmental periods, events, and processes and ends with a section on the mechanisms of nonnormal development and the classification of anomalies. Chapter 2 addresses gastrulation, the vertebrate body plan, and the placenta. Chapters 3 through 8 are organized by systems and include congenital anomalies. Chapter 9 is on the head and neck region. Changes in this second edition enhance the goals of the first edition by improving the communication of key points and making them more informative for clinical practice. These include more clinical content in general, plus blue clinical boxes in the text to emphasize key points. There are new topics, such as early pregnancy detection and twinning, and more on congenital anomalies, including exstrophy of the bladder, holoprosencephaly, and amelia.

Finally, this second edition provides an opportunity to focus on placing the content in a context of representation, diversity, and inclusion. While maintaining the Netter style, new and updated illustrations address racial and ethnic diversity by including broader representation of skin tones. Specific "Inclusion and Bias Consideration Points" at the start of many chapters also encourage readers to consider and reflect on the biases that frequently exist in teaching, learning, and clinical practice when it comes to embryology. These include points on the differences between sex and gender, particularly for the embryology of sex determination (Chapter 7, "The Urogenital System"), and comments on perspectives around disability and disability advocacy, including recognition of person-first vs. identity-first language, which is particularly important when discussing congenital conditions in many organ systems. We hope the changes in this second edition contribute to further reflection and discussion of how anatomy and embryology can work to provide better representation and inclusion for all people.

This annotated *Atlas* can serve as a bridge between the material presented in the classroom and the detail found in textbooks, and in a way that hopefully fosters diversity and inclusiveness. It can also be useful for board exam review. More than anything, this *Atlas* is about the art of Dr. Netter. The clarity, realism, and beauty of his illustrations make the study of embryology more enlightening and enjoyable.

-Larry R. Cochard, PhD

-Angelique N. Dueñas, PhD

ABOUT THE AUTHORS

Larry R. Cochard, PhD, is a retired Associate Professor of Medical Education and Assistant Professor of Cell and Molecular Biology in the Office of Medical Education and Faculty Development at the Northwestern University Feinberg School of Medicine, where he taught embryology, anatomy, and histology from 1982 to 2021. He has won numerous Outstanding Teacher awards at Northwestern as one of the top five teachers selected by the combined M1 and M2 classes. He is a three-time winner of the American Medical Women's Association Gender Equity Award for teaching, and a four-time winner of the George H. Joost award for M1 basic science teacher of the year. He is a biological anthropologist with research interests in the development and evolution of the primate skull.

Angelique N. Dueñas, PhD, is an Assistant Professor in the Department of Medical Education at the Northwestern University Feinberg School of Medicine, where she teaches embryology, anatomy, ultrasound, and medical education content in the MD and PA programs. She has won numerous Outstanding Teaching awards since joining Northwestern for her teaching in the anatomical sciences. She has a background in anatomy education research from her Master's of Modern Human Anatomy and Teaching Certificate in Anatomical Sciences Education (University of Colorado Anschutz Medical Campus), where her interest in embryology started. Her doctorate work (Hull York Medical School, York, England) focused on diversity, equity, and inclusion in medical and anatomy education, with particular emphasis on qualitative methodologies to better understand these principles.

ACKNOWLEDGMENTS

First Edition:

Many people made my job easier and made this a better book. I thank the following faculty and students at the Feinberg School of Medicine for providing helpful comments, edits, and/or answers to a continuous string of questions: Dr. James Baker, Dr. Bob Berry, Dr. Joel Charrow, Jeff Craft, Dr. Marian Dagosto, Aaron Hogue, Najeeb Khan, Dr. Jim Kramer, Kelly Ormond, Dr. Randy Perkins, Dr. Matt Ravosa, Dr. Brian Shea, Dr. Al Telser, and Dr. Jay Thomas. I also thank the following reviewers who were instrumental in helping to shape the content of the book. The first edition reviewers were:

- Wojciech Pawlina, MD, Mayo School of Medicine

- Thomas A. Marino, PhD, Temple University School of Medicine

- Daniel O. Graney, PhD, University of Washington School of Medicine

- Leslie Gartner, PhD, University of Maryland Dental School

- Bruce Carlson, MD, PhD, University of Michigan

- Andreas H. Weiglein, MD, Karl-Franzens Universität Graz

- Ronald W. Dudek, PhD, Brody School of MedicineEast Carolina University

I assume full responsibility for any errors or inaccuracies that may remain.

Contributing artists added new illustrations in the "Netter style" to both editions. That their plates blend so well in the book is a tribute to their skill. We thank them for their important role in carrying on the Netter tradition.

I am grateful to Angelique Dueñas for agreeing to coauthor this second edition and for being such a wonderful colleague in her first year at Northwestern Feinberg School of Medicine. Her academic interests in embryology plus inclusion and bias in education were a perfect fit for the book. We both thank Elyse O'Grady from Elsevier for initiating this second edition, and Marybeth Thiel for her editorial skill at helping us make this a more relevant and useful book.

The most important contributor to both editions of the book was my wife, Suzy. The project was so much easier because of her support, patience, and encouragement, and for that she has my profound gratitude.

Last but not least, I thank my students for their perceptive questions about embryology that have made me a better teacher. I also thank them for putting up with my insistence that the secret to understanding the embryo is understanding the difference between somatopleure and splanchnopleure!

-Larry R. Cochard, PhD

As noted, many people made our job easier and made this a better book. A special thanks to Elyse, Marybeth, and the whole Elsevier team, especially the artists. I commend their support and hard work to make this edition more representative for so many people.

I would also like to give special thanks to Larry Cochard for offering the opportunity to collaborate and contribute to this edition. For an early-career anatomist and fellow embryology enthusiast, this was a dream project!

A special acknowledgment to those who have supported me, professionally and personally, so that I felt empowered to take on this opportunity when offered. Dr. Lisa M.J. Lee (noted in the dedication) and Professor Gabrielle Finn—thank you for the years of mentorship and support. And to my family, particularly my parents (Ricardo and Janet), who encouraged me to follow my educational dreams.

And lastly, to my students, whose commitment to their education and future patients inspires me on the daily basis. Thanks for your questions, ideas on how to represent embryology better visually, and your enthusiastic engagement (even when I break out the Play-Doh to teach cardiac looping!).

-Angelique N. Dueñas

ABOUT THE ARTISTS

Frank H. Netter, MD

Frank H. Netter was born in 1906 in New York City. He studied art at the Art Students League and the National Academy of Design before entering medical school at New York University, where he received his MD degree in 1931. During his student years, Dr. Netter's notebook sketches attracted the attention of the medical faculty and other physicians, allowing him to augment his income by illustrating articles and textbooks. He continued illustrating as a sideline after establishing a surgical practice in 1933, but he ultimately opted to give up his practice in favor of a full-time commitment to art. After service in the United States Army during World War II, Dr. Netter began his long collaboration with the CIBA Pharmaceutical Company (now Novartis Pharmaceuticals). This 45-year partnership resulted in the production of the extraordinary collection of medical art so familiar to physicians and other medical professionals worldwide.

In 2005, Elsevier, Inc. purchased the Netter Collection and all publications from Icon Learning Systems. There are now more than 50 publications featuring the art of Dr. Netter available through Elsevier, Inc.

Dr. Netter's works are among the finest examples of the use of illustration in the teaching of medical concepts. The 13-book Netter Collection of Medical Illustrations, which includes the greater part of the more than 4000 paintings created by Dr. Netter, became and remains one of the most famous medical works ever published. Netter's *Atlas of Human Anatomy*, first published in 1989, presents the anatomical paintings from the Netter Collection. Now translated into 16 languages, it is the anatomy atlas of choice among students of the medical and health professions across the world.

The Netter illustrations are appreciated not only for their aesthetic qualities but, more importantly, for their intellectual content. As Dr. Netter wrote in 1949, "…clarification of a subject is the aim and goal of illustration. No matter how beautifully painted, how delicately and subtly rendered a subject may be, it is of little value as a medical illustration if it does not serve to make clear some medical point." Dr. Netter's planning, conception, point of view, and approach are what inform his paintings and what makes them so intellectually valuable.

Frank H. Netter, MD, physician and artist, died in 1991.

Learn more about the physician-artist whose work has inspired the Netter Reference collection: https://netterimages.com/artist-frank-h-netter.html

Carlos A.G. Machado, MD

Carlos Machado was chosen by Novartis to be Dr. Netter's successor. He continues to be the main artist who contributes to the Netter collection of medical illustrations.

Self-taught in medical illustration, cardiologist Carlos Machado has contributed meticulous updates to some of Dr. Netter's original plates and has created many paintings of his own in the style of Netter as an extension of the Netter Collection. Dr. Machado's photorealistic expertise and his keen insight into the physician–patient relationship inform his vivid and unforgettable visual style. His dedication to researching each topic and subject he paints places him among the premier medical illustrators at work today.

Learn more about his background and see more of his art at https://netterimages.com/artist-carlos-a-g-machado.html

CONTENTS

1

OVERVIEW OF DEVELOPMENTAL EVENTS, PROCESSES, AND ANOMALIES

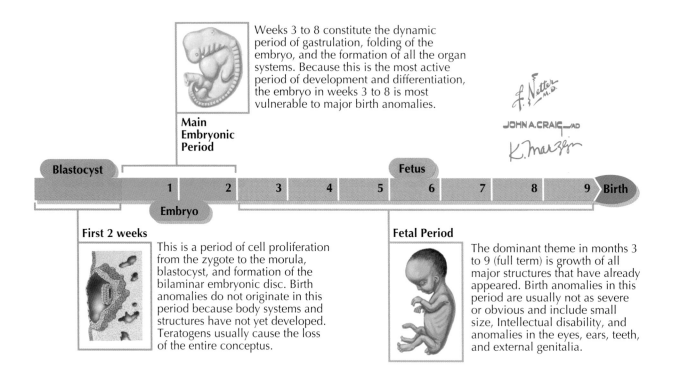

PRENATAL TIME SCALE (MONTHS)

Weeks 3 to 8 constitute the dynamic period of gastrulation, folding of the embryo, and the formation of all the organ systems. Because this is the most active period of development and differentiation, the embryo in weeks 3 to 8 is most vulnerable to major birth anomalies.

Main Embryonic Period

Blastocyst

Fetus

| 1 | 2 | 3 | 4 | 5 | 6 | 7 | 8 | 9 | Birth |

Embryo

First 2 weeks

This is a period of cell proliferation from the zygote to the morula, blastocyst, and formation of the bilaminar embryonic disc. Birth anomalies do not originate in this period because body systems and structures have not yet developed. Teratogens usually cause the loss of the entire conceptus.

Fetal Period

The dominant theme in months 3 to 9 (full term) is growth of all major structures that have already appeared. Birth anomalies in this period are usually not as severe or obvious and include small size, Intellectual disability, and anomalies in the eyes, ears, teeth, and external genitalia.

1.1 TIMELINE

PRIMORDIUM

The zygote is the beginning of human development.

OVERVIEW

Prenatal development can be divided into a period of cell division (weeks 1 and 2 after fertilization), an embryonic period (weeks 2 through 8), and a fetal period (weeks 9 through 38). In the first 2 weeks after fertilization, a blastocyst develops and sinks into the mucosal lining of the uterus during implantation. It consists of a two-layered embryonic disc of cells and three membranes that are external to it (trophoblast/chorion, amnion, and yolk sac). Most of the organ systems develop in the main embryonic period through week 8, and the embryo assumes a human appearance. The fetal period occupies the last 7 months. It is a period of growth and elaboration of organs that are already present. Three categories of genes (maternal effect, segmentation, and homeotic) establish patterns and tissue fates in the embryo, and dynamic interactions between cells characterize the differentiation and development of organs. Nonnormal development can be classified by the cause (e.g., genetic versus environmental), by the mechanism of the effect on a structure or tissue, by the relationship between anomalies, and by their severity.

INCLUSION AND BIAS CONSIDERATION: THE TERMINOLOGY OF "ABNORMALITIES"

This chapter aims to introduce basic embryonic processes and the bases of what were commonly called "abnormalities". An important part of this is to recognize the power of language and discourse in clinical communication. Although it is essential clinically to understand the bases of embryonic anomalies, particularly differentiating between the categorization of anomalies, it is important to always use terminology with sensitivity. Historically, presentation and research of congenital conditions has been used as a proxy to perpetuate stereotypes and biases against individuals affected by such conditions and to make assumptions about quality of life and patient care. It is important to understand the marginalization and treatment of these groups and to always be sensitive in the use of terminology. For example, some educators now prefer to use the terms "atypical", "nonnormal", "anomalous", or "variable" in embryology education to challenge perceptions of "normal versus abnormal."

CLINICAL POINT

Clinicians divide pregnancy into three equal trimesters: the first trimester (3 months) is for organ development, the second trimester is for organ system maturation, and the third trimester marks potential fetal viability outside the womb.

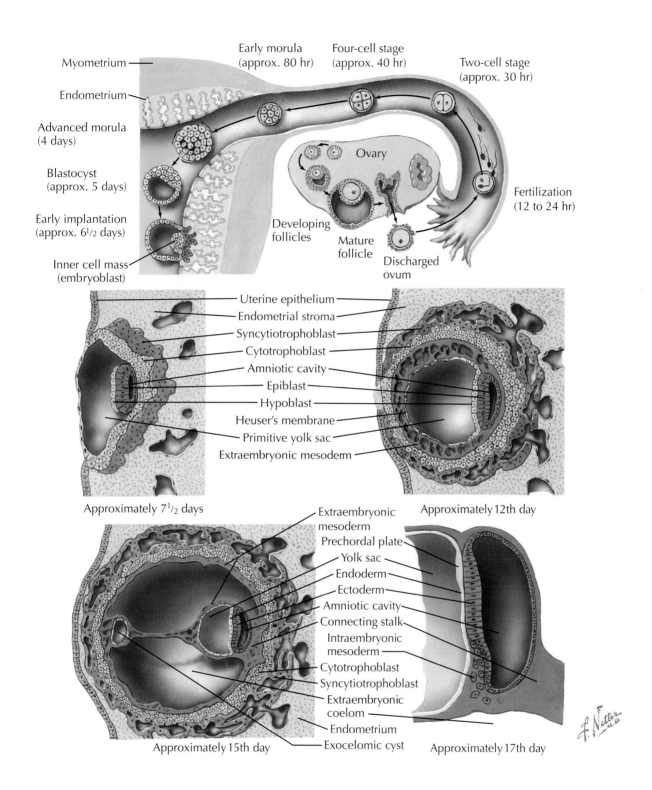

Myometrium

Endometrium

Advanced morula
(4 days)

Blastocyst
(approx. 5 days)

Early implantation
(approx. 6½ days)

Inner cell mass
(embryoblast)

Early morula
(approx. 80 hr)

Four-cell stage
(approx. 40 hr)

Two-cell stage
(approx. 30 hr)

Ovary

Developing
follicles

Mature
follicle

Discharged
ovum

Fertilization
(12 to 24 hr)

Uterine epithelium
Endometrial stroma
Syncytiotrophoblast
Cytotrophoblast
Amniotic cavity
Epiblast
Hypoblast
Heuser's membrane
Primitive yolk sac
Extraembryonic mesoderm

Approximately 7½ days

Approximately 12th day

Extraembryonic
mesoderm
Prechordal plate
Yolk sac
Endoderm
Ectoderm
Amniotic cavity
Connecting stalk
Intraembryonic
mesoderm
Cytotrophoblast
Syncytiotrophoblast
Extraembryonic
coelom
Endometrium
Exocelomic cyst

Approximately 15th day

Approximately 17th day

1.2 THE FIRST AND SECOND WEEKS

Cell division and the elaboration of structures that will be outside the embryo (extraembryonic) characterize the first 2 weeks. The **morula,** a ball of cells, becomes hollow to form a **blastocyst** that develops into a placenta and membranes that will surround the future embryo. The embryo is first identifiable as a mass of cells within the blastocyst late in the first week. By the end of week 2, the embryo will be a disc that is two cell layers thick. The **conceptus** (all the intraembryonic and extraembryonic products of fertilization) takes most of week 1 to travel down the uterine tubes to the uterine cavity. In week 2, the blastocyst sinks within the endometrial wall of the uterus (implantation).

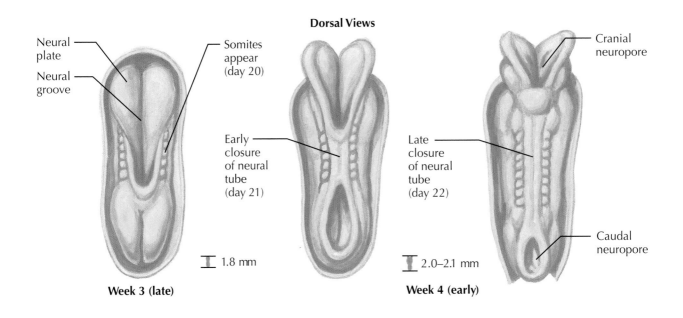

Dorsal Views

Neural plate

Neural groove

Somites appear (day 20)

Early closure of neural tube (day 21)

1.8 mm

Week 3 (late)

Cranial neuropore

Late closure of neural tube (day 22)

Caudal neuropore

2.0–2.1 mm

Week 4 (early)

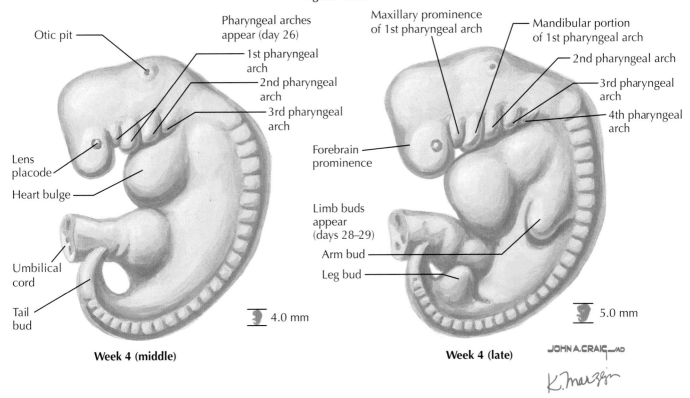

Sagittal Views

Otic pit

Pharyngeal arches appear (day 26)

1st pharyngeal arch

2nd pharyngeal arch

3rd pharyngeal arch

Lens placode

Heart bulge

Umbilical cord

Tail bud

4.0 mm

Week 4 (middle)

Maxillary prominence of 1st pharyngeal arch

Mandibular portion of 1st pharyngeal arch

2nd pharyngeal arch

3rd pharyngeal arch

4th pharyngeal arch

Forebrain prominence

Limb buds appear (days 28–29)

Arm bud

Leg bud

5.0 mm

Week 4 (late)

JOHN A.CRAIG—AD

K. marzyn

1.3 THE EARLY EMBRYONIC PERIOD

Prenatal ages in this book refer to **conceptual age**, which begins with fertilization or conception. Because the day of fertilization is usually unknown, clinicians use **gestational age**, which begins with the first day of the last normal menstrual period. This is 2 weeks earlier than fertilization (e.g., week 3 of conceptual age is week 5 of gestational age).

The embryonic period (weeks 3 through 8) begins with gastrulation in the bilaminar disc and ends with an embryo that looks very human. The embryonic disc folds into a cylinder to establish the basic characteristics of the vertebrate body plan, and the primordia of all the organ systems develop. It is a very dynamic period of differentiation, development, and morphological change. The cardiovascular system is the first organ system to function (day 21 or 22) as the embryo becomes too large for diffusion to address the metabolic needs of the embryonic tissues.

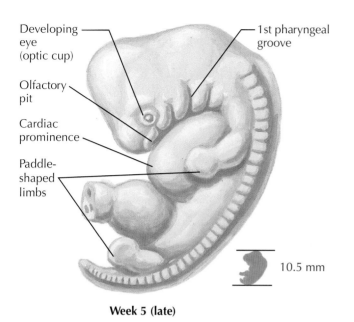

Developing eye (optic cup)

Olfactory pit

Cardiac prominence

Paddle-shaped limbs

1st pharyngeal groove

10.5 mm

Week 5 (late)

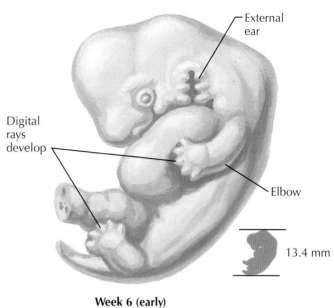

External ear

Digital rays develop

Elbow

13.4 mm

Week 6 (early)

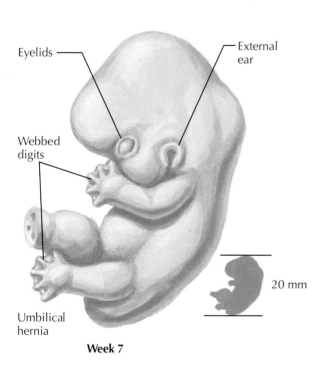

Eyelids

External ear

Webbed digits

Umbilical hernia

20 mm

Week 7

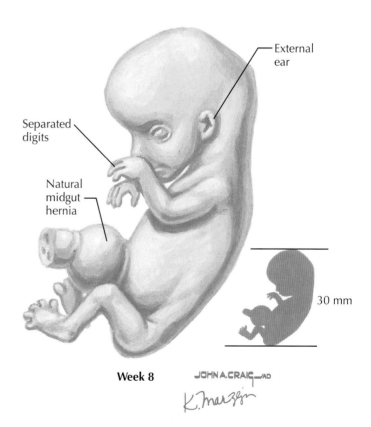

External ear

Separated digits

Natural midgut hernia

30 mm

Week 8

JOHN A. CRAIG—AD

K. Marzejon

1.4 THE LATE EMBRYONIC PERIOD

In the second half of the embryonic period, the human appearance of the embryo emerges. The neuropores have closed, the segmentation of the somites is no longer visible, and the pharyngeal arches are blending into a human-looking head. The upper and lower extremities are extending from the body, and fingers and toes develop. Eyes, ears, and a nose are visible, and the embryonic tail disappears with relative growth of the torso.

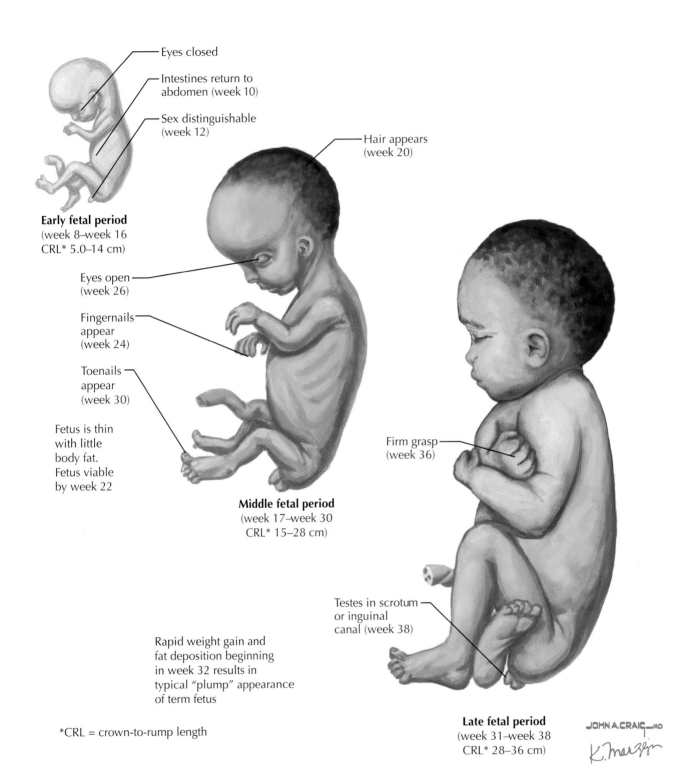

Eyes closed

Intestines return to abdomen (week 10)

Sex distinguishable (week 12)

Hair appears (week 20)

Early fetal period
(week 8–week 16
CRL* 5.0–14 cm)

Eyes open (week 26)

Fingernails appear (week 24)

Toenails appear (week 30)

Fetus is thin with little body fat. Fetus viable by week 22

Firm grasp (week 36)

Middle fetal period
(week 17–week 30
CRL* 15–28 cm)

Rapid weight gain and fat deposition beginning in week 32 results in typical "plump" appearance of term fetus

Testes in scrotum or inguinal canal (week 38)

*CRL = crown-to-rump length

Late fetal period
(week 31–week 38
CRL* 28–36 cm)

JOHN A. CRAIG—MD

K. marzyn

1.5 THE FETAL PERIOD

The theme of the 7-month fetal period is the growth and elaboration of structures already present. Movement of the fetus within the amniotic fluid is a crucial part of the process. The fluid is maternal tissue fluid that crosses the chorion and amnion. It is increasingly supplemented by fetal urine, which is more similar to blood plasma than urine because metabolic waste products in the blood are eliminated in the placenta. The fetus swallows up to 400 mL of amniotic fluid each day for the normal development of oral and facial structures and to provide a favorable environment for the development of the epithelia that line the airway and gastrointestinal tract. The fluid is absorbed into fetal tissues via the gastrointestinal tract.

Blastocyst with embryo within the uterine mucosa

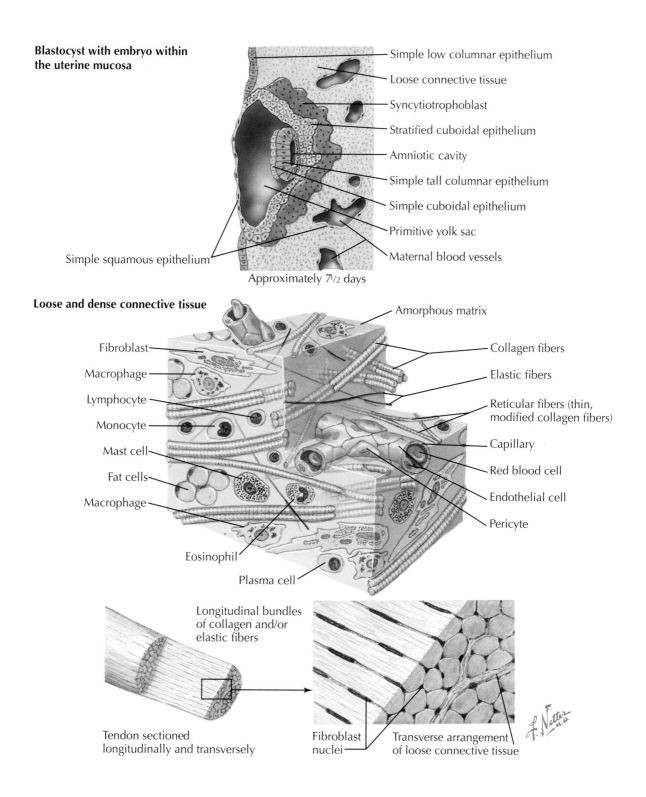

Simple low columnar epithelium

Loose connective tissue

Syncytiotrophoblast

Stratified cuboidal epithelium

Amniotic cavity

Simple tall columnar epithelium

Simple cuboidal epithelium

Primitive yolk sac

Maternal blood vessels

Simple squamous epithelium

Approximately 7½ days

Loose and dense connective tissue

Amorphous matrix

Fibroblast

Macrophage

Lymphocyte

Monocyte

Mast cell

Fat cells

Macrophage

Collagen fibers

Elastic fibers

Reticular fibers (thin, modified collagen fibers)

Capillary

Red blood cell

Endothelial cell

Pericyte

Eosinophil

Plasma cell

Longitudinal bundles of collagen and/or elastic fibers

Tendon sectioned longitudinally and transversely

Fibroblast nuclei

Transverse arrangement of loose connective tissue

1.6 SAMPLES OF EPITHELIA AND CONNECTIVE TISSUE

Histology is the microscopic study of cells, tissues, and organs. Every tissue in the body is classified as nerve, muscle, **epithelium,** or **connective tissue.** Epithelia line body surfaces and have cells in tight contact with each other. Epithelia are classified as simple (one cell layer thick) or stratified; in addition, they are classified according to the shape of the cells on the surface (e.g., squamous [flat], cuboidal, columnar). Connective tissue cells are dispersed in some type of extracellular matrix. **Dense connective tissue** is dense with collagen fibers and contains a higher ratio of matrix to **fibroblasts,** the cells that secrete and maintain the matrix. **Loose connective tissue** has relatively more cells than dense connective tissue and a greater variety of fibers, cells, and matrix molecules.

A. Cross section of skin

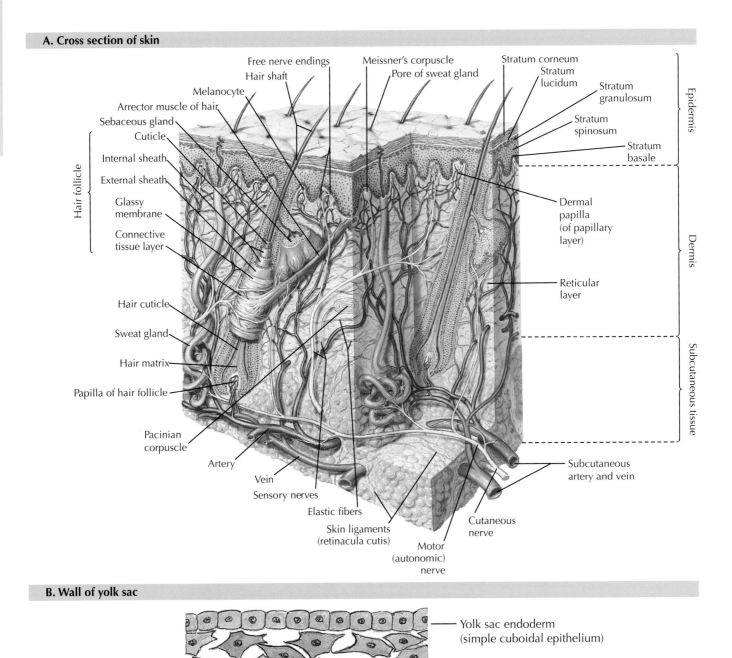

B. Wall of yolk sac

1.7 SKIN AND EMBRYONIC CONNECTIVE TISSUE

The **epidermis** of skin is a stratified, squamous epithelium with a protective, keratinized layer of dead cells on the surface. The **dermis** is dense, irregular connective tissue where the collagen fibers are arranged in "irregular" bundles. The fascia beneath the skin (subcutaneous) is loose connective tissue with a high fat content. The epidermis develops from the surface ectoderm of the embryo; the connective tissue layers are derived from loose, undifferentiated embryonic connective tissue called mesenchyme (demonstrated in Fig. 1.7B, the wall of the yolk sac). **Mesenchyme** is a cellular connective tissue with stellate-shaped cells.

A. Neurulation. The classic and perhaps most-studied example of induction is the formation of the neural tube, where the surface ectoderm (neural plate) is induced by the notochord and paraxial columns.

B. Complex induction: eye development. The eye requires at least eight inductive interactions, most of which are specific and require the participation of both tissues in a particular role.

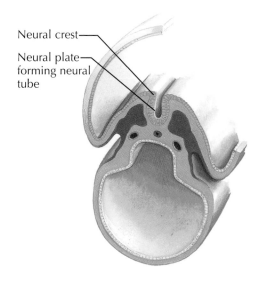

Neural crest

Neural plate forming neural tube

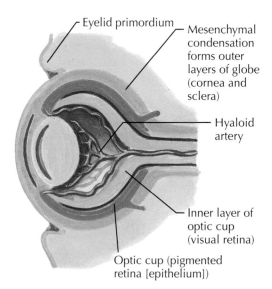

Eyelid primordium

Mesenchymal condensation forms outer layers of globe (cornea and sclera)

Hyaloid artery

Inner layer of optic cup (visual retina)

Optic cup (pigmented retina [epithelium])

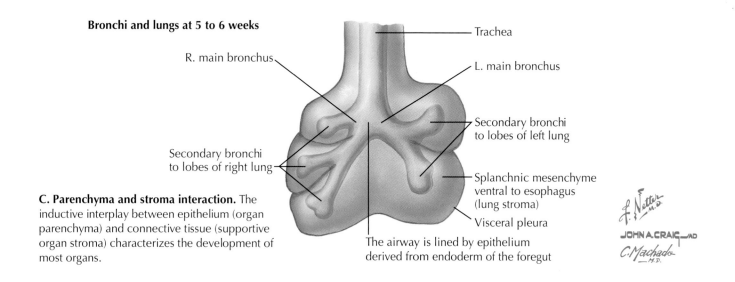

Bronchi and lungs at 5 to 6 weeks

R. main bronchus

Secondary bronchi to lobes of right lung

Trachea

L. main bronchus

Secondary bronchi to lobes of left lung

Splanchnic mesenchyme ventral to esophagus (lung stroma)

Visceral pleura

The airway is lined by epithelium derived from endoderm of the foregut

C. Parenchyma and stroma interaction. The inductive interplay between epithelium (organ parenchyma) and connective tissue (supportive organ stroma) characterizes the development of most organs.

1.8 INDUCTION

Induction is the interaction between two separate histological tissues or primordia in the embryo that results in morphological differentiation. One tissue usually induces the other, but one or both can participate in subsequent organogenesis. The signal varies. It may be a molecule or an extracellular matrix secreted by one of the tissues and encountered by the other, or induction may require direct cellular contact between the two embryonic rudiments. Some inductions (e.g., neural tube formation) are nonspecific. A variety of factors can cause the response; the inducing tissue plays no unique role.

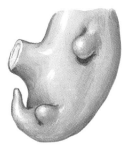
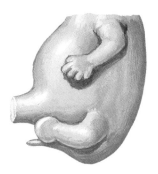

A. Upper and lower limb buds at 5 and 6 weeks. An obvious function of apoptosis is the disappearance of a large number of tissues and structures in development. Fingers and toes form by the elimination of tissue between them.

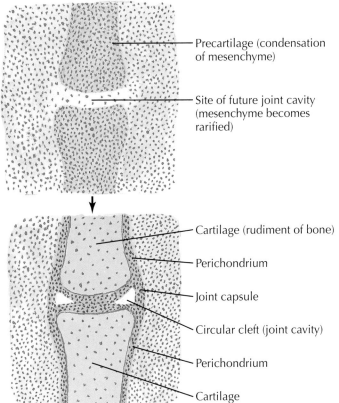

Precartilage (condensation of mesenchyme)

Site of future joint cavity (mesenchyme becomes rarified)

Cartilage (rudiment of bone)

Perichondrium

Joint capsule

Circular cleft (joint cavity)

Perichondrium

Cartilage

B. Formation of a joint cavity between two developing bones. Apoptosis plays an important role in cavitation and the shaping of structures. The lumen of vessels, ducts, hollow organs, and other spaces form via apoptosis.

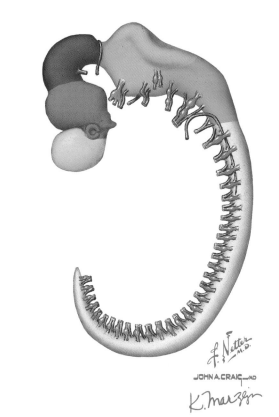

C. Cranial and spinal nerves at 36 days. Another important role of apoptosis is the cell selection process that occurs in the development of most organs. This is particularly significant in the nervous system, where huge numbers of neurons die to allow for the proper connections and functions of the remaining cells.

1.9 APOPTOSIS

Apoptosis is programmed cell death, an extremely important process of normal development. It is initiated in mitochondria in response to a variety of stimuli. Cytochrome c and other molecules are released into the cytoplasm, triggering a cascade of reactions involving a number of cysteine proteases called **caspases.** The result is the condensation of chromatin in the nucleus and the degradation of DNA. There may also be caspase-independent mechanisms for apoptosis that act in very early development.

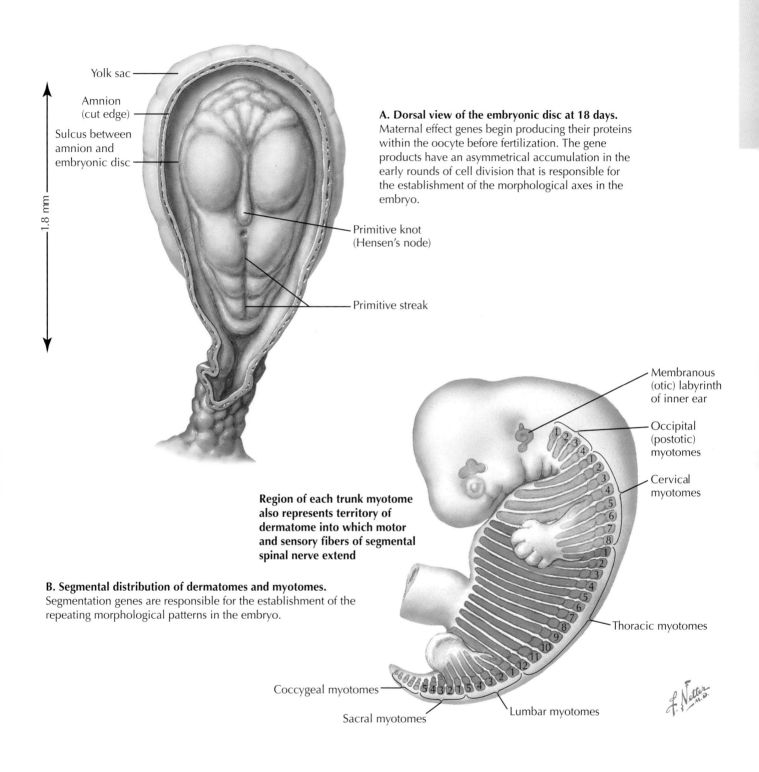

Yolk sac

Amnion (cut edge)

Sulcus between amnion and embryonic disc

1.8 mm

A. Dorsal view of the embryonic disc at 18 days.
Maternal effect genes begin producing their proteins within the oocyte before fertilization. The gene products have an asymmetrical accumulation in the early rounds of cell division that is responsible for the establishment of the morphological axes in the embryo.

Primitive knot (Hensen's node)

Primitive streak

Membranous (otic) labyrinth of inner ear

Occipital (postotic) myotomes

Cervical myotomes

Region of each trunk myotome also represents territory of dermatome into which motor and sensory fibers of segmental spinal nerve extend

B. Segmental distribution of dermatomes and myotomes.
Segmentation genes are responsible for the establishment of the repeating morphological patterns in the embryo.

Thoracic myotomes

Coccygeal myotomes

Sacral myotomes

Lumbar myotomes

1.10 GENETIC DETERMINATION OF EMBRYONIC AXES AND SEGMENTS

The establishment of a bilaterally symmetrical, segmented body plan with craniocaudal and dorsoventral axes is a hallmark of chordate (and vertebrate) development. These features are the result of three gene categories: **maternal effect, segmentation**, and **homeotic genes.** Their products are mostly transcription factors that regulate the expression of other genes. Many of these genes contain a 183-base-pair **homeobox,** a phylogenetically conservative segment whose product is the DNA-binding component of the transcription factor. These three gene groups act in sequence in a complex cascade involving regulatory gene interactions within each group, from one group to the next, and with structural genes.

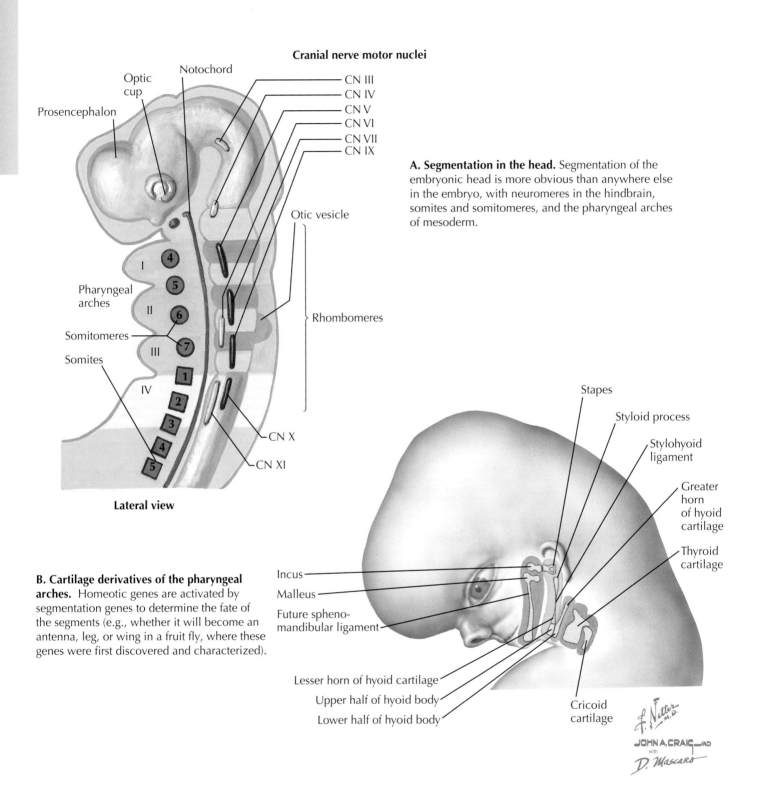

Cranial nerve motor nuclei

Optic cup
Prosencephalon
Notochord
CN III
CN IV
CN V
CN VI
CN VII
CN IX

Pharyngeal arches
Somitomeres
Somites

I
II
III
IV

4
5
6
7
1
2
3
4
5

Otic vesicle
Rhombomeres

CN X
CN XI

Lateral view

A. Segmentation in the head. Segmentation of the embryonic head is more obvious than anywhere else in the embryo, with neuromeres in the hindbrain, somites and somitomeres, and the pharyngeal arches of mesoderm.

Stapes
Styloid process
Stylohyoid ligament
Greater horn of hyoid cartilage
Thyroid cartilage

Incus
Malleus
Future spheno-mandibular ligament

Lesser horn of hyoid cartilage
Upper half of hyoid body
Lower half of hyoid body

Cricoid cartilage

B. Cartilage derivatives of the pharyngeal arches. Homeotic genes are activated by segmentation genes to determine the fate of the segments (e.g., whether it will become an antenna, leg, or wing in a fruit fly, where these genes were first discovered and characterized).

1.11 SEGMENTATION AND SEGMENT FATES

Segmentation is expressed throughout the embryo in the formation of cranial and spinal nerves, the vertebral column and ribs, early muscle development, and patterns of blood vessel formation. The pharyngeal arches of mesoderm in the embryonic head are the most externally visible segments. Segmentation genes of the *Hox* gene family (and others) play a major role in arch development, and they extend their effects to the cranial somites and segments of the hindbrain (rhombomeres). Homeotic genes are required to determine the fate of the segments. Examples shown in Fig. 1.11B include the development of ear ossicles, the hyoid bone, cartilages of the larynx, etc., from mesoderm in each pharyngeal arch.

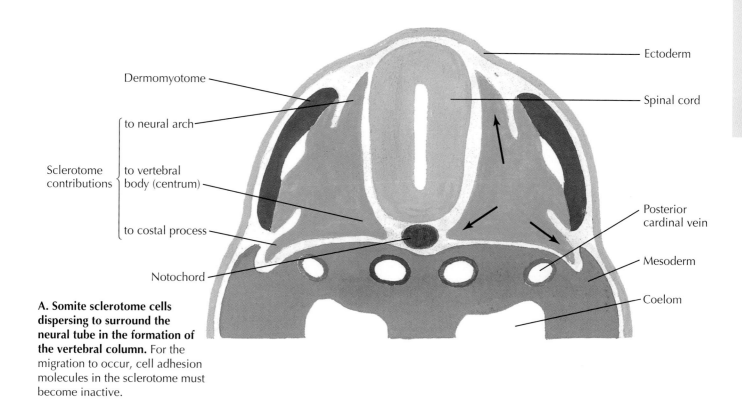

Dermomyotome

Sclerotome contributions
- to neural arch
- to vertebral body (centrum)
- to costal process

Notochord

Ectoderm

Spinal cord

Posterior cardinal vein

Mesoderm

Coelom

A. Somite sclerotome cells dispersing to surround the neural tube in the formation of the vertebral column. For the migration to occur, cell adhesion molecules in the sclerotome must become inactive.

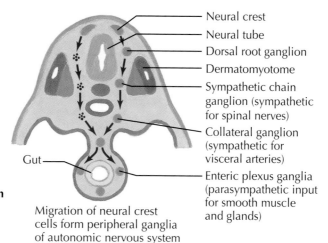

Neural crest
Neural tube
Dorsal root ganglion
Dermatomyotome
Sympathetic chain ganglion (sympathetic for spinal nerves)
Collateral ganglion (sympathetic for visceral arteries)

Gut

Enteric plexus ganglia (parasympathetic input for smooth muscle and glands)

Migration of neural crest cells form peripheral ganglia of autonomic nervous system

B. The migration of neural crest cells to form autonomic ganglia. The deposition of hyaluronic acid in the migration pathway is one of the first steps in a migration event.

1.12 CELL ADHESION AND CELL MIGRATION

Most events in embryogenesis involve the association, disassociation, and migration of cells. The interrelated processes involve dynamic changes in the molecules expressed in cell membranes. **Cell adhesion molecules** (CAMs) cause cells to aggregate. Their inactivation is a requirement of the initiation of cell migration, but control of the migration pathway is very complex. Trails of connective tissue fibers often help guide cells, a process termed **contact guidance.** Chemical signals may attract cells, and an inhibitory effect of cells bordering the path may also play a role. The deposition of **hyaluronic acid,** a connective tissue protein that binds water, creates a favorable environment for cell migration.

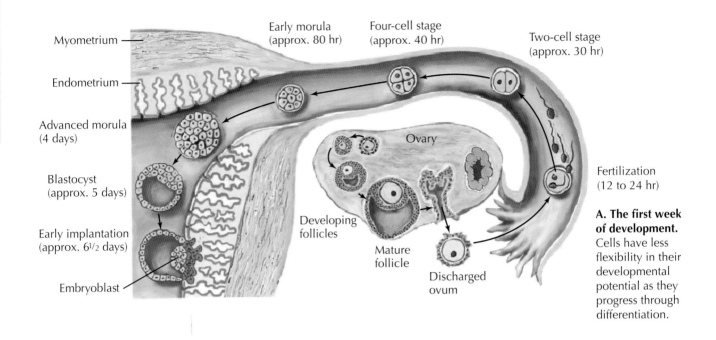

Myometrium

Endometrium

Advanced morula
(4 days)

Blastocyst
(approx. 5 days)

Early implantation
(approx. 6½ days)

Embryoblast

Early morula
(approx. 80 hr)

Four-cell stage
(approx. 40 hr)

Two-cell stage
(approx. 30 hr)

Ovary

Developing
follicles

Mature
follicle

Discharged
ovum

Fertilization
(12 to 24 hr)

**A. The first week
of development.**
Cells have less
flexibility in their
developmental
potential as they
progress through
differentiation.

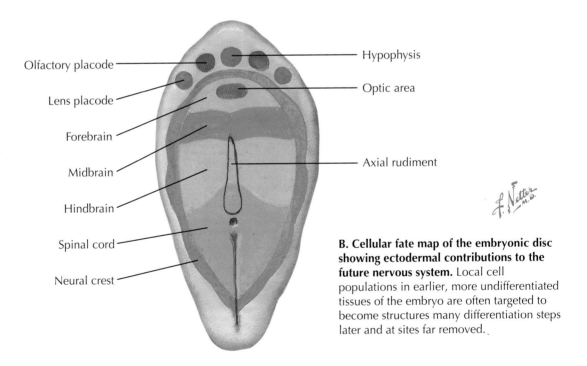

Olfactory placode

Lens placode

Forebrain

Midbrain

Hindbrain

Spinal cord

Neural crest

Hypophysis

Optic area

Axial rudiment

**B. Cellular fate map of the embryonic disc
showing ectodermal contributions to the
future nervous system.** Local cell
populations in earlier, more undifferentiated
tissues of the embryo are often targeted to
become structures many differentiation steps
later and at sites far removed.

1.13 CELL DIFFERENTIATION AND CELL FATES

Cells in the first few days before the embryo develops are **toti-potent**, meaning each is capable of forming a normal embryo or developing into any of the more than 200 cell types in the body. Cells in the blastocyst, including the early embryo, are **pluripotent**, capable of forming a variety of cell types but not a whole individual. They are genetically programmed to follow more specific developmental paths. Some undifferentiated **stem cells** remain in adult organs as a source of new cells. These **multipotent** cells can be cultured to form entirely different tissues than in their organ of origin but are thought to have less flexibility in differentiation than embryonic stem cells; they are therefore less attractive for therapeutic and embryonic research.

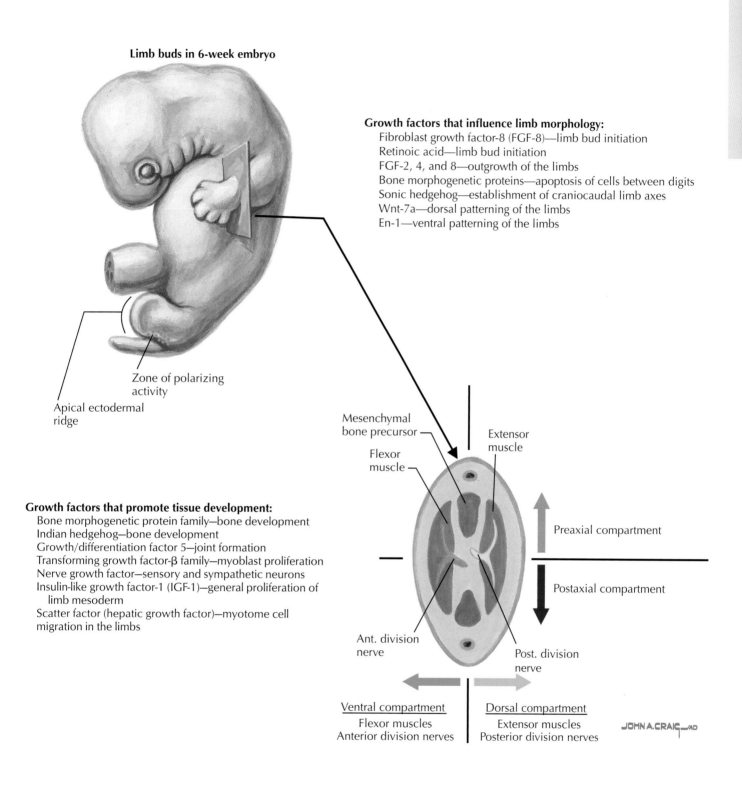

Limb buds in 6-week embryo

Growth factors that influence limb morphology:
Fibroblast growth factor-8 (FGF-8)—limb bud initiation
Retinoic acid—limb bud initiation
FGF-2, 4, and 8—outgrowth of the limbs
Bone morphogenetic proteins—apoptosis of cells between digits
Sonic hedgehog—establishment of craniocaudal limb axes
Wnt-7a—dorsal patterning of the limbs
En-1—ventral patterning of the limbs

Zone of polarizing activity

Apical ectodermal ridge

Growth factors that promote tissue development:
Bone morphogenetic protein family—bone development
Indian hedgehog—bone development
Growth/differentiation factor 5—joint formation
Transforming growth factor-β family—myoblast proliferation
Nerve growth factor—sensory and sympathetic neurons
Insulin-like growth factor-1 (IGF-1)—general proliferation of limb mesoderm
Scatter factor (hepatic growth factor)—myotome cell migration in the limbs

Mesenchymal bone precursor

Flexor muscle

Extensor muscle

Preaxial compartment

Postaxial compartment

Ant. division nerve

Post. division nerve

Ventral compartment
Flexor muscles
Anterior division nerves

Dorsal compartment
Extensor muscles
Posterior division nerves

JOHN A. CRAIG—AD

1.14 GROWTH FACTORS

Growth factors are a group of more than 50 proteins that bind to specific cell receptors to stimulate cell division, differentiation, and other functions related to the control of tissue proliferation. They are inducers that can act alone or in combination, but they can affect only cells that express their receptors. Some can stimulate only one cell type (e.g., nerve growth factor), whereas others have broad specificity. Other functions include various roles in cell function, migration, survival, and inhibition of proliferation. Other types of molecules, like steroid hormones, can have effects similar to growth factors.

The Classification of Errors of Morphogenesis

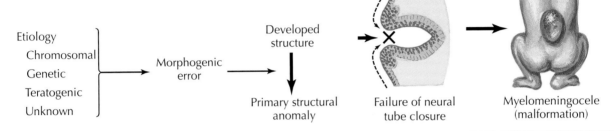

Categories of anomalies

Anomalous formation of tissue → Malformation or malformation sequence

Excessive forces on normal tissue → Deformation or deformation sequence

Destruction of normal tissue → Disruption or disruption sequence

Malformation. Structural anomaly resulting from error in tissue formation

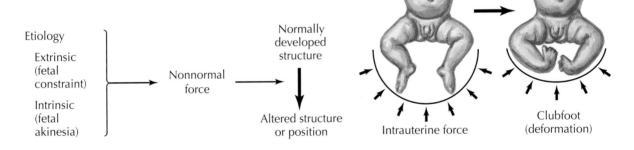

Etiology
Chromosomal
Genetic
Teratogenic
Unknown

→ Morphogenic error →

Developed structure
↓
Primary structural anomaly

Failure of neural tube closure

Myelomeningocele (malformation)

Deformation. Alteration in shape or position of normally developed structure

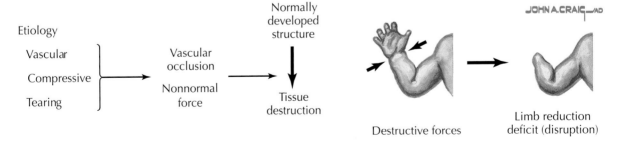

Etiology

Extrinsic (fetal constraint)

Intrinsic (fetal akinesia)

→ Nonnormal force →

Normally developed structure
↓
Altered structure or position

Intrauterine force

Clubfoot (deformation)

Disruption. Destruction of previously normally developed structure

Etiology

Vascular

Compressive

Tearing

→ Vascular occlusion

Nonnormal force →

Normally developed structure
↓
Tissue destruction

JOHN A.CRAIG—AD

Destructive forces

Limb reduction deficit (disruption)

1.15 CLASSIFICATION OF NONNORMAL PROCESSES

There are two broad categories in the classification of developmental anomalies. Those that result from either the nonnormal development of a tissue or structure or from the secondary deformation or disruption of a normal structure. The first type of malformation can be genetic or produced by external teratogens. The second category includes excessive forces exerted on a structure from any source, internal or external.

Syndrome

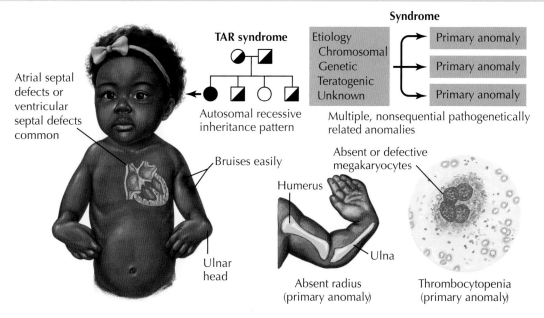

TAR syndrome

Atrial septal defects or ventricular septal defects common

Bruises easily

Ulnar head

Autosomal recessive inheritance pattern

Humerus

Absent or defective megakaryocytes

Ulna

Absent radius (primary anomaly)

Thrombocytopenia (primary anomaly)

Syndrome

Etiology
Chromosomal
Genetic
Teratogenic
Unknown

Primary anomaly

Primary anomaly

Primary anomaly

Multiple, nonsequential pathogenetically related anomalies

TAR syndrome. Includes two anomalies: thrombocytopenia (T) and absent radius (AR). May be associated with congenital heart anomalies; autosomal recessive transmission

Sequence

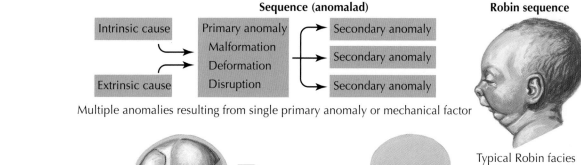

Sequence (anomalad)

Intrinsic cause

Extrinsic cause

Primary anomaly
Malformation
Deformation
Disruption

Secondary anomaly

Secondary anomaly

Secondary anomaly

Multiple anomalies resulting from single primary anomaly or mechanical factor

Robin sequence

Typical Robin facies with micrognathia

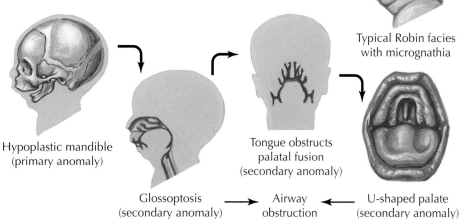

Hypoplastic mandible (primary anomaly)

Tongue obstructs palatal fusion (secondary anomaly)

Glossoptosis (secondary anomaly) → Airway obstruction ← U-shaped palate (secondary anomaly)

Sequence of anomalies initiated by hypoplastic mandible that causes glossoptosis. Resulting palatal defect with glossoptosis may obstruct airway

Paul Kim
JOHN A. CRAIG—AD

1.16 CLASSIFICATION OF MULTIPLE ANOMALIES: SYNDROME VERSUS A SEQUENCE

A syndrome is a number of primary pathogenetically related anomalies from a single cause. A sequence has a primary cause but leads to a cascade of secondary effects. A syndrome is referred to as a disease if the cause is known.

Classification of Malformations

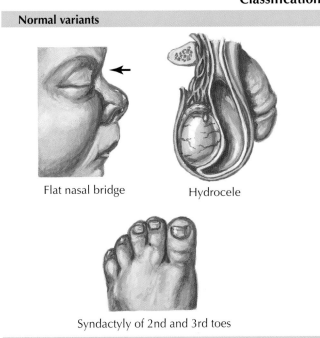

Normal variants

Flat nasal bridge

Hydrocele

Syndactyly of 2nd and 3rd toes

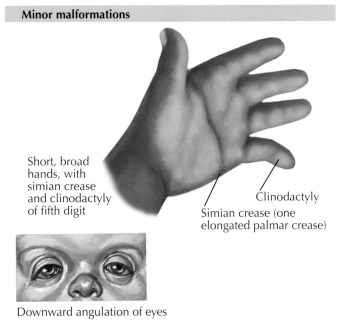

Minor malformations

Short, broad hands, with simian crease and clinodactyly of fifth digit

Clinodactyly

Simian crease (one elongated palmar crease)

Downward angulation of eyes

Major malformations

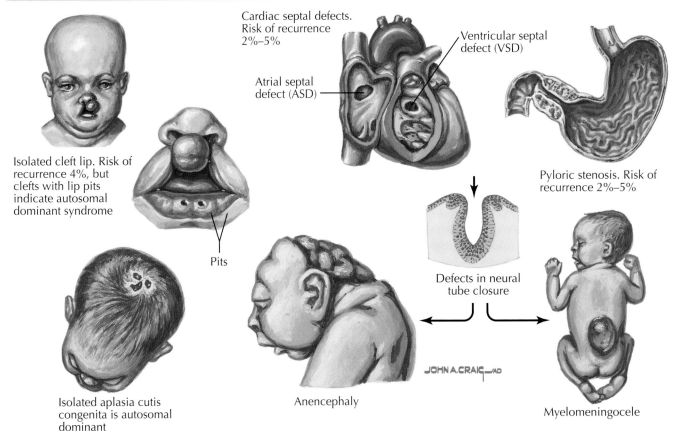

Cardiac septal defects. Risk of recurrence 2%–5%

Ventricular septal defect (VSD)

Atrial septal defect (ASD)

Isolated cleft lip. Risk of recurrence 4%, but clefts with lip pits indicate autosomal dominant syndrome

Pits

Pyloric stenosis. Risk of recurrence 2%–5%

Defects in neural tube closure

JOHN A.CRAIG—AD

Isolated aplasia cutis congenita is autosomal dominant

Anencephaly

Myelomeningocele

Major and minor malformations may occur as isolated entities or as components of multiple malformation syndrome. Risk of recurrence refers to future pregnancies where normal parents have an affected infant. It depends on the cause of the defect.

1.17 NORMAL VERSUS MAJOR VERSUS MINOR MALFORMATIONS

Variations present in more than 4% of the population are considered normal variations. Minor and major malformations occur in less than 4% of the population and are distinguished from each other by using functional and/or cosmetic criteria. Major and minor malformations may occur as isolated entities or as components of multiple malformation syndromes. The presence of two or more minor anomalies in a newborn may indicate an undetected major anomaly.

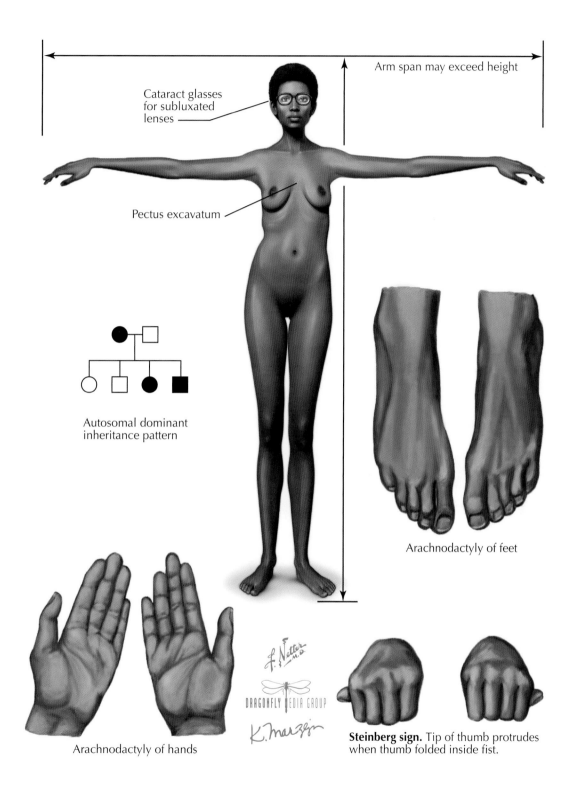

Cataract glasses for subluxated lenses

Arm span may exceed height

Pectus excavatum

Autosomal dominant inheritance pattern

Arachnodactyly of feet

Arachnodactyly of hands

Steinberg sign. Tip of thumb protrudes when thumb folded inside fist.

1.18 MARFAN SYNDROME

Marfan syndrome is a **multiple malformation syndrome of postnatal onset** that is inherited in an autosomal dominant pattern. Many cases are linked to advanced paternal age. Although characterized by notable body proportions, subluxated lenses, and a sunken or everted sternum, Marfan syndrome is a progressive connective tissue disorder. The most severe consequences are often in the cardiovascular system, where aneurysms of the aorta and other arteries may result from defective connective tissue in their walls.

Apert Syndrome

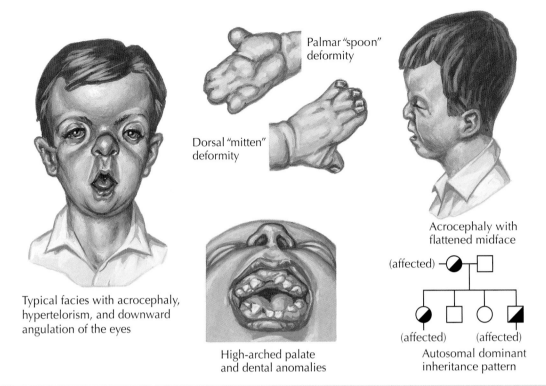

Typical facies with acrocephaly, hypertelorism, and downward angulation of the eyes

Palmar "spoon" deformity

Dorsal "mitten" deformity

High-arched palate and dental anomalies

Acrocephaly with flattened midface

(affected)

(affected)   (affected)

Autosomal dominant inheritance pattern

Cornelia de Lange Syndrome

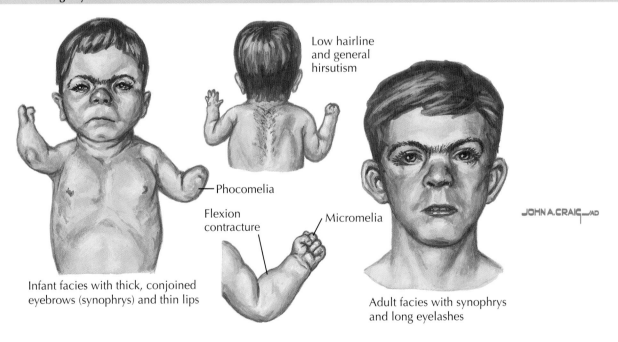

Infant facies with thick, conjoined eyebrows (synophrys) and thin lips

Low hairline and general hirsutism

Phocomelia

Flexion contracture

Micromelia

Adult facies with synophrys and long eyelashes

JOHN A.CRAIG—AD

1.19 APERT AND CORNELIA DE LANGE SYNDROMES

Apert and Cornelia de Lange syndromes are **multiple malformation syndromes of prenatal onset.** Like Marfan syndrome, they are inherited as autosomal dominant mutations, although chromosomal aberrations may be present in Cornelia de Lange syndrome. In syndromes with prenatal onset and serious defects, affected individuals usually do not reproduce, and the syndromes arise as new mutations. Limb malformations, intellectual disability, and the facial characteristics shown typify Cornelia de Lange syndrome. Premature fusion of the coronal suture is a primary anomaly in Apert syndrome. The skull is wide and flat, with palate and dental anomalies. Digits in the hands and feet are fused. Intelligence is often normal.

Conditions that cause intrauterine crowding can lead to nonnormal fetal positions and thus cause constraint anomalies

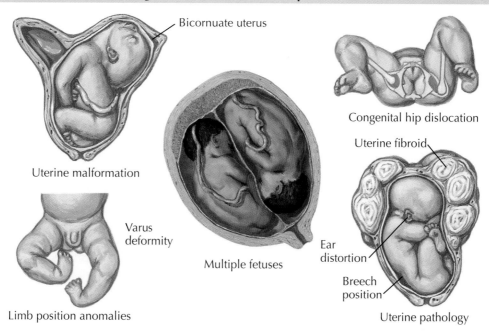

Bicornuate uterus

Uterine malformation

Congenital hip dislocation

Uterine fibroid

Varus deformity

Multiple fetuses

Ear distortion

Breech position

Limb position anomalies

Uterine pathology

Constraint-related growth deficiency is transient. Given room, small infants catch up rapidly.

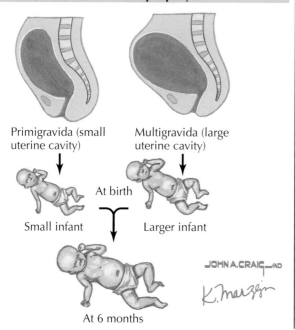

Primigravida (small uterine cavity)

Multigravida (large uterine cavity)

At birth

Small infant

Larger infant

At 6 months

JOHN A. CRAIG—AD

K. marzjn

Early engagement of fetal head may limit sutural growth and result in craniosynostotic skull anomalies.

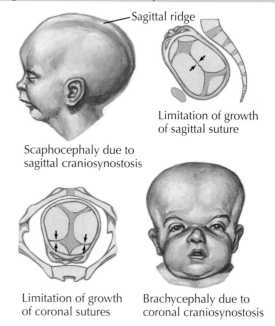

Sagittal ridge

Limitation of growth of sagittal suture

Scaphocephaly due to sagittal craniosynostosis

Limitation of growth of coronal sutures

Brachycephaly due to coronal craniosynostosis

1.20 EXAMPLES OF DEFORMATIONS

Extrinsic deformations are usually related to some type of constraint from uterine pathology or multiple fetuses. Intrinsic deformations are derived from a variation in the fetus (e.g., bone anomalies caused by neural or muscle pathology, as in clubfoot). Extrinsic constraint may have a single effect or a sequence of effects. The prognosis for deformations is usually excellent. Once the fetus is free of the constraining environment, normal growth and morphology are usually restored.

Potter Sequence

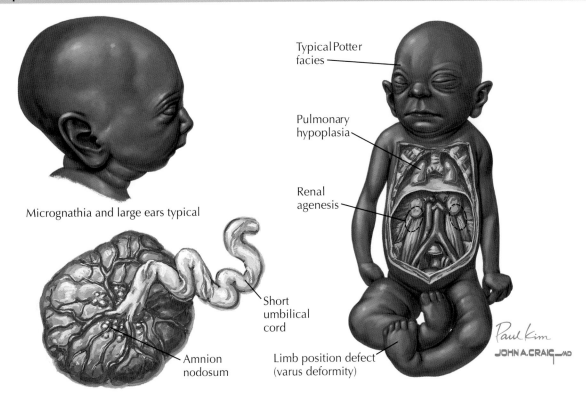

Typical Potter facies

Pulmonary hypoplasia

Renal agenesis

Micrognathia and large ears typical

Short umbilical cord

Amnion nodosum

Limb position defect (varus deformity)

Paul Kim
JOHN A. CRAIG—AD

Events in Potter sequence

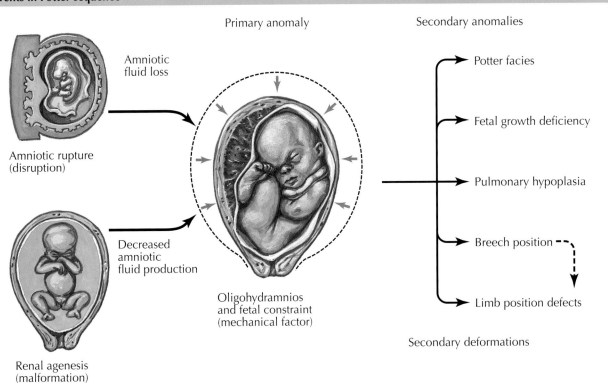

Primary anomaly

Secondary anomalies

Amniotic fluid loss

Amniotic rupture (disruption)

Decreased amniotic fluid production

Renal agenesis (malformation)

Oligohydramnios and fetal constraint (mechanical factor)

Potter facies

Fetal growth deficiency

Pulmonary hypoplasia

Breech position

Limb position defects

Secondary deformations

1.21 EXAMPLE OF A DEFORMATION SEQUENCE

The primary cause in this example of a deformation sequence is a reduction in the amount of amniotic fluid (oligohydramnios) that results in several secondary deformation effects (listed on the right in the figure). Multiple factors can trigger the primary cause. Shown here is oligohydramnios caused by renal agenesis (a malformation) or amniotic rupture (a disruption).

Thalidomide

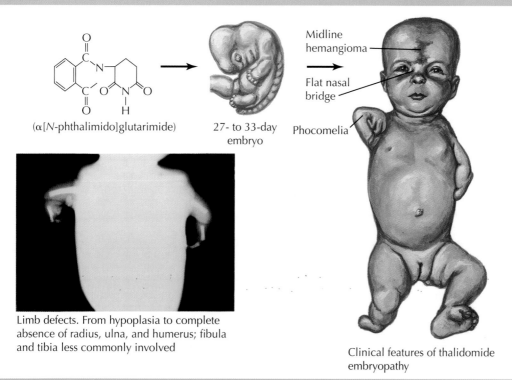

(α[*N*-phthalimido]glutarimide)

27- to 33-day embryo

Midline hemangioma

Flat nasal bridge

Phocomelia

Limb defects. From hypoplasia to complete absence of radius, ulna, and humerus; fibula and tibia less commonly involved

Clinical features of thalidomide embryopathy

Retinoic acid

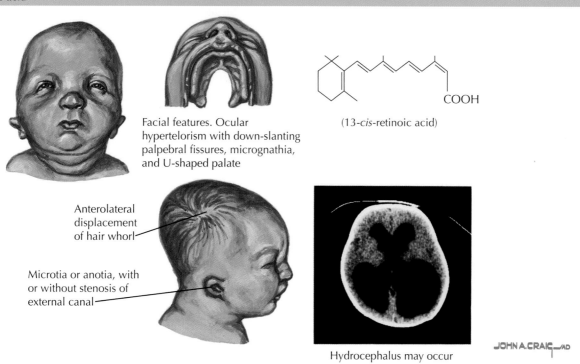

Facial features. Ocular hypertelorism with down-slanting palpebral fissures, micrognathia, and U-shaped palate

(13-*cis*-retinoic acid)

Anterolateral displacement of hair whorl

Microtia or anotia, with or without stenosis of external canal

Hydrocephalus may occur

JOHN A. CRAIG—AD

1.22 DRUG-INDUCED EMBRYOPATHIES

Although alcohol is the most common teratogen in humans, thalidomide has one of the most specific mechanisms of action (disruption of blood vessels in the embryonic limb buds). The epidemic of defects it produced between 1959 and 1962 led to research that opened the field of study of drug and chemical agent effects on morphogenesis. Thalidomide, a popular sleeping medication, was discovered to affect the developing embryo in small doses and during a very specific time frame to produce the characteristic anomalies shown. Retinoic acid became a common treatment for acne and psoriasis in the 1980s. Both retinoic acid and its cousin, vitamin A, were known teratogens, but many women who were treated with the medication did not know they were pregnant.

Terminology

Anomaly	(G., "irregularity") In embryology and anatomy, an unusual structure that is the result of nonnormal development.
Apoptosis	Programmed cell death initiated in mitochondria and usually involving changes in a number of caspase proteins. The result is degradation of DNA and breakup of the cell.
Blastocyst	(G., "germ" + "bladder") Fluid-filled ball of cells that consists of an inner cell mass destined to become the embryo and an outer trophoblast that will be a surrounding membrane (chorion) and the embryonic/fetal contribution to the placenta.
Carnegie stages	A numerical system for characterizing developmental stages. The stages range from 1–23 and cover days 1–56.
Conceptual age	The age of an embryo or fetus that starts with conception (fertilization).
Conceptus	All the products of fertilization, including the embryo, amnion, chorion, yolk sac, allantois, and umbilical cord.
Crown–rump (CR) length	A convenient measure of size of the embryo and fetus, which have varying degrees of curvature. Taken as the maximum, straight-line distance between the top of the head and bottom of the "rump."
Embryo	The developing human through the first 2 months when all the organ systems are forming.
Etiology	(G., "cause" + "discourse") The study of the causes of diseases or anomalies. Pathogenesis.
Facies	(L., "Face, surface, or expression") In development, it is the characteristic appearance of a newborn related to congenital anomalies.
Fascia	A layer of connective tissue surrounding muscles, nerves, and vessels or separating tissue layers. It can be thick, loose connective tissue, like the fat-filled superficial fascia under the skin, or dense and sheetlike.
Fetus	The developing human from months 3 through 9 (to term).
Fibroblasts	Cells that secrete and maintain the dense and loose connective tissue matrix, including all the fibers.
Gestational age	Clinical age of an embryo or fetus that begins with the first day of the last normal menstrual period rather than the date of conception, which is usually unknown. It is 2 weeks longer than conceptual age.
Growth factor	An unsatisfactory term derived in the late 1950's from the identification of a series of proteins that promotes the growth of specific tissues in culture. "Growth" does not characterize the variety of molecular processes and mechanisms in development. Not all "growth factors" are proteins (e.g., retinoic acid), and more recent factors have been identified and named from gene expression studies.
Homeobox	A phylogenetically conservative gene segment of 183 base pairs in many segmentation and homeotic genes (its name is derived from its discovery in the latter). The product, the homeodomain, is a protein segment that binds to DNA as part of the transcription factor function of these regulatory genes.
Homeotic genes	A family of genes, usually transcription factors, that plays a role in determining the fate of body segments in the embryo. They are identified by mutations that cause one segment to become another (e.g., a leg will become an antenna in a fly).
Hyperplasia	(G., hyper- "formation") Nonnormal enlargement of an organ or structure because of an increase in the number of cells.
Hypertrophy	(G., hyper- "nutrition") Nonnormal enlargement of an organ or structure because of an increase in the size of its cells.
Hypoplasia	Underdevelopment of an organ or structure.
Keratin	A large family of proteins that forms intracellular filaments and is the major component of hair; nails; and the outer, protective layer of the skin epidermis (epithelium).

Terminology—cont'd

Lamina propria	Histological layer of loose connective tissue beneath the epithelium lining the lumen of a hollow organ.
Lanugo hair	(L., wooly, down) Fine, soft fetal hair that appears around week 12.
LNMP	Last normal menstrual period. Clinicians measure gestational development starting with the first day of the last normal menstrual period. This is 2 weeks longer than conceptual age, which starts with fertilization or conception.
Lumen	(L., "light") Space within a blood vessel or hollow organ.
Malformation	Anomaly caused by an intrinsic disruption in a primordium or process.
Malformation sequence	A number of secondary malformations that are a result of a primary malformation.
Mesenchyme	Usually considered undifferentiated embryonic connective tissue derived from primitive streak mesoderm or neural crest. Definitions vary depending on whether they are from a histological, embryological, or anatomical point of view.
Mesoderm	(G., "middle skin") First interior cells of the embryonic disc that are the product of gastrulation. They are initially in the form of mesenchyme, but some cells quickly condense into longitudinal epithelial columns, a second type of mesoderm.
Monozygotic twins	"Identical" twins resulting from the separation of cells into two distinct populations after fertilization. Heterozygotic twins are from the fertilization of two separate ova.
Morula	(L., "little mulberry") Mass of cells that is the product of early cell division after fertilization.
Multipotent	Capability of adult or some other stem cells to differentiate into a number of cell types but with less flexibility than embryonic totipotent or multipotent stem cells.
Oligohydramnios	(G., "little water in the amnion") Reduction in the amount of amniotic fluid that surrounds and protects the fetus. It is often a clinical sign of renal agenesis because amniotic fluid is fetal urine produced by the kidneys.
Parenchyma	Epithelial cells of an organ that are metabolically active in the organ's function (e.g., secretory cells in a gland or absorptive enterocytes in the intestine).
Pluripotent	Capability of cells of the blastocyst and early embryo to differentiate into many cell lines, but not a whole individual.
Primordium	(L., "origin") First cellular indication of an organ or structure.
Quickening	Fetal movements felt by the mother.
Reticular fibers	Small-caliber collagen fibers with sugar groups that are predominant in the stroma of lymphatic organs. They are also present in general connective tissue matrix along with larger collagen fibers and elastic fibers.
Somites	Epithelial blocks of mesoderm that flank the neural tube and give rise to bone (from the sclerotome of a somite), muscle (from the myotome), and connective tissue (from the dermatome). They can serve as convenient indicators of developmental stages from 20–30 days (e.g., "4-somite stage").
Stem cell	Undifferentiated cell in the embryo or adult that is capable of forming many cell types. The earlier in development, the more flexibility for differentiation.
Stroma	The supporting, connective tissue framework of an organ.
Syndrome	(G., "running together") Combination of primary symptoms and anomalies that results from a particular genetic or environmental cause and is not a sequence of secondary anomalies.
Teratology	Study of nonnormal development. A "teratogen" is an agent that causes birth anomalies.
Totipotent	Capability of the cells formed soon after fertilization to each develop into a whole human being or any of its cells.

Continued

Terminology—cont'd

Transcription	The making of messenger RNA from DNA in chromosomes in the cell nucleus, the first step in the creation of proteins. The initiation and regulation of transcription is a fundamental process controlling cell and tissue differentiation.
Translation	The "conversion" of the sequence of nucleotide bases in messenger RNA into protein amino acid sequences via transfer RNA in ribosomes.
Trimester	Clinical division of the prenatal period into three 3-month segments. The organ systems develop in the first trimester, and the fetus is potentially viable after the second.
Trophic	(G., "nourishing") An influence on an organ or structure that promotes its general growth and sustenance.
Tropic	(G., "a turn, turning") Developmental response of a cell or structure to an external stimulus, such as growing toward a chemical secretion.
Vernix caseosa	(L., "varnish") A greasy, protective covering of the fetal skin that develops at week 18. It consists of dead epidermal cells, the secretion of sebaceous glands, and lanugo hair.
Zygote	(G., "union") Cell product of fertilization, the union of the sperm and egg. It is the beginning of development.

G., Greek; L., Latin.

2

EARLY EMBRYONIC DEVELOPMENT AND THE PLACENTA

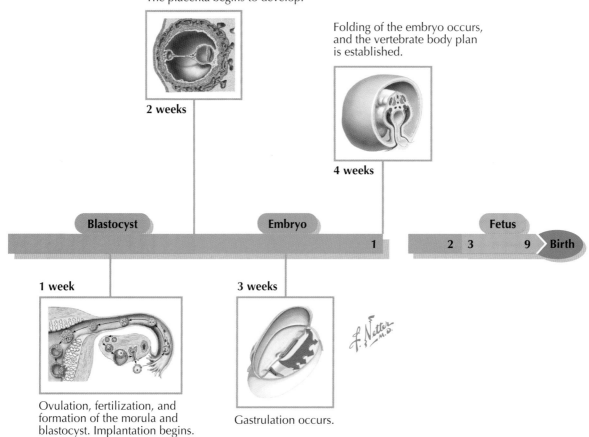

PRENATAL TIME SCALE (MONTHS)

Implantation completed.
The amnion, chorion, and yolk sac form.
The placenta begins to develop.

2 weeks

Folding of the embryo occurs,
and the vertebrate body plan
is established.

4 weeks

Blastocyst

Embryo

Fetus

1

2 3 9 Birth

1 week

3 weeks

Ovulation, fertilization, and
formation of the morula and
blastocyst. Implantation begins.

Gastrulation occurs.

2.1 TIMELINE

EARLY EMBRYONIC PRIMORDIA:

Inner cell mass, ectoderm, endoderm, primitive streak and node (knot) of ectoderm, and mesoderm derived from the latter two ectodermal structures.

PRIMORDIA OF THE GASTRULA AND CYLINDRICAL EMBRYO:

Notochord, somites (from paraxial columns), intermediate mesoderm, lateral plate enclosing the intraembryonic coelom, somatopleure, splanchnopleure, gut tube and mesenteries, cardiogenic mesoderm, neural crest, and neural tube.

PLAN

The embryonic gastrula, a trilaminar disc of ectoderm, endoderm, and mesoderm, is continuous with the amnion above it and yolk sac below. Coeloms form in the lateral plate mesoderm, dividing it into a somatic component with the ectoderm (somatopleure) and a splanchnic component with the endoderm (splanchnopleure). As the trilaminar embryonic disc folds into a cylinder, the endoderm folds into a gut tube extending the length of the embryo with a surrounding coelom that separates it from the somatopleure body wall. Segmentation is established in the paraxial columns and developing nervous system. By the end of the first month, all the basic organ and tissue relationships seen in the adult are established.

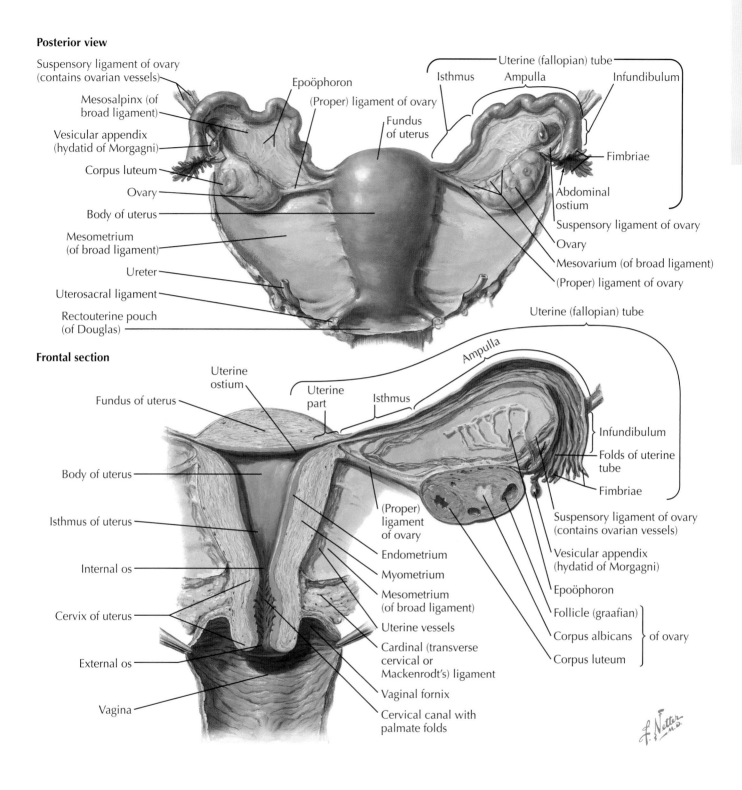

Posterior view

Suspensory ligament of ovary (contains ovarian vessels)

Mesosalpinx (of broad ligament)

Vesicular appendix (hydatid of Morgagni)

Corpus luteum

Ovary

Body of uterus

Mesometrium (of broad ligament)

Ureter

Uterosacral ligament

Rectouterine pouch (of Douglas)

Epoöphoron

(Proper) ligament of ovary

Fundus of uterus

Uterine (fallopian) tube

Isthmus   Ampulla   Infundibulum

Fimbriae

Abdominal ostium

Suspensory ligament of ovary

Ovary

Mesovarium (of broad ligament)

(Proper) ligament of ovary

Frontal section

Uterine (fallopian) tube

Ampulla

Fundus of uterus

Uterine ostium

Uterine part

Isthmus

Infundibulum

Folds of uterine tube

Fimbriae

Body of uterus

Isthmus of uterus

Internal os

Cervix of uterus

External os

Vagina

(Proper) ligament of ovary

Endometrium

Myometrium

Mesometrium (of broad ligament)

Uterine vessels

Cardinal (transverse cervical or Mackenrodt's) ligament

Vaginal fornix

Cervical canal with palmate folds

Suspensory ligament of ovary (contains ovarian vessels)

Vesicular appendix (hydatid of Morgagni)

Epoöphoron

Follicle (graafian)

Corpus albicans   } of ovary

Corpus luteum

2.2 ADULT UTERUS, OVARIES, AND UTERINE TUBES

The uterus, uterine tubes, and ovaries are enclosed by the **broad ligament (mesometrium)**, a transverse fold of visceral peritoneum across the pelvic floor. The upper part of this mesentery is the **mesosalpinx,** the mesentery of the uterine tubes. A posterior extension of the broad ligament investing each ovary and fibrous ovarian ligament is the **mesovarium**. The uterine tubes terminate in finger-like **fimbriae** that envelop the ovary at the time of ovulation. Like most hollow organs, the uterus has a thick wall of smooth muscle, the **myometrium**, and an inner mucosal lining of loose connective tissue and epithelium, the **endometrium**, where development takes place.

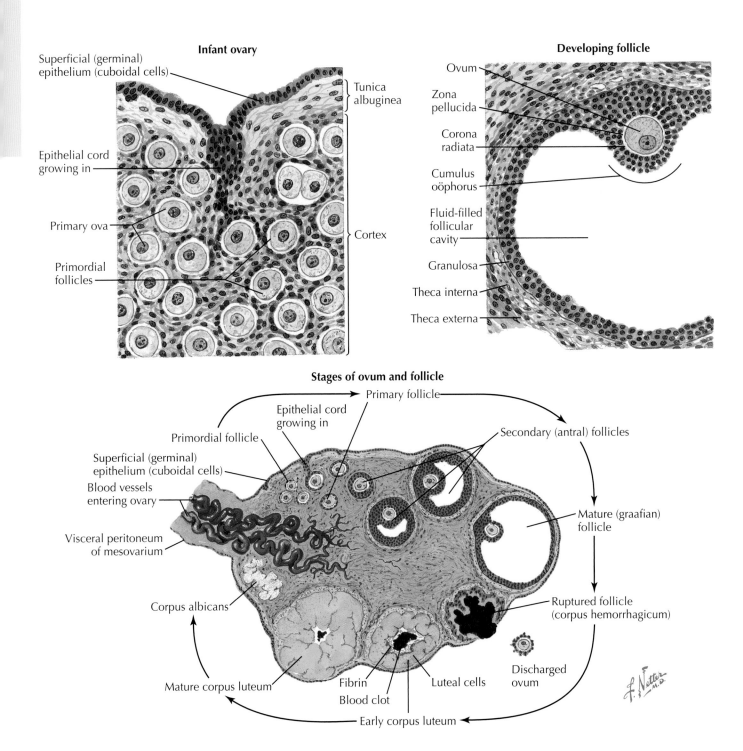

Infant ovary

Superficial (germinal) epithelium (cuboidal cells)

Tunica albuginea

Epithelial cord growing in

Primary ova

Primordial follicles

Cortex

Developing follicle

Ovum

Zona pellucida

Corona radiata

Cumulus oöphorus

Fluid-filled follicular cavity

Granulosa

Theca interna

Theca externa

Stages of ovum and follicle

Primary follicle

Epithelial cord growing in

Primordial follicle

Superficial (germinal) epithelium (cuboidal cells)

Blood vessels entering ovary

Visceral peritoneum of mesovarium

Secondary (antral) follicles

Mature (graafian) follicle

Corpus albicans

Mature corpus luteum

Fibrin

Blood clot

Early corpus luteum

Luteal cells

Ruptured follicle (corpus hemorrhagicum)

Discharged ovum

2.3 OVARY, OVA, AND FOLLICLE DEVELOPMENT

The ovary is an exocrine and endocrine organ composed of loose connective tissue, a fibrous capsule, and a **germinal epithelium** continuous with the peritoneum of the mesovarium. Its exocrine process is ovulation. Each ovary has approximately 400,000 oocytes at birth, and each month in the reproductive years, a few begin to develop in hormone-secreting **follicles.** Typically, only one follicle reaches maturity and ruptures to release the oocyte from the ovary. After ovulation, the follicle becomes the **corpus luteum.** Follicular hormones control the timing of ovulation, and the corpus luteum prepares the uterus for pregnancy. If pregnancy occurs, the corpus luteum greatly enlarges to maintain the pregnancy and develop the mammary glands (in conjunction with placental hormones).

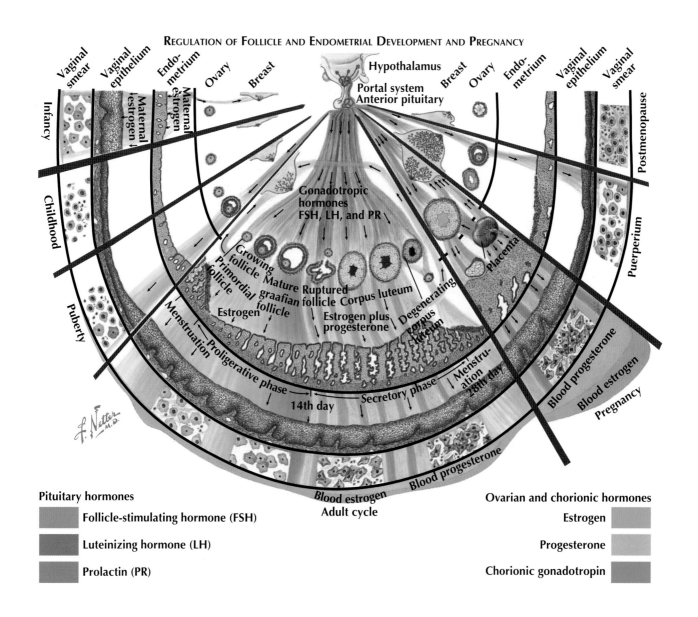

REGULATION OF FOLLICLE AND ENDOMETRIAL DEVELOPMENT AND PREGNANCY

Pituitary hormones

- Follicle-stimulating hormone (FSH)
- Luteinizing hormone (LH)
- Prolactin (PR)

Ovarian and chorionic hormones

- Estrogen
- Progesterone
- Chorionic gonadotropin

2.4 THE MENSTRUAL CYCLE AND PREGNANCY

Gonadotropic hormones from the hypothalamus cause the anterior lobe of the pituitary gland (pars distalis) to release **follicle-stimulating hormone** (FSH) and **luteinizing hormone** (LH). These hormones stimulate the development of ovarian follicles, which in turn secrete **estrogen**. Rising estrogen levels trigger a surge of LH. This results in ovulation and the development of the corpus luteum,

which begins to secrete **progesterone** and estrogen. Progesterone builds up the endometrial wall in preparation for implantation (pregnancy). Progesterone also inhibits LH, so if no pregnancy occurs, the corpus luteum causes its own demise because its hormone secretion inhibits the hormone that promotes its development. If a pregnancy occurs, the placenta produces **human chorionic gonadotropin** (hCG) to maintain the corpus luteum and pregnancy.

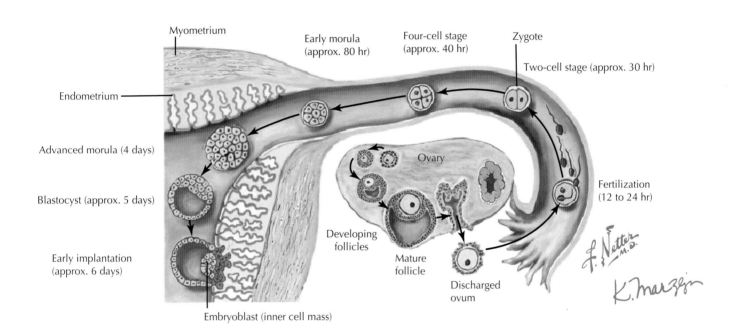

Myometrium · Early morula (approx. 80 hr) · Four-cell stage (approx. 40 hr) · Zygote · Two-cell stage (approx. 30 hr) · Endometrium · Ovary · Advanced morula (4 days) · Blastocyst (approx. 5 days) · Fertilization (12 to 24 hr) · Early implantation (approx. 6 days) · Developing follicles · Mature follicle · Discharged ovum · Embryoblast (inner cell mass)

2.5 OVULATION, FERTILIZATION, AND MIGRATION DOWN THE UTERINE TUBE

Ovulation occurs when a maturing egg (**ovum**) is released from an **ovarian follicle** at the surface of the ovary. **Fimbriae** of the uterine tube cover the ovary and guide the ovum into the uterine tube. **Conception**, or **fertilization**, occurs in the distal third of the uterine tube. A **zygote** forms when the sperm and egg nuclei unite. Cell division results in two-, four-, and eight-cell stages in the uterine tube. By 3 to 4 days, a tight ball of cells termed the **morula** is ready to enter the uterine cavity. Near the end of the first week, the morula becomes the fluid-filled **blastocyst** with an **inner cell mass** (embryoblast) and outer **trophoblast**. The blastocyst adheres to the uterine mucosa (usually high up on the posterior wall) and sinks within it during **implantation.**

Sites of ectopic implantation

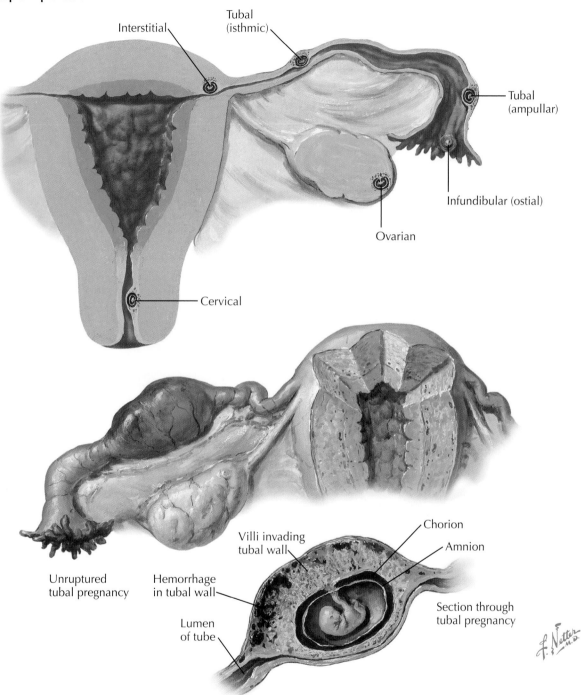

Interstitial

Tubal (isthmic)

Tubal (ampullar)

Infundibular (ostial)

Ovarian

Cervical

Unruptured tubal pregnancy

Hemorrhage in tubal wall

Villi invading tubal wall

Lumen of tube

Chorion

Amnion

Section through tubal pregnancy

2.6 ECTOPIC PREGNANCY

An ectopic pregnancy results from the implantation of the blastocyst in an abnormal location. It can occur on the surface of the ovary or anywhere along the path of migration into the uterine cavity. Implantation can occur at any location within the uterus, including the cervix, although that location is extremely rare. The most common ectopic implantation site (95%) is within the uterine tube.

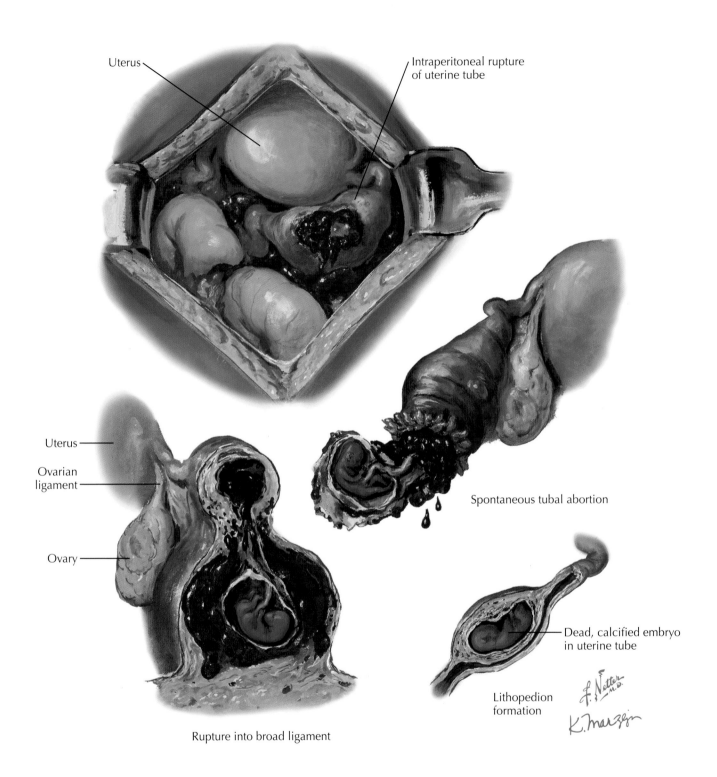

Uterus

Intraperitoneal rupture
of uterine tube

Spontaneous tubal abortion

Uterus

Ovarian
ligament

Ovary

Dead, calcified embryo
in uterine tube

Lithopedion
formation

Rupture into broad ligament

2.7 TUBAL PREGNANCY

Tubal pregnancies are common ectopic sites that can lead to maternal mortality if undetected. Unlike the uterus, the uterine tubes are not capable of expanding, and the likelihood of tubal rupture and hemorrhage increases from the second through the fifth month.

CLINICAL POINT

Symptoms of a tubal pregnancy may include blood passing out of the end of the uterine tube into the rectouterine pouch or other abdominal locations, resulting in peritoneal pain. Blood may also enter the endometrial cavity, presenting as a **pseudosac** that may be confused with an intrauterine **gestational sac** (chorionic sac), an early indicator of a normal intrauterine pregnancy.

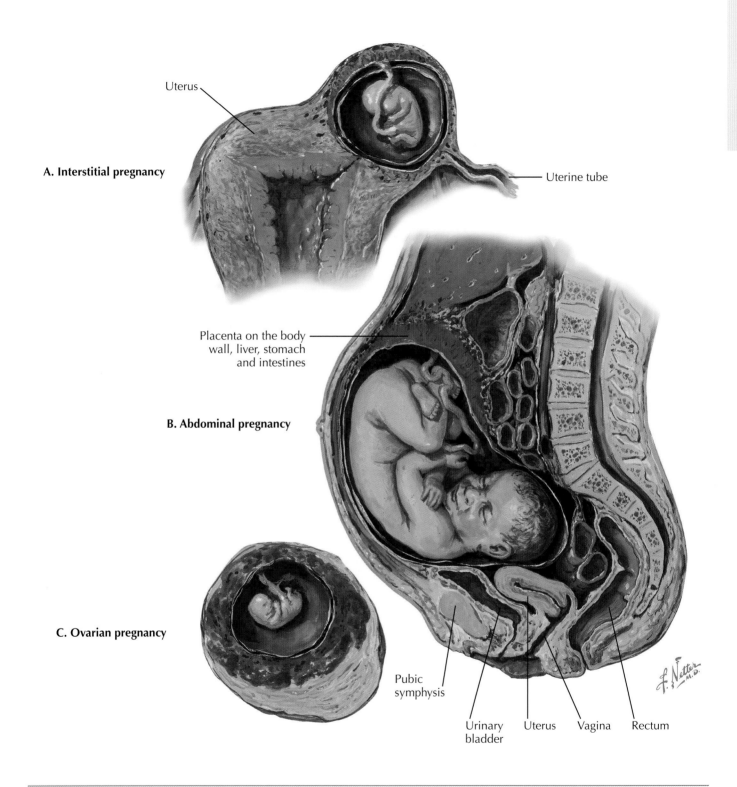

A. Interstitial pregnancy

Uterus

Uterine tube

Placenta on the body wall, liver, stomach and intestines

B. Abdominal pregnancy

C. Ovarian pregnancy

Pubic symphysis

Urinary bladder

Uterus

Vagina

Rectum

2.8 INTERSTITIAL, ABDOMINAL, AND OVARIAN PREGNANCY

Fig. 2.8A shows an ectopic pregnancy in the interstitial, uterine part of the uterine tube. Because the uterine tubes are not physically connected to the ovary, it is possible for a fertilized oocyte or spontaneously aborted conceptus in the distal uterine tube to escape into the pelvic or abdominal cavity with implantation on the ovary (Fig. 2.8C), uterus, urinary bladder, or any abdominal organ or mesentery (Fig. 2.8B). A placenta can form on most tissues or structures, and development can proceed to term outside of the uterus. This is extremely rare, and abdominal pregnancies may have considerable bleeding because of gastrointestinal organ movement and the unstable environment for the placenta.

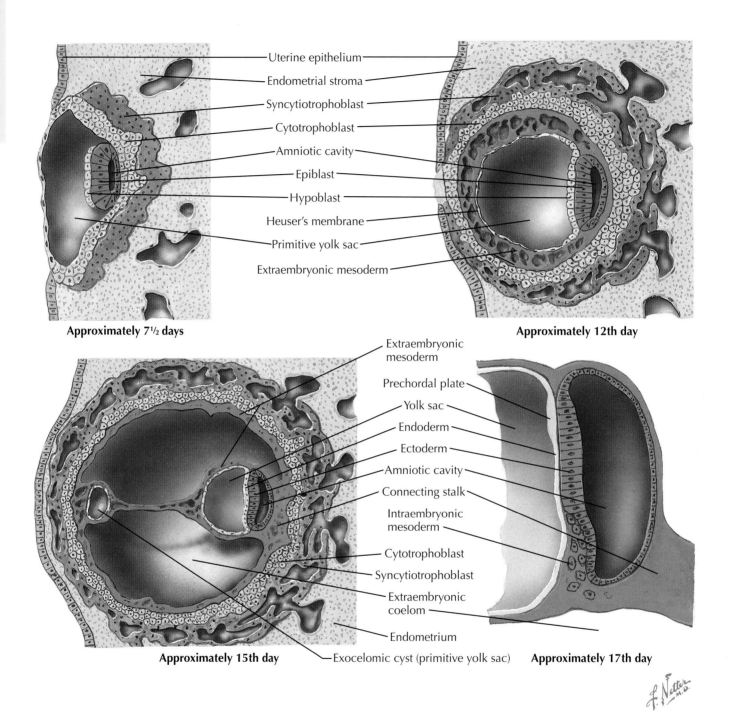

Uterine epithelium
Endometrial stroma
Syncytiotrophoblast
Cytotrophoblast
Amniotic cavity
Epiblast
Hypoblast
Heuser's membrane
Primitive yolk sac
Extraembryonic mesoderm

Approximately 7½ days

Approximately 12th day

Extraembryonic mesoderm
Prechordal plate
Yolk sac
Endoderm
Ectoderm
Amniotic cavity
Connecting stalk
Intraembryonic mesoderm
Cytotrophoblast
Syncytiotrophoblast
Extraembryonic coelom
Endometrium

Approximately 15th day   Exocelomic cyst (primitive yolk sac)   **Approximately 17th day**

2.9 IMPLANTATION AND EXTRAEMBRYONIC MEMBRANE FORMATION

The trophoblast develops two layers: an outer **syncytiotrophoblast** (or syntrophoblast) and inner **cytotrophoblast.** The inner cell mass develops into two cell types: a columnar epithelial **epiblast** and cuboidal **hypoblast.** The epiblast cell mass becomes hollow to form the fluid-filled primitive amniotic cavity. The hypoblast cells form a simple squamous primitive yolk sac (Heuser's membrane). A second wave of hypoblast cell migration displaces the primitive yolk sac. Extraembryonic mesoderm coats the old blastocyst cavity to complete the extraembryonic membranes. The trophoblast is now the three-layered **chorion.** Mesoderm and endoderm (former hypoblast cells) form the definitive yolk sac. Mesoderm and ectoderm (former epiblast cells) form the definitive amnion.

Formation of Intraembryonic Mesoderm from the Primitive Streak and Node (Knot)

Ectoderm

Amniotic cavity

Notochord

Primitive knot (node)

Primitive streak

Extraembryonic mesoderm

Endoderm

Migration of cells from the primitive streak to form the intraembryonic mesoderm

Yolk sac cavity

Cupola of yolk sac

Oropharyngeal membrane

Oropharyngeal membrane

Notochord

Paraxial column

Intermediate column

Lateral plate

Appearance of the neural plate

Notochord

Spreading of intraembryonic mesoderm

Cloacal membrane

C. Machado
—M.D.

2.10 **GASTRULATION**

Gastrulation is the production of intraembryonic mesoderm from thickenings of ectoderm—the primitive streak and primitive knot (or node). The latter forms a midline cord of mesoderm, the notochord. The primitive streak gives rise to the rest of the intraembryonic mesoderm, including the cardiogenic mesoderm in front of the oropharyngeal membrane. Gastrulation is complete when the intraembryonic mesoderm condenses into columns flanking the notochord: paraxial columns (future somites), intermediate mesoderm, and lateral plates. The mesoderm between the columns is in the form of mesenchyme, the loose embryonic connective tissue that surrounds structures in the embryo. The primitive streak and node recede toward the tail end of the embryo and disappear.

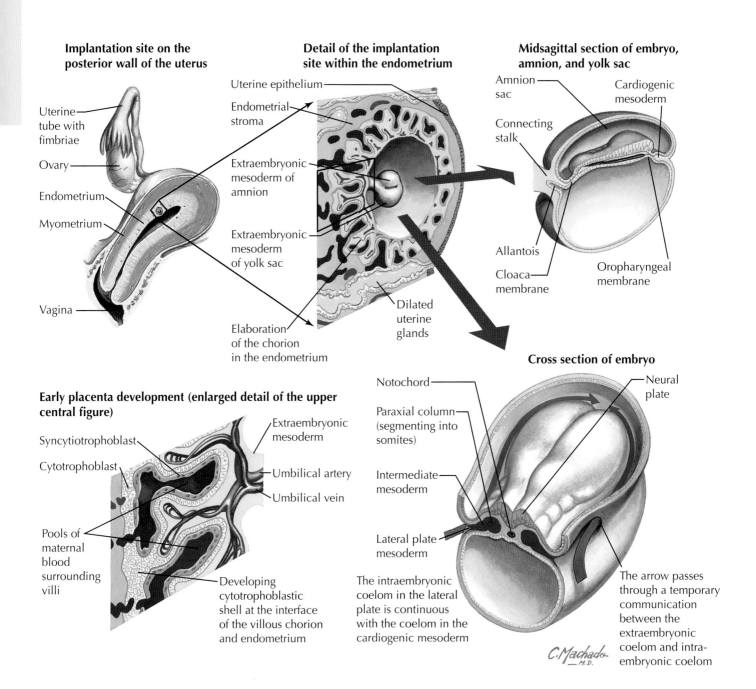

Implantation site on the posterior wall of the uterus

Uterine tube with fimbriae

Ovary

Endometrium

Myometrium

Vagina

Detail of the implantation site within the endometrium

Uterine epithelium

Endometrial stroma

Extraembryonic mesoderm of amnion

Extraembryonic mesoderm of yolk sac

Elaboration of the chorion in the endometrium

Dilated uterine glands

Midsagittal section of embryo, amnion, and yolk sac

Amnion sac

Cardiogenic mesoderm

Connecting stalk

Allantois

Cloaca membrane

Oropharyngeal membrane

Early placenta development (enlarged detail of the upper central figure)

Syncytiotrophoblast

Cytotrophoblast

Extraembryonic mesoderm

Umbilical artery

Umbilical vein

Pools of maternal blood surrounding villi

Developing cytotrophoblastic shell at the interface of the villous chorion and endometrium

Cross section of embryo

Notochord

Neural plate

Paraxial column (segmenting into somites)

Intermediate mesoderm

Lateral plate mesoderm

The intraembryonic coelom in the lateral plate is continuous with the coelom in the cardiogenic mesoderm

The arrow passes through a temporary communication between the extraembryonic coelom and intra-embryonic coelom

C. Machado ＿M.D.

2.11 NEURULATION AND EARLY PLACENTA AND COELOM DEVELOPMENT

Concurrent with gastrulation are the first steps in the formation of the nervous system, heart, placenta, umbilical cord, and intra-embryonic coelom (body cavities). Primordia include neural plate ectoderm in front of the primitive streak, cardiogenic mesoderm in front of the oral membrane, and a hollowing of the lateral plate to form an intraembryonic coelom. The placenta develops from the chorion. The connecting stalk between the embryo and placenta shifts toward the tail end of the embryo to form the umbilical cord. Oral and cloacal membranes are sites of the future mouth and anus, respectively. The allantois is a vestigial extraembryonic membrane in humans consisting of an endodermal evagination of the yolk sac into the mesoderm of the connecting stalk.

Midsagittal section of folding gastrula

Notochord in gastrula

Amnion

Oropharyngeal membrane

Connecting stalk

Cardiogenic mesoderm

Allantois

Yolk sac

Cloacal membrane

Foregut

Midgut

Stomodeum

Developing heart tube and pericardial cavity

Hindgut

C. Machado — M.D.

Cross section of folding gastrula

Connecting stalk

Amnion (*cut*)

Neural plate

Paraxial column

Intermediate mesoderm

Communication between extraembryonic and intraembryonic coeloms

Lateral plate

Notochord

Yolk sac

Neural crest

Embryonic endoderm forming gastrointestinal (gut) tube

Neural plate forming neural tube

Somite

Somatic mesoderm of lateral plate

Intermediate mesoderm

Intraembryonic coelom

Amnion tucking around the sides of the folding embryo

Notochord

Splanchnic mesoderm of lateral plate

2.12 FOLDING OF THE GASTRULA

Shaping of the gastrula occurs as the amnion tucks around and under the elongated embryo on all sides. The endoderm of the embryo (roof of the yolk sac) is compressed into a tube by this process. The remainder of the yolk sac extends out of the embryo ventrally and is pushed against the connecting stalk by the amnion. Most of the transverse folding involves an extension of the lateral plate and enlargement of the coelom, which divides the ventral part of the embryo into gut and body wall components. The amnion also tucks around the head and tail ends of the embryo.

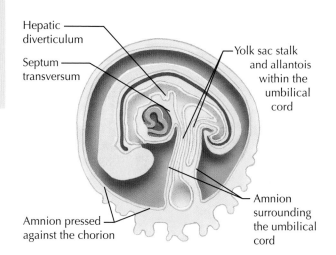

Hepatic diverticulum

Septum transversum

Yolk sac stalk and allantois within the umbilical cord

Amnion surrounding the umbilical cord

Amnion pressed against the chorion

Cross section of folding gastrula

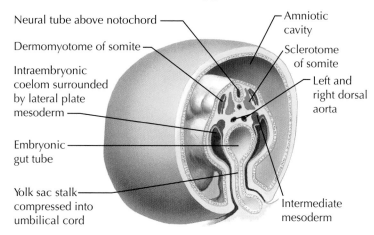

Neural tube above notochord

Dermomyotome of somite

Intraembryonic coelom surrounded by lateral plate mesoderm

Embryonic gut tube

Yolk sac stalk compressed into umbilical cord

Amniotic cavity

Sclerotome of somite

Left and right dorsal aorta

Intermediate mesoderm

Vertebrate body plan after 4 weeks

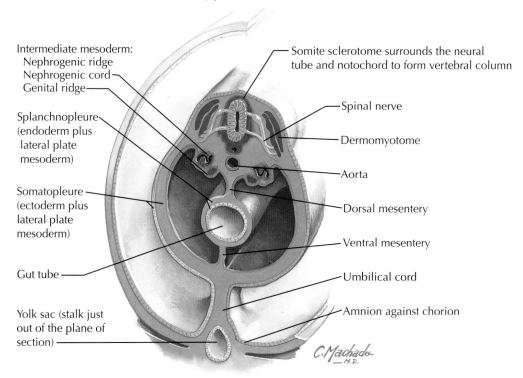

Intermediate mesoderm:
Nephrogenic ridge
Nephrogenic cord
Genital ridge

Splanchnopleure (endoderm plus lateral plate mesoderm)

Somatopleure (ectoderm plus lateral plate mesoderm)

Gut tube

Yolk sac (stalk just out of the plane of section)

Somite sclerotome surrounds the neural tube and notochord to form vertebral column

Spinal nerve

Dermomyotome

Aorta

Dorsal mesentery

Ventral mesentery

Umbilical cord

Amnion against chorion

C. Machado
M.D.

2.13 THE VERTEBRATE BODY PLAN

The vertebrate body plan is established after folding of the gastrula. By the end of the fourth week (bottom), the lateral plate is now a thin coating of the coelomic cavities. With the surface ectoderm, it forms **somatopleure**, the basis of the lateral and ventral body wall. The endoderm and mesoderm from the lateral plate form **splanchnopleure**, the primordium of the gut tube and visceral organs that develop from it. Each somite differentiates into a **myotome** that will form muscle, a **dermatome** relating to the surface ectoderm, and a bone-forming **sclerotome** that condenses around the neural tube. The somite myotomes connect with the spinal nerves, and the ventral part (hypomere) will migrate into the somatopleure.

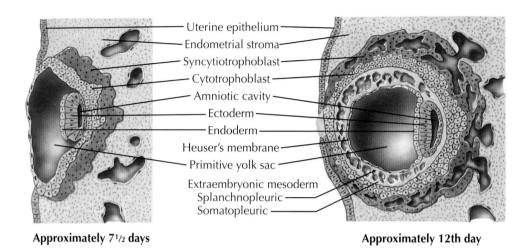

Approximately 7½ days

- Uterine epithelium
- Endometrial stroma
- Syncytiotrophoblast
- Cytotrophoblast
- Amniotic cavity
- Ectoderm
- Endoderm
- Heuser's membrane
- Primitive yolk sac
- Extraembryonic mesoderm
  - Splanchnopleuric
  - Somatopleuric

Approximately 12th day

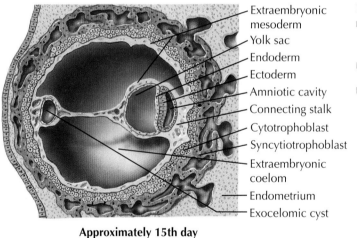

Approximately 15th day

- Extraembryonic mesoderm
- Yolk sac
- Endoderm
- Ectoderm
- Amniotic cavity
- Connecting stalk
- Cytotrophoblast
- Syncytiotrophoblast
- Extraembryonic coelom
- Endometrium
- Exocelomic cyst

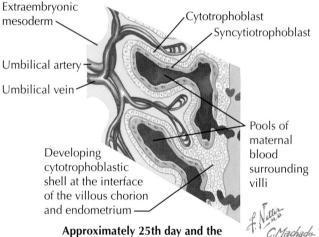

- Extraembryonic mesoderm
- Umbilical artery
- Umbilical vein
- Cytotrophoblast
- Syncytiotrophoblast
- Pools of maternal blood surrounding villi
- Developing cytotrophoblastic shell at the interface of the villous chorion and endometrium

Approximately 25th day and the establishment of placental circulation

2.14 FORMATION OF THE PLACENTA

All three layers of the chorion invade the endometrium to form branching, finger-like **villi**. The **syncytiotrophoblast** is in direct contact with maternal blood, and the mesoderm forms the connective tissue core of the villi and their blood vessels. The **cytotrophoblast** disappears midway through pregnancy to help thin the placental membrane between fetal and maternal blood.

CLINICAL POINT

The syncytiotrophoblast synthesizes hormones from fetal and maternal precursors. **Protein hormones** include hCG, human placental lactogen, human chorionic thyrotropin, and human chorionic corticotropin. hCG prevents menstruation by maintaining the corpus luteum. Placental **steroid hormones**, including **progesterone** and **estrogens**, help the corpus luteum maintain the later stages of pregnancy.

Early fetal development and membrane formation in relation to the uterus as a whole (schematic)

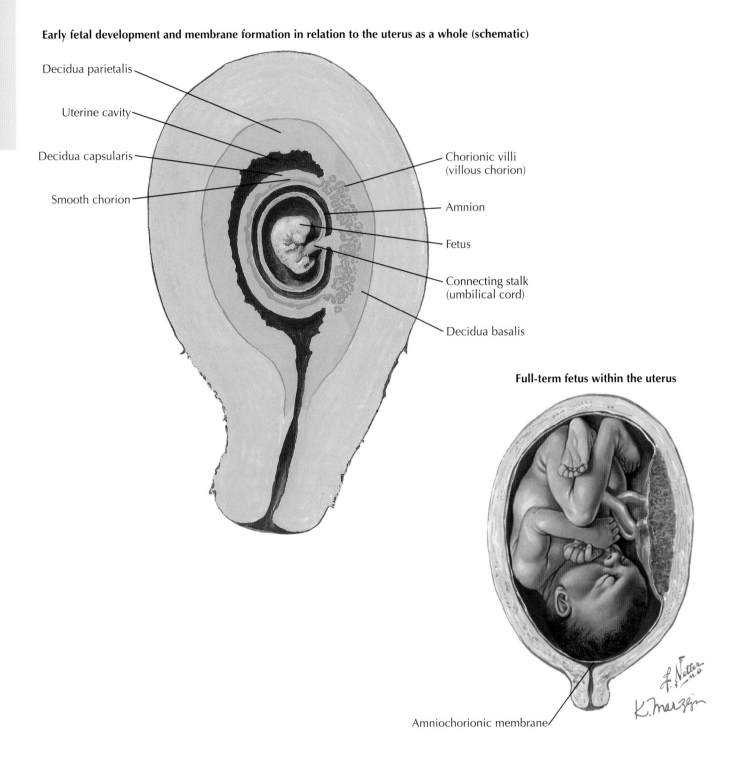

Decidua parietalis

Uterine cavity

Decidua capsularis

Smooth chorion

Chorionic villi
(villous chorion)

Amnion

Fetus

Connecting stalk
(umbilical cord)

Decidua basalis

Full-term fetus within the uterus

Amniochorionic membrane

2.15 THE ENDOMETRIUM AND FETAL MEMBRANES

Fetal development is entirely within the decidua (mucosal wall of the uterus or **endometrium**). The decidua is named according to its relationship to the placenta and fetal membranes. The **decidua parietalis** is uninvolved with the fetus and placenta on the anterior uterine wall. The **decidua capsularis** is the thin layer or "capsule" of endometrium over the **smooth chorion** and amnion. The **decidua basalis** is the maternal contribution to the placenta. The **villous chorion** is the fetal component of the placenta. The decidua capsularis disappears, and the fused **amniochorionic membrane** is pressed against the decidua parietalis, obliterating the uterine cavity. This membrane ruptures during labor or, if the rupture is premature, it may cause labor.

Development of the placenta: chorionic villi

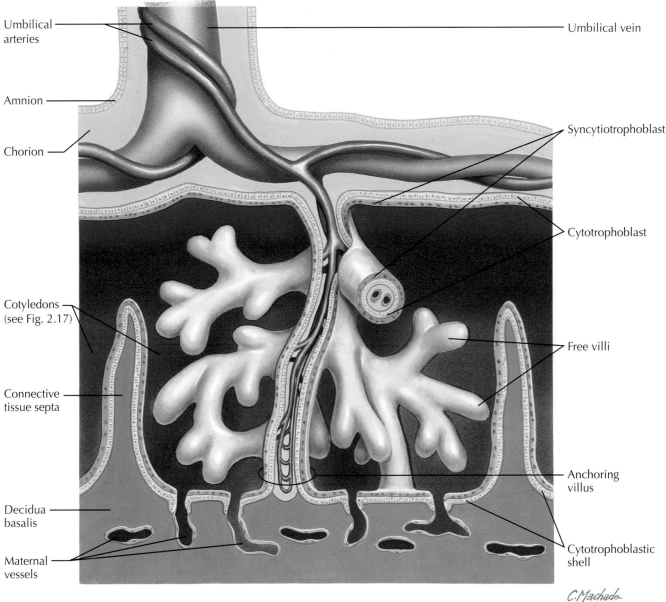

Umbilical arteries

Amnion

Chorion

Cotyledons (see Fig. 2.17)

Connective tissue septa

Decidua basalis

Maternal vessels

Umbilical vein

Syncytiotrophoblast

Cytotrophoblast

Free villi

Anchoring villus

Cytotrophoblastic shell

C. Machado
_M.D._

2.16 PLACENTAL STRUCTURE

The **chorionic plate** is on the fetal surface of the placenta. Extending from it with placental branches of the umbilical vessels are **stem villi** that branch extensively to form the free villi, where metabolic exchange occurs. The syntrophoblast is the outer layer of the villi, except at the ends of the **anchoring villi**, which connects the villous chorion to the decidua basalis. Here the cytotrophoblast layer extends through the syntrophoblast to form the **cytotrophoblastic shell** at the interface between fetal and maternal components of the placenta. Decidual spiral arteries open through this shell to directly bathe the chorionic villi in maternal blood. The placental membrane (formerly the "maternal-fetal blood barrier") separating maternal and fetal blood consists of these components early in pregnancy: syncytiotrophoblast, cytotrophoblast, villi mesenchyme, and fetal blood vessel epithelium and its basal lamina. The placental membrane thins in later pregnancy by the elimination of the cytotrophoblast and the pressing of fetal blood vessels against the syntrophoblast, where they share a basal lamina. This gets maternal and fetal blood as close together as possible for more efficient metabolic exchange.

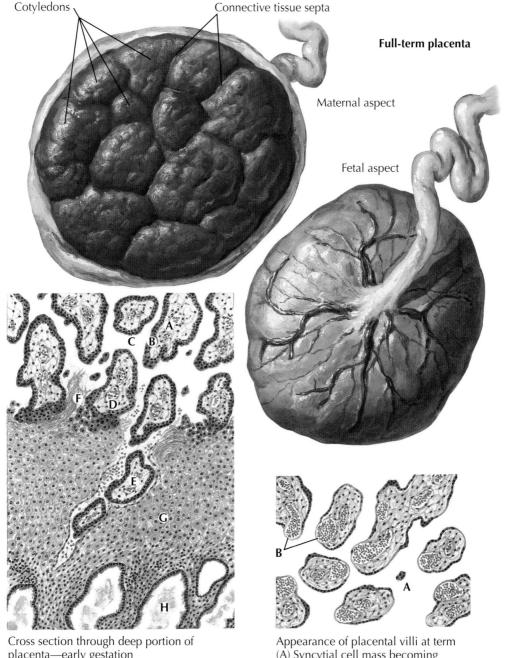

Cotyledons

Connective tissue septa

Full-term placenta

Maternal aspect

Fetal aspect

Cross section through deep portion of
placenta—early gestation
(A) Villus, (B) trophoblast, (C) intervillous
space, (D) anchoring villus, (E) villus invading
blood vessel, (F) fibrinoid degeneration,
(G) decidua basalis, (H) gland

Appearance of placental villi at term
(A) Syncytial cell mass becoming
trophoblastic embolus, (B) fetal blood vessel
endothelium against a thinned
syncytiotrophoblast, where they share a basal
lamina. The cytotrophoblast has disappeared

2.17 EXTERNAL PLACENTAL STRUCTURE; PLACENTAL MEMBRANE

SUBSTANCES THAT CROSS THE PLACENTAL MEMBRANE
Beneficial:
- Metabolic gases (O_2, CO_2)
- Fetal urea, uric acid, bilirubin
- Water and electrolytes
- Vitamins, glucose, amino acids, free fatty acids
- Fetal and maternal red blood cells (later months)
- Steroid hormones
- IgG immunoglobulins
  Harmful:

- Carbon monoxide
- Most viruses (including HIV, polio, measles)
- Most drugs (including alcohol, cocaine, nicotine, caffeine, anesthetics, anticancer drugs)
- Treponema pallidum (syphilis) and Toxoplasma gondii (parasite)
- Anti-Rh antibodies (IgG)

SUBSTANCES THAT DO NOT CROSS THE PLACENTAL MEMBRANE
- Most bacteria
- Most proteins (cross very slowly), protein hormones, insulin
- IgM immunoglobulins
- Maternal triglycerides, cholesterol, and phospholipids
- Some drugs (e.g., heparin, curare, methyldopa)

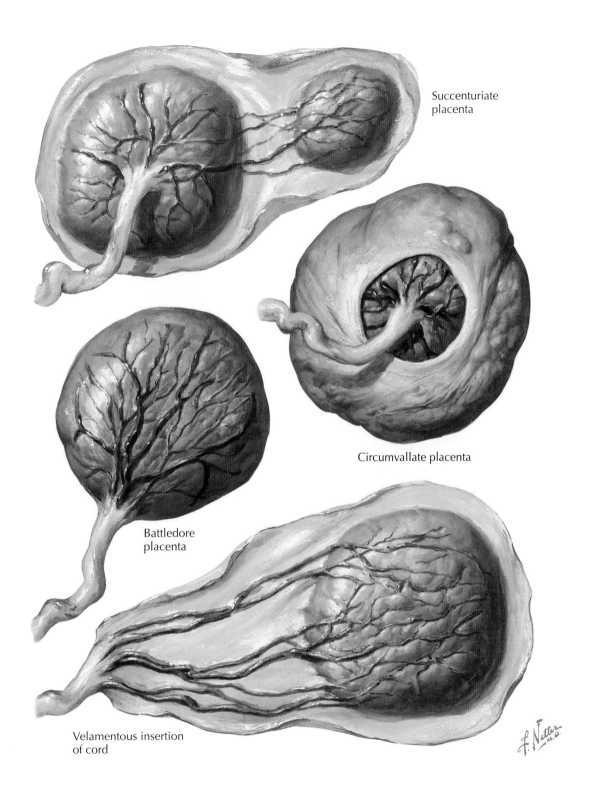

Succenturiate placenta

Circumvallate placenta

Battledore placenta

Velamentous insertion of cord

2.18 PLACENTAL VARIATIONS

A placenta can have accessory lobes with vascular connections between them (succenturiate placenta), or there can be no vascular connections (placenta spuria—not shown). The umbilical cord may be inserted at the margin of the placenta to give it a club-like appearance (battledore placenta). In a more extreme type of marginal insertion, the umbilical cord is attached to the chorion and amnion instead of the placenta (velamentous insertion of cord), and the vessels branch between the membranes before they extend over the placenta. In a circumvallate placenta, the membranes extend over the placenta to form a ring before doubling back toward the margin. Most variations are of no consequence, although velamentous insertion of the cord can result in serious bleeding.

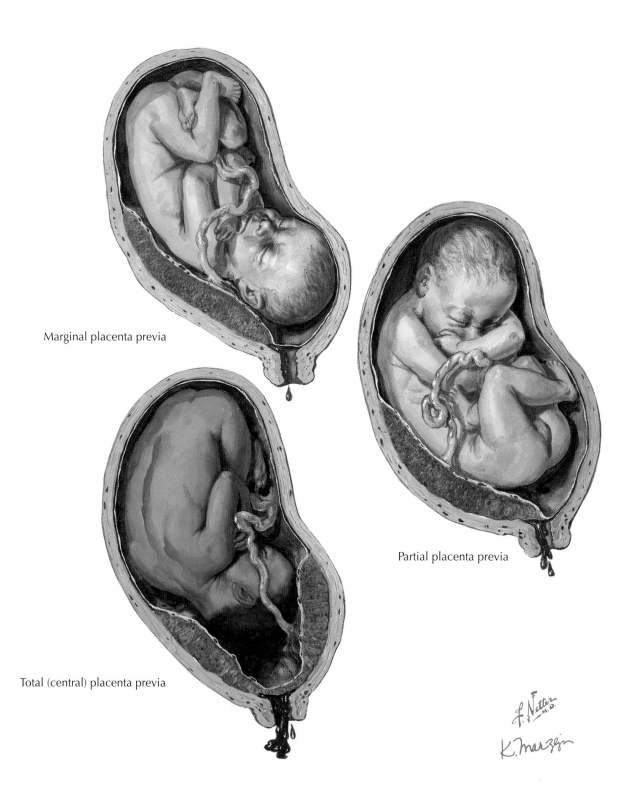

Marginal placenta previa

Partial placenta previa

Total (central) placenta previa

2.19 PLACENTA PREVIA

If implantation is in the lower part of the uterus, the placenta will partially or totally cover the internal os of the cervix. It can block the birth canal and is a common cause of bleeding in the third trimester. Hemorrhage from placenta previa can be fatal to the fetus or even the mother.

A. First appearance of the gestational sac (chorionic sac). Transvaginal axial image, 2 ½ weeks. Key on the left. *(Reused with permission from Hertzberg BS, Middleton WD. Ultrasound: The Requisites, 3rd Ed., Elsevier, 2015.)*

Endometrium

Gestational sac

↓ ↓ ↓ = Uterine cavity

Embryo   Amnion

Embryo   Decidua basalis (placenta)

Uterus myometrium

Secondary yolk sac

Gestational sac

Decidua capsularis

Primary yolk sac

Decidua parietalis   Uterine cavity

SAG UT   4.0-

B. Appearance of the yolk sac and embryo. Transvaginal sagittal image, 4 weeks. Transvaginal sagittal image, 4 weeks, on the right. Key on the left (gestational sac detail) a bit earlier. Note in the image the **double decidual sign** of the darker decidua capsularis against the lighter decidua parietalis with the collapsed uterine cavity in between. *(Radiology reused with permission from Lazarus E, Levine D. The First Trimester in Diagnostic Ultrasound, edited by Rumack CM, Levine D. Elsevier, 2017, 1048-1087.)*

2.20 EARLY DETECTION OF PREGNANCY

The first indication of a pregnancy is a detectable blood level of human chorionic gonadotropin within 6 to 12 days after ovulation. Pregnancy can be confirmed by confirmation of a **gestational sac** (chorion) in the endometrium with transvaginal ultrasound. A 1- to 2-mm gestational sac is detectable as early as 2 ½ weeks after conception (Fig. 2.20A) but can be confused with a **pseudosac**, which is an accumulation of blood or fluid in the endometrial (uterine) cavity, or other cyst-like structure. A yolk sac is visible in a 10-mm gestational sac in the third week (Fig. 2.20B). This is the first unequivocal confirmation of a gestational sac and intrauterine pregnancy. The embryo and amnion show up at 4+ weeks.

CLINICAL POINT

Another diagnostic feature of pregnancy in the third week is a **double decidual sign** consisting of a thickened band of decidua capsularis surrounding the gestational sac bulging against the decidua parietalis on the other side of the collapsed endometrial cavity (Fig. 2.20B). Contributing to the echogenicity of the double decidual sign is the **decidual reaction** of the decidua capsularis and basalis. Progesterone and induction from the conceptus cause the endometrial stromal cells to enlarge with lipid and glycogen and produce cytokines that cause edema and the infiltration leukocytes that suppress a maternal immune reaction to the conceptus. Also effected are changes in uterine arteries and the trophoblast that facilitate placenta formation.

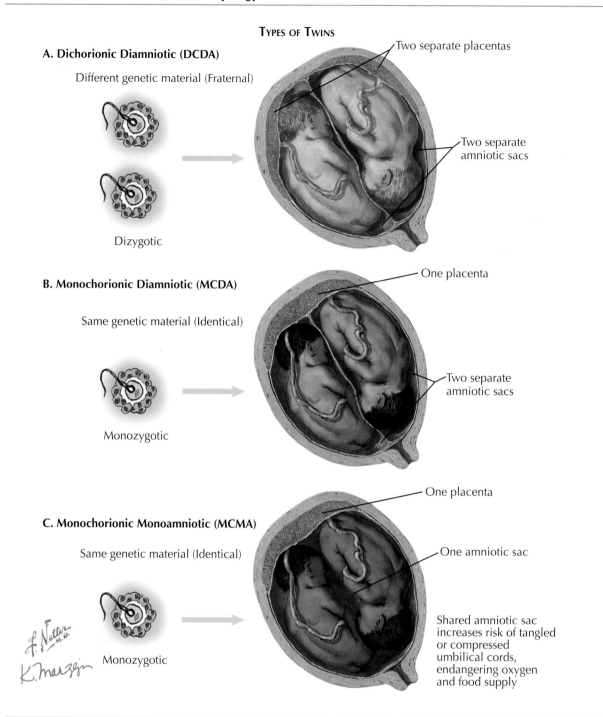

TYPES OF TWINS

A. Dichorionic Diamniotic (DCDA)

Different genetic material (Fraternal)

Dizygotic

Two separate placentas

Two separate amniotic sacs

B. Monochorionic Diamniotic (MCDA)

Same genetic material (Identical)

Monozygotic

One placenta

Two separate amniotic sacs

C. Monochorionic Monoamniotic (MCMA)

Same genetic material (Identical)

Monozygotic

One placenta

One amniotic sac

Shared amniotic sac increases risk of tangled or compressed umbilical cords, endangering oxygen and food supply

2.21 TWINNING

Most twins (70%) are dizygotic (nonidentical) twins that originate from two ova fertilized by two sperm, often associated with higher levels of FSH in the maternal serum. There are two implantations and the development of two genetically distinct embryos with two chorions, two amnions, and two placentas (Fig. 2.21A). Monozygotic (identical) twins result from a single zygote, with division of the embryoblast occurring during the first 2 weeks of development. More than 60% of monozygotic twins result from division of the inner cell mass of the blastocyst after the chorion has started to develop (Fig. 2.21B). There are one chorion and one placenta but two amnions. If division occurs before the blastocyst, placentation and extraembryonic membranes will be the same as in dizygotic twins. Division later will result in two embryos enclosed by a single amnion (Fig. 2.21C) or incomplete division of the embryos, the embryonic basis of conjoined twins. The mechanism of division anywhere in the timeline is not well understood.

CLINICAL POINT

The incidence of dizygotic twinning varies between populations but is relatively stable for monozygotic twinning, although the incidence in the latter is two to five times greater with in vitro fertilization. The incidence of congenital anomalies in monozygotic twins is two to three times higher, likely a mechanical artifact of the division event. Complications can also result from abnormal connections of blood vessels between the two placentas. Twinning, in general, increases the risk of placenta previa and can have many adverse cardiovascular effects in the mother.

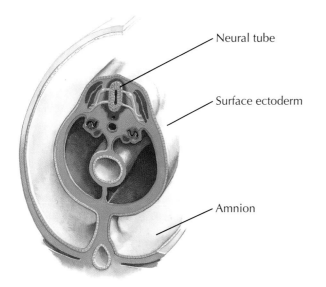

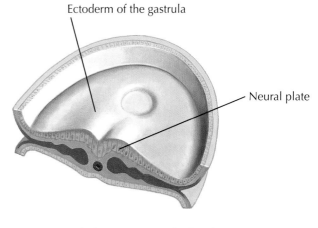

CHART 2.1   ECTODERMAL DERIVATIVES

Primordia	Derivatives or Fate
Surface ectoderm	Epidermis of the skin
	Sweat, sebaceous, and mammary glands
	Nails and hair
	Tooth enamel
	Lacrimal glands
	Conjunctiva
	External auditory meatus
(Stomodeum and nasal placodes)	Oral and nasal epithelium
	Anterior pituitary
(Otic placodes)	Inner ear
(Lens placodes)	Lens of eye
Neural tube	Central nervous system
	Somatomotor neurons
	Branchiomotor neurons
	Presynaptic autonomic neurons
	Retina/optic nerves
	Posterior pituitary
Neural crest	Peripheral sensory neurons
	Postsynaptic autonomic neurons
	All ganglia
	Adrenal medulla cells
	Melanocytes
	Bone, muscle, and connective tissue in the head and neck
Amnion	Protective bag (with chorion) around fetus

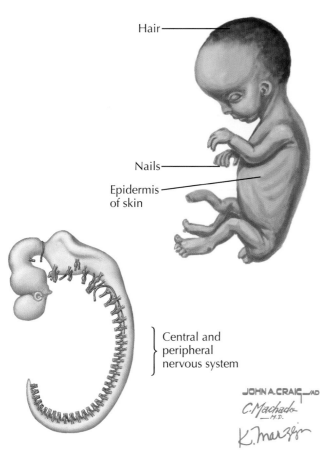

JOHN A. CRAIG—AD
C. Machado—M.D.
K. Marzin

2.22 SUMMARY OF ECTODERMAL DERIVATIVES

Ectoderm gives rise to the nervous system and the outer covering of the body. It forms the epithelial component of the skin—the epidermis—and all of the glands, continuations, invaginations, and structures that develop from it. Hair and nails consist of protein-filled ("keratinized") cells that are similar in composition to the keratinized layer of squamous cells on the surface of the epidermis. Placodes are thickenings of surface ectoderm in the head, and the stomodeum is an invagination of ectoderm that lines the oral cavity. An unusual fate of ectoderm is the formation of connective tissue and muscle from neural crest cells in the head and neck. Ectoderm and all other cells and tissues in the body originally come from the embryonic epiblast.

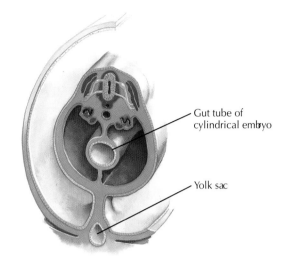

Gut tube of cylindrical embryo

Yolk sac

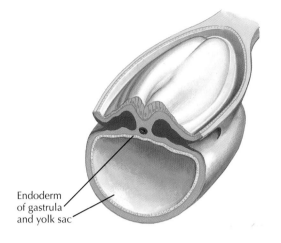

Endoderm of gastrula and yolk sac

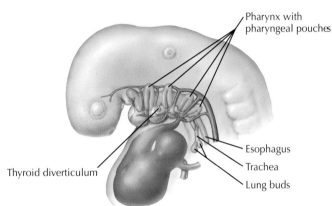

Pharynx with pharyngeal pouches

Thyroid diverticulum

Esophagus

Trachea

Lung buds

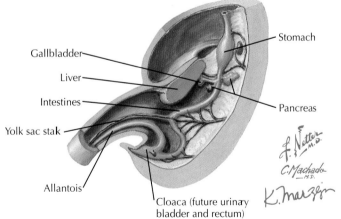

Gallbladder

Liver

Intestines

Yolk sac stalk

Allantois

Stomach

Pancreas

Cloaca (future urinary bladder and rectum)

CHART 2.2   ENDODERMAL DERIVATIVES

Primordia	Epithelial Derivatives or Fate
Gut tube endoderm	GI tract (enterocytes) Mucosal glands of GI tract Parenchyma of GI organs (liver, pancreas) Airway lining (larynx, trachea, bronchial tree) Thyroid gland Tonsils
Cloaca (part of hindgut)	Rectum and anal canal Bladder, urethra, and related glands Vestibule Lower vagina
Pharyngeal pouches (part of foregut)	Auditory tube and middle ear epithelium Palatine tonsil crypts Thymus gland Parathyroid glands C cells of the thyroid gland
Yolk sac	Embryonic blood cell production (mesoderm) Pressed into umbilical cord, then disappears
Allantois (from yolk sac, then cloaca)	Embryonic blood cell production (mesoderm) Vestigial, fibrous urachus Umbilical cord part disappears

GI, Gastrointestinal.

2.23 SUMMARY OF ENDODERMAL DERIVATIVES

Endoderm is derived from the embryonic epiblast in a wave of cellular migration that displaces the hypoblast. After folding of the gastrula into a cylinder, the endoderm is shaped into an epithelial, gastrointestinal tube extending from the stomodeum to the cloacal membrane. Most internal glands and organs develop as buds or evaginations of the endodermal tube (e.g., thyroid gland, liver, pancreas) or from the tube itself (e.g., stomach, intestines). The simple cuboidal endoderm gives rise to the epithelial linings (parenchyma) of these organs. Included is the lining of the airway—the larynx, trachea, and bronchial tree.

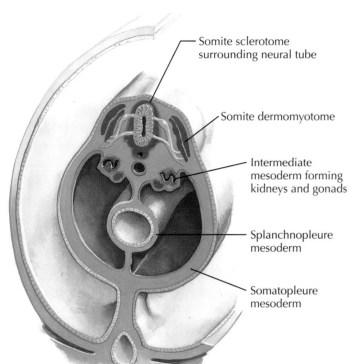

Somite sclerotome surrounding neural tube

Somite dermomyotome

Intermediate mesoderm forming kidneys and gonads

Splanchnopleure mesoderm

Somatopleure mesoderm

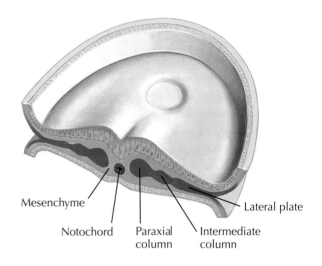

Mesenchyme

Notochord   Paraxial column   Intermediate column

Lateral plate

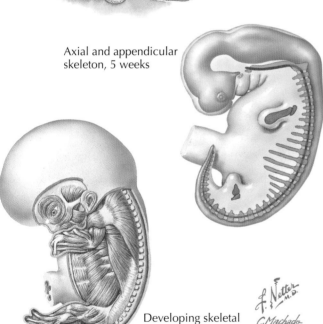

Axial and appendicular skeleton, 5 weeks

Developing skeletal muscles, 8 weeks

CHART 2.3   MESODERMAL DERIVATIVES

Primordia	Derivatives or Fate
Notochord	Nucleus pulposus of an intervertebral disc Induces neurulation
Paraxial columns (somites)	Skeletal muscle Bone Connective tissue (e.g., dorsal dermis, dura mater)
Intermediate mesoderm	Gonads Kidneys and ureters Uterus and uterine tubes Upper vagina Ductus deferens, epididymis, and related tubules Seminal vesicles and ejaculatory ducts
Lateral plate mesoderm	Dermis (ventral) Superficial fascia and related tissues (ventral) Bones and connective tissues of limbs Pleura and peritoneum GI tract connective tissue stroma
Cardiogenic mesoderm	Heart Pericardium

GI, Gastrointestinal.

2.24 SUMMARY OF MESODERMAL DERIVATIVES

Mesoderm originates from the ectoderm of the primitive streak and primitive node during gastrulation. Cardiogenic mesoderm is also from the primitive streak—the heart and pericardium have no endodermal contributions. Mesoderm is in the form of dense, cellular, craniocaudal columns surrounded by loose embryonic connective tissue (mesenchyme). They give rise to bone, muscle, connective tissue, urogenital organs, and the pleural and peritoneal linings of the body cavities. The head is not well developed at the time of gastrulation, so most of the mesoderm in the head and neck comes from the ectodermal neural crest instead of the mesodermal columns (except for somites that do extend into the head).

Terminology

Allantois	The fourth extraembryonic membrane that extends from the yolk sac into the connecting stalk (future umbilical cord), then shifts to the hindgut cloaca. With the yolk sac, it is the first source of embryonic blood cells in mammals. In egg-laying animals, it lines the inner surface of the egg for gas exchange.
Chorion	Extraembryonic membrane derived from the trophoblast of the blastocyst. The smooth chorion and amnion surround the fetus as its protective "bag." The villous chorion is the fetal component of the placenta.
Chorionic plate	The chorionic membrane on the fetal surface of the placenta that gives rise to the stem villi. The umbilical vessels extend from the umbilical cord to the villi through the chorionic plate.
Coelom (celom)	Early embryonic cavity that develops within the lateral plate mesoderm. Intraembryonic coelom will form the pleural and abdominopelvic cavities. The extraembryonic coelom is the interior of the chorionic cavity outside of the embryo.
Corona radiata	Cumulus oophorus cells that are released from the follicle and ovary with the ovum during ovulation. The cells attached to the ovum give the appearance of a "crown" around it.
Corpus luteum	(L., "yellow body") The endocrine gland in the ovary that is formed from a follicle after release of the ovum at ovulation. It produces progesterone (and estrogen) to prepare the endometrium for pregnancy. If pregnancy does not occur, it degenerates into a corpus albicans ("white body") that eventually disappears.
Cotyledons	(G., "a cup-shaped hollow") Irregularly shaped lobes visible on the maternal surface of the placenta circumscribed by deep clefts and decidual septa.
Cumulus oophorus	Mound of stratum granulosum cells that surround an oocyte in an ovarian follicle.
Cytotrophoblastic shell	The cellular plate that attaches the chorionic villi of the placenta to the decidua basalis of the endometrium. It is derived from cytotrophoblast cells that migrate through the external syntrophoblast layer at the maternal ends of anchoring villi.
Decidual reaction	Reaction of maternal connective tissue cells in the decidua basalis to implantation. They swell with glycogen and lipid and produce immunosuppressive molecules to prevent a maternal immune reaction to the conceptus-derived cytotrophoblastic shell of the placenta.
Double decidual sign	An ultrasound indicator of pregnancy along with visualization of the gestational sac (chorion). It consists of echogenicity differences between the decidua capsularis (and basalis) and the adjacent decidua parietalis, due in large part to the decidual reaction in the former.
Ectopic	(G., "displaced") A general term for an organ or structure that ends up in an abnormal location. An ectopic pregnancy results from abnormal implantation sites (e.g., uterine tubes, abdominal cavity).
Epiblast	Columnar cells of the inner cell mass of the blastocyst that constitute the primary ectoderm.
Endometrium	(G., "inside of the uterus") The mucosa of the uterus consisting of simple columnar epithelium and very cellular, loose connective tissue with simple tubular glands. Also called decidua (L., "falling off") because much of the mucosa is shed during menstruation.
Exocoelomic cyst	The remnant of the primary yolk sac (Heuser's membrane) that is displaced by a second wave of endodermal cell migration from the hypoblast that forms the definitive yolk sac.
Extraembryonic	The tissues and structures that are outside the embryo. These mostly consist of the extraembryonic membranes: chorion, amnion, yolk sac, and allantois.
Extraembryonic mesoderm	The mesoderm that appears between the primary yolk sac and cytotrophoblast then cavitates to line the old blastocyst cavity and complete extraembryonic membrane formation. Its origin is controversial. Various studies have it derived from the cytotrophoblast, yolk sac, or epiblast.
Fimbriae	(L., "fringe") Finger-like projections at the end of the uterine tubes that envelop the ovary at the time of ovulation and sweep the ovum into the ostium of the uterine tube.
Follicle (ovarian)	An ovarian follicle is a fluid-filled, cellular envelope surrounding an ovum that enlarges and moves to the surface of the ovary in preparation for ovulation. It is supportive and nutritive for the egg and secretes hormones.

Terminology—cont'd

Gastrulation	The production of intraembryonic mesoderm in the third week that makes the bilaminar embryonic disc of ectoderm and endoderm a trilaminar disc (gastrula).
Gestational sac	This is the early, fluid-filled chorion with its covering of decidua capsularis detectable within the endometrium via ultrasound. It is diagnostic of an intrauterine pregnancy, particularly when the yolk sac is visible within it (and later the amnion and embryo).
Heuser's (exocoelomic) membrane	The primary yolk sac formed as endodermal cells migrate to line the inner surface of the cytotrophoblast with a layer of simple squamous epithelium.
Hypoblast	Simple cuboidal epithelium of the inner cell mass of the blastocyst that constitutes the primary endoderm. It is displaced by a second wave of migration of hypoblast cells that form the definitive yolk sac coated with extraembryonic mesoderm.
Intermediate mesoderm	Primitive streak mesoderm in the gastrula that gives rise to the gonads, kidneys, and tubules and ducts of the urogenital system. It is "intermediate" between the paraxial columns and lateral plate mesoderm.
Lithopedion	(G., "stone child") A dead fetus that has become calcified or hard.
Mesoderm	(G., "middle skin") The inner tissue of the gastrula between the ectoderm and endoderm. It differentiates into two forms: mesenchyme (loose embryonic connective tissue) and the very cellular mesodermal columns (notochord, paraxial columns, intermediate mesoderm, and lateral plate). Extraembryonic mesoderm is the middle layer between the trophoblast and amnion/yolk sac.
Morula	(L., "little mulberry") A product of conception, a morula is the ball of cells 3–4 days after fertilization that is ready to enter the uterine cavity.
Notochord	Midline mesoderm originating during gastrulation from the ectodermal primitive knot (node). It induces neurulation, and its only structural derivative is the nucleus pulposus of an intervertebral disc.
Notochordal canal	The hollow center that develops in the notochordal process. It communicates with the amniotic cavity via the primitive pit in the primitive knot (node).
Oropharyngeal membrane	Also called the oral membrane, it is a circular area at the head end of the gastrula where the ectoderm and endoderm remain in tight contact with no intervening mesoderm. It ends up at the junction of the oral cavity and pharynx, where it breaks down. Its equivalent at the tail end of the embryo is the cloacal membrane.
Prechordal plate	Endodermal cells of the future oropharyngeal membrane at the cranial end of the bilaminar disc. It limits the cranial extension of the notochordal process mesoderm during gastrulation.
Pseudosac	Accumulation of blood/fluid within the endometrial/uterine cavity as seen via ultrasound that may be mistaken for a gestational sac (chorion). One source can be blood from a tubal pregnancy.
Villi (placental)	Finger-like projections of the chorion that are the structural and functional units of the placenta. Most are free villi bathed in maternal blood. They originate from large stem villi on the fetal side of the placenta. Anchoring villi extend from the stem villi to the cytotrophoblastic shell that attaches to the decidua basalis.
Yolk sac (umbilical vesicle)	Endodermal sac extending ventrally from the embryo. It is the secondary yolk sac that displaces the primary yolk sac (Heuser's membrane). It is the first source of embryonic blood cells.
Zona pellucida	The eosinophilic layer of glycoproteins surrounding the ovum cell membrane that will play a role in preventing additional sperm from penetrating the cell membrane after fertilization.

3

THE NERVOUS SYSTEM

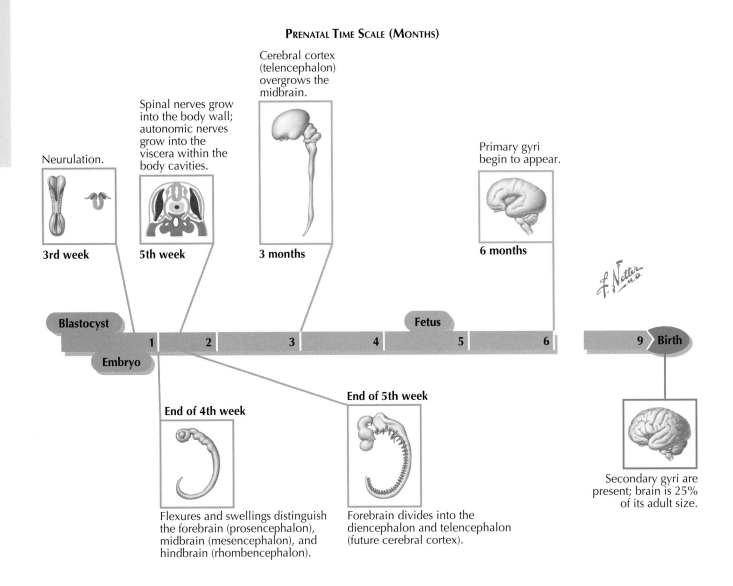

PRENATAL TIME SCALE (MONTHS)

Cerebral cortex
(telencephalon)
overgrows the
midbrain.

Spinal nerves grow
into the body wall;
autonomic nerves
grow into the
viscera within the
body cavities.

Primary gyri
begin to appear.

Neurulation.

3rd week   5th week   3 months   6 months

Blastocyst

| 1 | 2 | 3 | 4 | 5 | 6 | 9 | Birth |

Embryo   Fetus

End of 4th week   End of 5th week

Flexures and swellings distinguish
the forebrain (prosencephalon),
midbrain (mesencephalon), and
hindbrain (rhombencephalon).

Forebrain divides into the
diencephalon and telencephalon
(future cerebral cortex).

Secondary gyri are
present; brain is 25%
of its adult size.

3.1 TIMELINE

PRIMORDIA
Ectodermal neural plate, which forms the neural tube and neural crest.

PLAN
The anatomy of the adult nervous system can appear to be complex, but the pattern established in the embryo is simple and logical with a few basic organizing principles. The dorsal half of the spinal cord and brain stem is sensory; the ventral half is motor. The 12 pairs of cranial nerves and 31 pairs of spinal nerves are mostly mixed nerves (motor and sensory) that innervate the body tissues in segmental fashion. The types and functions of the nerves are in large part related to whether they grow into somatopleure (the developing body wall) or splanchnopleure (the developing visceral compartment). The cell bodies for the motor neurons supplying skeletal muscles are located within the central nervous system (CNS); the cell bodies for sensory neurons (and postganglionic autonomic neurons) are in ganglia outside the CNS. With a few exceptions, the territoriality of the segmental peripheral

nerves is retained in the adult. The nervous system may seem complex because of the absolute and differential growth of structures, plexus formation, migration of structures, nerve branching, and other phenomena, but the simple plan in the embryo is in large part retained.

INCLUSION AND BIAS CONSIDERATION: NEUROCOGNITIVE DEVELOPMENT
This chapter describes some of the essential embryology as it relates to the nervous system and neurocognitive elements. As such, it is important to keep in mind the language surrounding cognitive disabilities. Work with individuals on a case-by-case basis to understand the preferred language of the individuals. For example, some may prefer person-first language (for example, a person with Down syndrome), as this places emphasis on the person rather than the disability. However, others advocate for identity-first language, particularly when they feel that disability plays a role in identity and positive culture. Again, always use sensitivity in language when discussing neurocognitive development, and, when possible, ask people their language preferences.

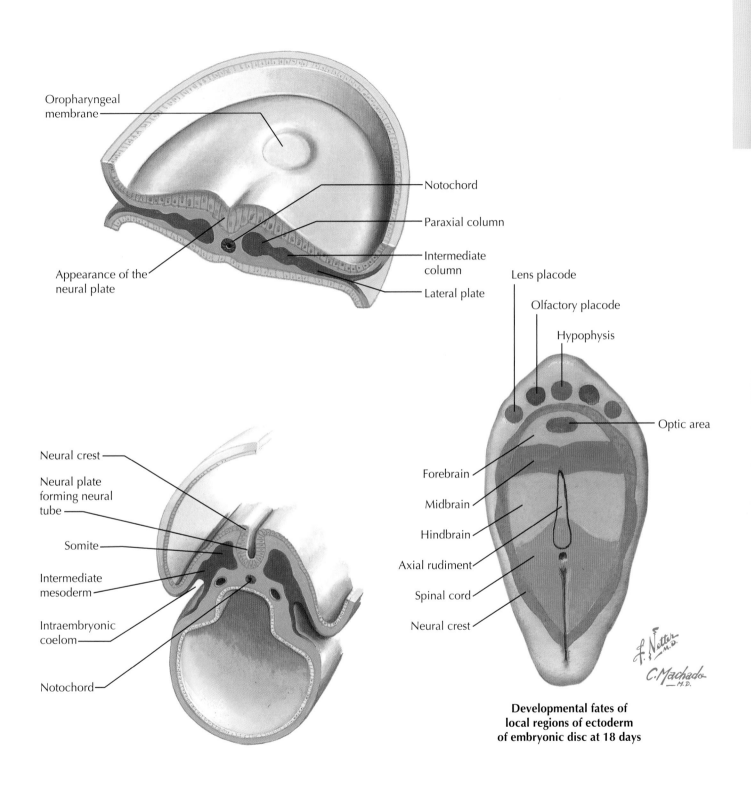

Oropharyngeal membrane

Notochord

Paraxial column

Intermediate column

Lateral plate

Appearance of the neural plate

Lens placode

Olfactory placode

Hypophysis

Optic area

Neural crest

Neural plate forming neural tube

Somite

Intermediate mesoderm

Intraembryonic coelom

Notochord

Forebrain

Midbrain

Hindbrain

Axial rudiment

Spinal cord

Neural crest

Developmental fates of local regions of ectoderm of embryonic disc at 18 days

3.2 FORMATION OF THE NEURAL PLATE

As the primitive streak recedes toward the tail of the embryo near the end of gastrulation, the mesodermal notochord and paraxial columns begin to induce the formation of the **neural plate**, a thickening of the overlying surface ectoderm cranial to the primitive streak.

Contributions of the neural ectoderm to the future brain, spinal cord, and neural crest are shown in the figure on the right. Because of the way the neural plate invaginates to form the neural tube, the dorsal, sensory components of the tube are lateral on the neural plate, and the ventral, motor components of the tube are medial.

Embryo at 20 days (dorsal view)

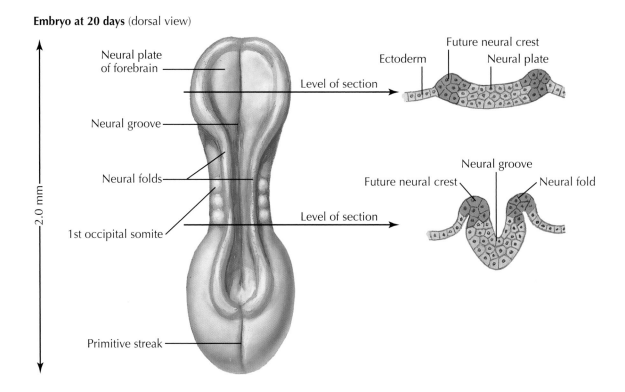

Neural plate of forebrain

Neural groove

Neural folds

1st occipital somite

Primitive streak

2.0 mm

Ectoderm

Future neural crest

Neural plate

Level of section

Future neural crest

Neural groove

Neural fold

Level of section

Embryo at 21 days (dorsal view)

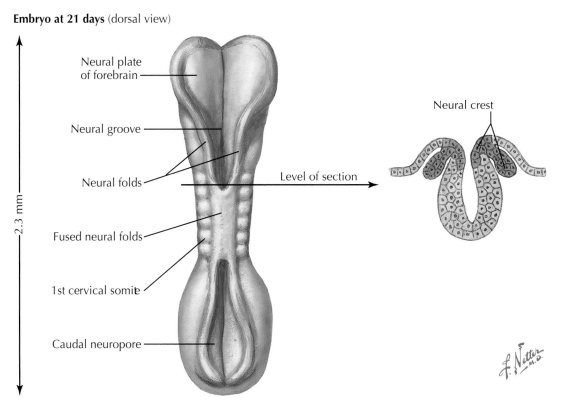

Neural plate of forebrain

Neural groove

Neural folds

Fused neural folds

1st cervical somite

Caudal neuropore

2.3 mm

Neural crest

Level of section

3.3 NEURULATION

In response to induction by the notochord and paraxial mesoderm, the surface ectoderm thickens and begins to sink and fold in on itself near the junction of the future brain and spinal cord in the middle of the embryo. The ectodermal neural crests on each side approach each other and fuse as the tube sinks beneath the surface. Some of these cells will pinch off and migrate to form ganglia throughout the trunk and a variety of other tissues in the head and neck. Neurulation advances both cranially and caudally. In many mammals, particularly in species with large tails, there is a secondary neurulation of midline primitive streak mesoderm in the sacral or coccygeal region beyond the caudal neuropore. The mesenchyme condenses, forms a central canal, and connects with the caudal neural tube. Abnormal secondary neurulation may contribute to tethered cord syndrome, an abnormally low positioning of the inferior portion of the spinal cord below L1.

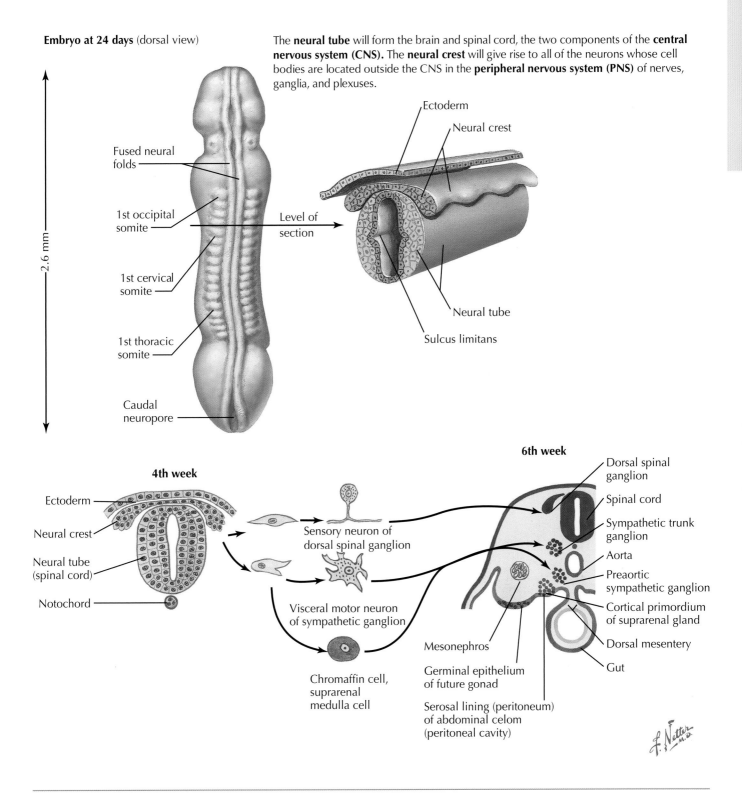

Embryo at 24 days (dorsal view)

The **neural tube** will form the brain and spinal cord, the two components of the **central nervous system (CNS).** The **neural crest** will give rise to all of the neurons whose cell bodies are located outside the CNS in the **peripheral nervous system (PNS)** of nerves, ganglia, and plexuses.

2.6 mm

Fused neural folds

1st occipital somite

1st cervical somite

1st thoracic somite

Caudal neuropore

Level of section

Ectoderm

Neural crest

Neural tube

Sulcus limitans

6th week

4th week

Ectoderm

Neural crest

Neural tube (spinal cord)

Notochord

Sensory neuron of dorsal spinal ganglion

Visceral motor neuron of sympathetic ganglion

Chromaffin cell, suprarenal medulla cell

Mesonephros

Germinal epithelium of future gonad

Serosal lining (peritoneum) of abdominal celom (peritoneal cavity)

Dorsal spinal ganglion

Spinal cord

Sympathetic trunk ganglion

Aorta

Preaortic sympathetic ganglion

Cortical primordium of suprarenal gland

Dorsal mesentery

Gut

3.4 NEURAL TUBE AND NEURAL CREST

Derivatives of the neural tube include:
- Neurons of the CNS
- Supporting cells of the CNS
- Somatomotor neurons of the peripheral nervous system (PNS)
- Presynaptic autonomic neurons of the PNS

Derivatives of the neural crest include:
- Sensory neurons in the PNS
- Postsynaptic autonomic neurons
- Schwann (neurilemma) cells
- Adrenal medulla cells
- Head mesenchyme
- Melanocytes in the skin
- Arachnoid and pia mater of meninges (dura mater from mesoderm)

Spinal bifida occulta

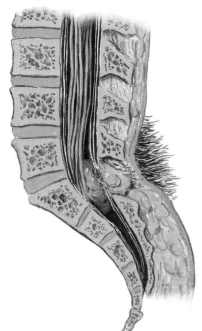

Dermal sinus

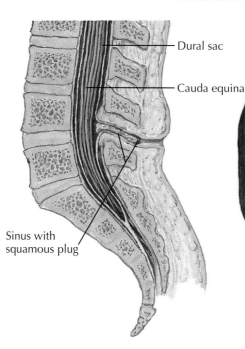

- Dural sac
- Cauda equina

Sinus with squamous plug

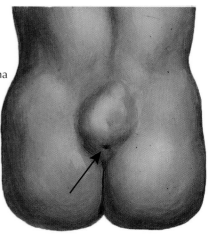

Surface correlations of spina bifida occulta may include a tuft of hair (far left figure), a fat pad and sinus (center figure and arrow above), or a dimple in the middle of the fat pad (above)

Types of spina bifida aperta with protrusion of spinal contents

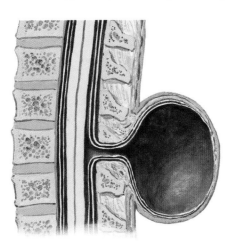

Meningocele

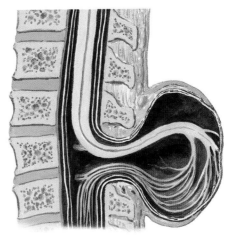

Meningomyelocele

3.5 DEFECTS OF THE SPINAL CORD AND VERTEBRAL COLUMN

Many nervous system defects occur when the neural tube fails to develop properly. **Spina bifida** is an incomplete vertebral arch that results when the neural tube fails to sink completely beneath the surface of the embryo, and somite sclerotome cells cannot migrate over it to complete the vertebral arch. The spinal cord may be exposed on the surface with severe functional deficits (**myeloschisis**); it may be completely normal in function with few visible manifestations (**spina bifida occulta**), or there may be a variety of intermediate conditions. In **meningocele**, the spinal cord is normal, but a swelling of meninges with cerebrospinal fluid (CSF) projects through the defect. If part of the spinal cord is included, it is a **meningomyelocele**.

CLINICAL POINT

Neural tube defects result in elevated levels of alpha-fetoprotein (AFP), the fetal equivalent of adult serum albumin, in the amniotic fluid and maternal serum and urine. AFP measurements can serve as screening tests for neural tube (and other) defects, although they usually serve as confirmation of detection by ultrasound, which is more reliable.

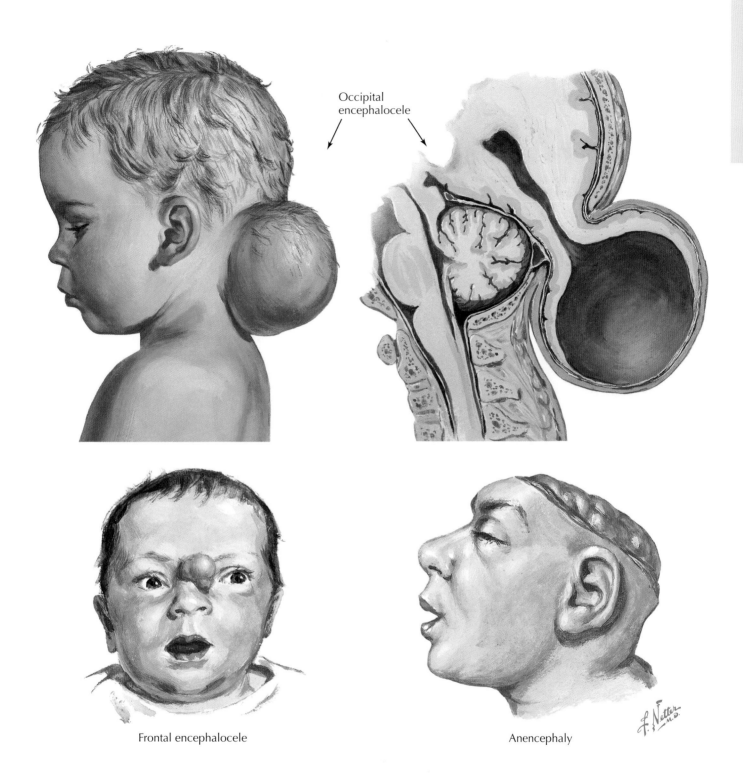

Occipital encephalocele

Frontal encephalocele

Anencephaly

3.6 DEFECTS OF THE BRAIN AND SKULL

Neural tube defects in the head have effects similar to those in spina bifida, but the skull and brain are involved instead of the vertebral column and spinal cord. The occipital bone (or other midline cranial bones) may fail to ossify, and meninges project through the defect (**encephalocele**) with or without brain tissue. An extreme neural tube defect is failure of the anterior neuropore to close, resulting in absence of most of the brain and neurocranium (**anencephaly**). This is the most common major malformation in stillborn fetuses. An **Arnold-Chiari malformation** is the most common cerebellar defect (1/1000 births). Part of the cerebellum and medulla herniate through the foramen magnum, blocking the flow of CSF (**communicating hydrocephalus**).

Two postganglionic autonomic neurons of a sympathetic or parasympathetic ganglion

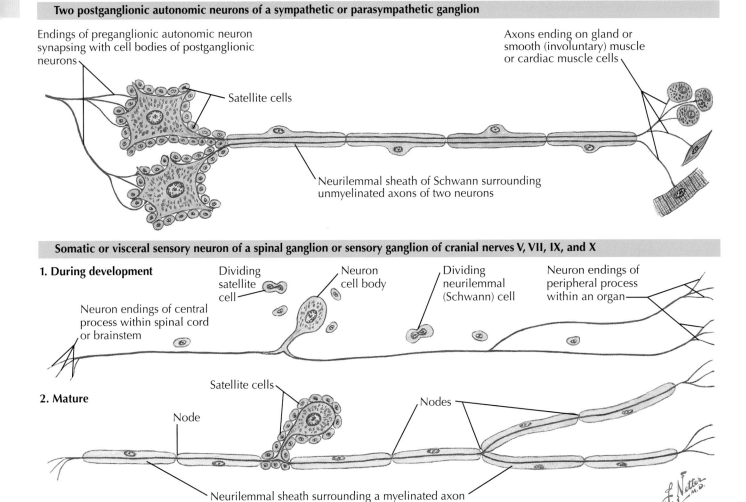

Endings of preganglionic autonomic neuron synapsing with cell bodies of postganglionic neurons

Satellite cells

Axons ending on gland or smooth (involuntary) muscle or cardiac muscle cells

Neurilemmal sheath of Schwann surrounding unmyelinated axons of two neurons

Somatic or visceral sensory neuron of a spinal ganglion or sensory ganglion of cranial nerves V, VII, IX, and X

1. During development

Dividing satellite cell

Neuron cell body

Dividing neurilemmal (Schwann) cell

Neuron endings of peripheral process within an organ

Neuron endings of central process within spinal cord or brainstem

2. Mature

Satellite cells

Nodes

Node

Nodes

Neurilemmal sheath surrounding a myelinated axon

3.7 NEURON DEVELOPMENT

A nerve cell (fiber), or **neuron**, is the functional unit of the nervous system. Nerve cell bodies are derived from the neural tube or the neural crest. Nerve cell processes—**axons** and **dendrites**—sprout from the cell bodies and often grow considerable distances to the tissues and structures they innervate. The axons of motor nerves to muscles or glands grow from the CNS or autonomic ganglia; the processes from peripheral sensory neurons grow from spinal (dorsal root) and cranial ganglia to their sensory territories and into the CNS. A sheath of supporting cells envelops most neurons. These are **satellite cells** around cell bodies and **Schwann (neurilemma) cells** around the peripheral cell processes in nerves.

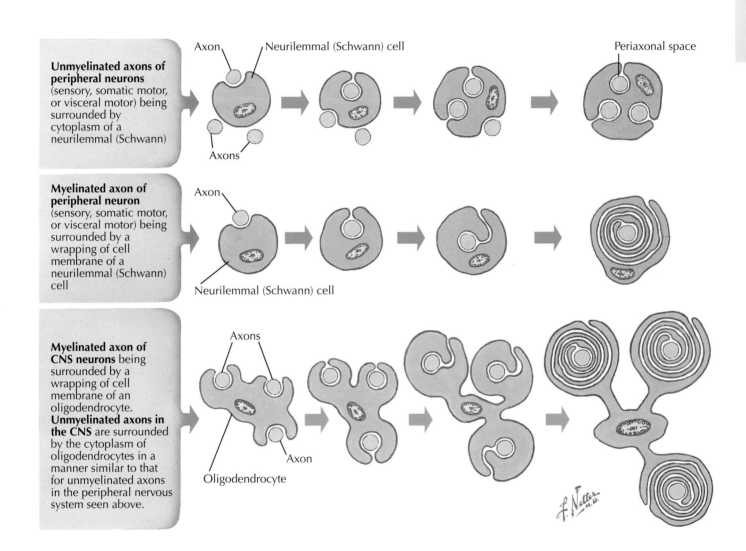

Unmyelinated axons of peripheral neurons (sensory, somatic motor, or visceral motor) being surrounded by cytoplasm of a neurilemmal (Schwann)

Axon — Neurilemmal (Schwann) cell

Periaxonal space

Axons

Myelinated axon of peripheral neuron (sensory, somatic motor, or visceral motor) being surrounded by a wrapping of cell membrane of a neurilemmal (Schwann) cell

Axon

Neurilemmal (Schwann) cell

Myelinated axon of CNS neurons being surrounded by a wrapping of cell membrane of an oligodendrocyte. **Unmyelinated axons in the CNS** are surrounded by the cytoplasm of oligodendrocytes in a manner similar to that for unmyelinated axons in the peripheral nervous system seen above.

Axons

Axon

Oligodendrocyte

3.8 DEVELOPMENT OF THE CELLULAR SHEATH OF AXONS

Oligodendrocytes are equivalent to Schwann cells in the CNS. Axon sheaths are either **myelinated** or **unmyelinated**. Myelinated sheaths are designed for fast nerve conduction (e.g., in somatic nerves). The supporting cell wraps its membrane around the neuron process, and myelination results from the higher contribution of cell membrane relative to cytoplasm in the sheath. Unmyelinated sheaths (e.g., in slow-conducting autonomic neurons) are enveloped by supporting cells, but not in spiral fashion. In the myelinated axons of peripheral nerves, one Schwann cell will surround only one axon.

Embryo at 24 days (dorsal view)

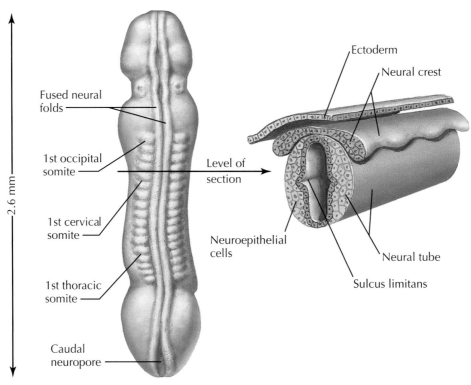

Development of the neural tube layers in the spinal cord

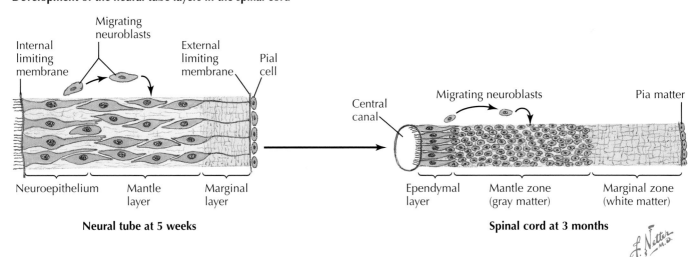

3.9 DEVELOPMENT OF THE SPINAL CORD LAYERS

The neuroepithelium gives rise to three layers. The inner **ependymal zone** will become the ependymal epithelium lining the diminishing central canal of the spinal cord. The **intermediate (mantle) zone** will develop into the gray matter of the spinal cord, the location of nerve cell bodies. The outer **marginal zone** will become white matter as neuron cell processes grow into it from the mantle layer. These axons will extend from the spinal cord to the brain as sensory tracts or descend from the brain to spinal cord levels as motor tracts. **Glial cells** and rich capillary networks are found in both the mantle and marginal zones.

5¹/₂ weeks (transverse section)

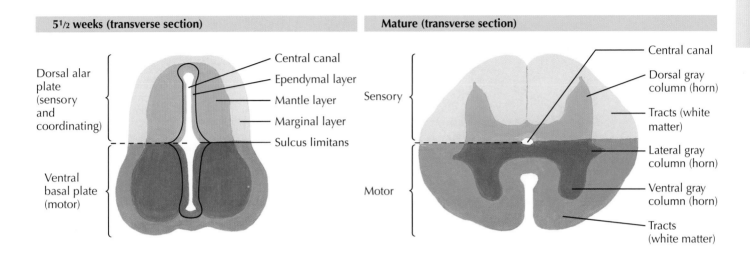

Dorsal alar plate (sensory and coordinating)

Ventral basal plate (motor)

Central canal
Ependymal layer
Mantle layer
Marginal layer
Sulcus limitans

Mature (transverse section)

Sensory

Motor

Central canal
Dorsal gray column (horn)
Tracts (white matter)
Lateral gray column (horn)
Ventral gray column (horn)
Tracts (white matter)

Differentiation and growth of neurons at 26 days

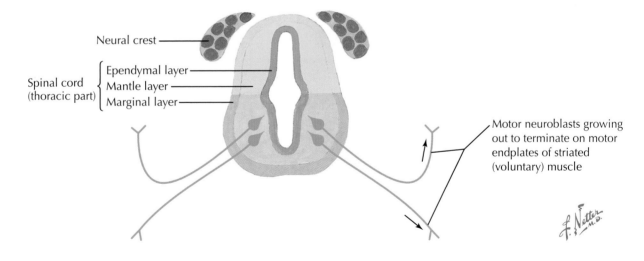

Neural crest

Spinal cord (thoracic part)
Ependymal layer
Mantle layer
Marginal layer

Motor neuroblasts growing out to terminate on motor endplates of striated (voluntary) muscle

3.10 ALAR AND BASAL PLATES

The sulcus limitans is a longitudinal groove on each side of the central canal that divides the neural tube into a dorsal **alar plate** and ventral **basal plate**. The alar plate contains the cell bodies of neurons with sensory functions in the dorsal horn of gray matter. They receive input from sensory neurons in the spinal nerves. Somatic and autonomic motor neurons develop in the ventral and lateral horns of gray matter in the basal plate. Their axons leave the spinal cord as the ventral roots of spinal nerves. The neuron processes within the white matter are organized into tracts (funiculi) that relate to specific functions. Ascending sensory tracts and descending motor tracts overlap with each other and do not segregate neatly into alar and basal plates.

Differentiation and growth of neurons at 28 days (right side of diagram shows newly acquired neurons only)

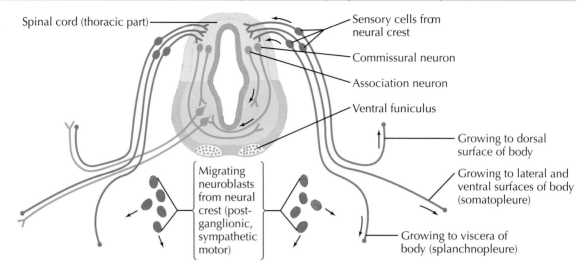

Spinal cord (thoracic part)

Sensory cells from neural crest

Commissural neuron

Association neuron

Ventral funiculus

Growing to dorsal surface of body

Growing to lateral and ventral surfaces of body (somatopleure)

Migrating neuroblasts from neural crest (post-ganglionic, sympathetic motor)

Growing to viscera of body (splanchnopleure)

Differentiation and growth of neurons at 5 to 7 weeks (right side of diagram shows neurons acquired since 28th day only)

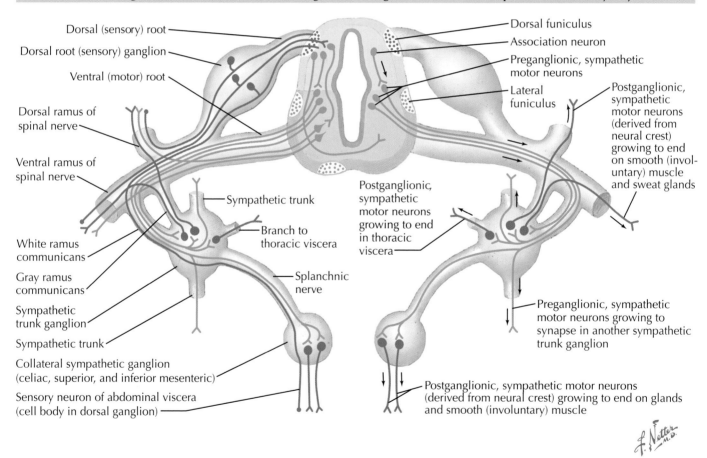

Dorsal (sensory) root

Dorsal root (sensory) ganglion

Ventral (motor) root

Dorsal ramus of spinal nerve

Ventral ramus of spinal nerve

White ramus communicans

Gray ramus communicans

Sympathetic trunk ganglion

Sympathetic trunk

Collateral sympathetic ganglion (celiac, superior, and inferior mesenteric)

Sensory neuron of abdominal viscera (cell body in dorsal ganglion)

Sympathetic trunk

Branch to thoracic viscera

Splanchnic nerve

Dorsal funiculus

Association neuron

Preganglionic, sympathetic motor neurons

Lateral funiculus

Postganglionic, sympathetic motor neurons (derived from neural crest) growing to end on smooth (involuntary) muscle and sweat glands

Postganglionic, sympathetic motor neurons growing to end in thoracic viscera

Preganglionic, sympathetic motor neurons growing to synapse in another sympathetic trunk ganglion

Postganglionic, sympathetic motor neurons (derived from neural crest) growing to end on glands and smooth (involuntary) muscle

3.11 DEVELOPMENT OF THE PERIPHERAL NERVOUS SYSTEM

Dorsal sensory roots and ventral motor roots form the spinal nerves that innervate the body wall of bone, muscle, connective tissue, and skin. At 28 days, the sensory and motor cell processes are growing into the dorsal and ventral aspects of the body wall via the **dorsal and ventral rami** of spinal nerves.

Autonomic neuron processes leave the spinal nerves to go to the viscera via **splanchnic nerves** (or rejoin spinal nerves). Sympathetic neurons will synapse with a second neuron in the **sympathetic trunk** or **collateral (preaortic) ganglia**. Parasympathetic neurons (in the vagus and pelvic splanchnic nerves) will synapse in scattered ganglia within the walls of visceral organs.

Autonomic Development

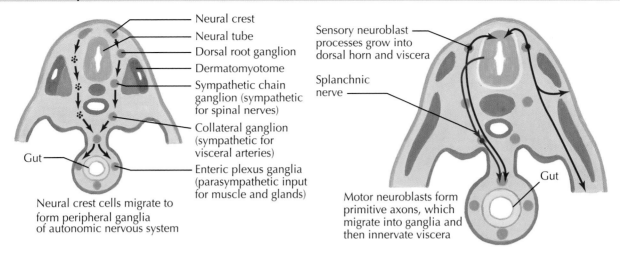

Neural crest cells migrate to form peripheral ganglia of autonomic nervous system

Autonomic nervous system mostly innervates splanchnopleure (viscera) but also body wall arteries

Somatic Development

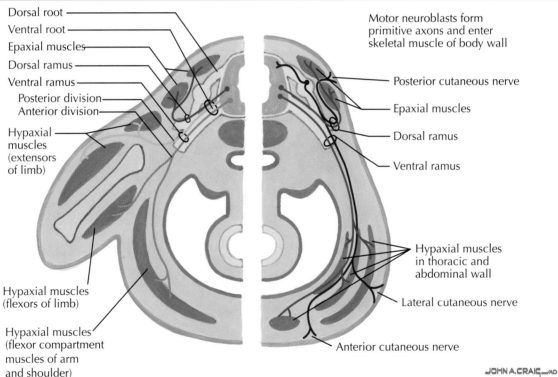

Innervation of somatopleure (body wall) derivatives by the somatic nervous system *(spinal nerves)*.
On the left is the organization of motor innervation to the back *(blue neurons)* and limbs *(yellow and green neurons)*.
On the right is motor innervation to trunk muscles *(light blue)* and sensory innervation in cutaneous nerves *(dark blue)*.
Sensory nerve processes are found in all nerves to muscle in addition to cutaneous nerves.
Sympathetic fibers supplying arterial smooth muscle are also in every spinal nerve branch.

3.12 SOMATIC VERSUS SPLANCHNIC NERVES

The embryonic basis of the division of the PNS into spinal (somatic) nerves and splanchnic autonomic nerves is the distinction between **somatopleure** and **splanchnopleure**. The former develops from ectoderm and the somatic part of lateral plate mesoderm. Somite hypoblasts migrate into the somatopleure to form the lateral and ventral aspects of the body wall, including the limbs. Visceral organs develop from splanchnopleure derived from endoderm and lateral plate mesoderm. The ventral rami migrate into somatopleure; splanchnic nerves grow into splanchnopleure. Thoracic and lumbar splanchnic nerves have sympathetic and visceral sensory neurons. Pelvic splanchnic nerves (S2, S3, and S4) are parasympathetic and visceral sensory.

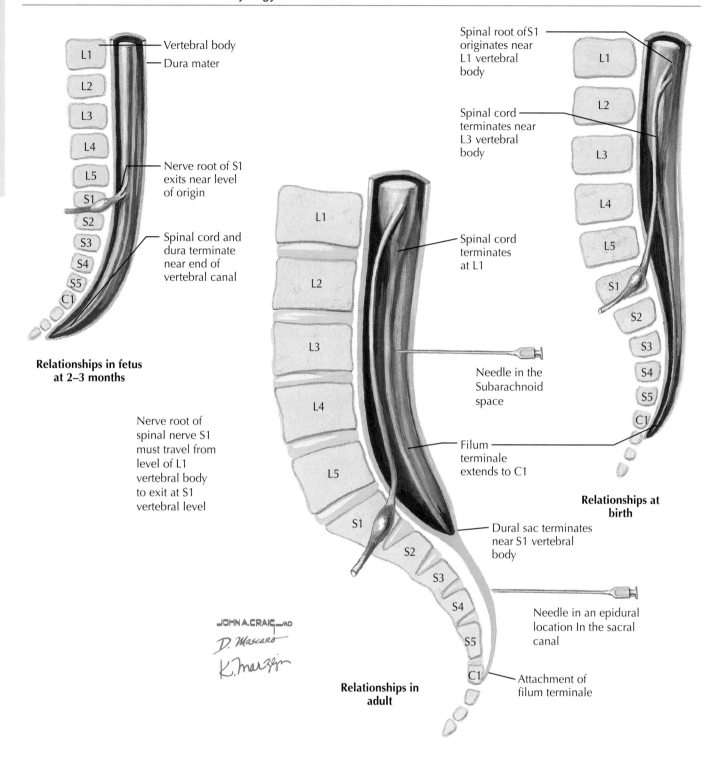

Vertebral body
Dura mater

Nerve root of S1
exits near level
of origin

Spinal cord and
dura terminate
near end of
vertebral canal

**Relationships in fetus
at 2–3 months**

Nerve root of
spinal nerve S1
must travel from
level of L1
vertebral body
to exit at S1
vertebral level

Spinal root of S1
originates near
L1 vertebral
body

Spinal cord
terminates near
L3 vertebral
body

Spinal cord
terminates
at L1

Needle in the
Subarachnoid
space

Filum
terminale
extends to C1

**Relationships at
birth**

Spinal cord
terminates
at L1

Dural sac terminates
near S1 vertebral
body

Needle in an epidural
location In the sacral
canal

Attachment of
filum terminale

**Relationships in
adult**

JOHN A.CRAIG—AD
D. Mascaro
K. marzin

3.13 GROWTH OF THE SPINAL CORD AND VERTEBRAL COLUMN

The spinal cord and vertebral column are approximately the same length at the end of the embryonic period. The vertebral column grows at a relatively faster rate through the fetal and postnatal periods of growth until the lower end of the spinal cord is at the L1–L2 vertebral level in the adult. Lumbar and thoracic spinal nerve roots must pass inferiorly in the vertebral canal as the cauda equina ("horse's tail") within the subarachnoid space to reach their appropriate level of exit from the vertebral column via the intervertebral foramina. The dural sac and subarachnoid space end at upper sacral levels. Lower sacral nerve roots leave the dural sac to pass inferiorly in the sacral canal to exit dorsal and ventral sacral foramina.

CLINICAL POINT

Spinal anesthesia. The clinically significant result of the differential growth of the spinal cord, dural sac, and vertebral column is that a needle can be passed into the subarachnoid space (to sample CSF or inject anesthetic) below the level of L2 without danger of piercing the spinal cord. A needle in the sacral canal below S1/S2 (e.g., for a sacral nerve block) will be in an epidural location.

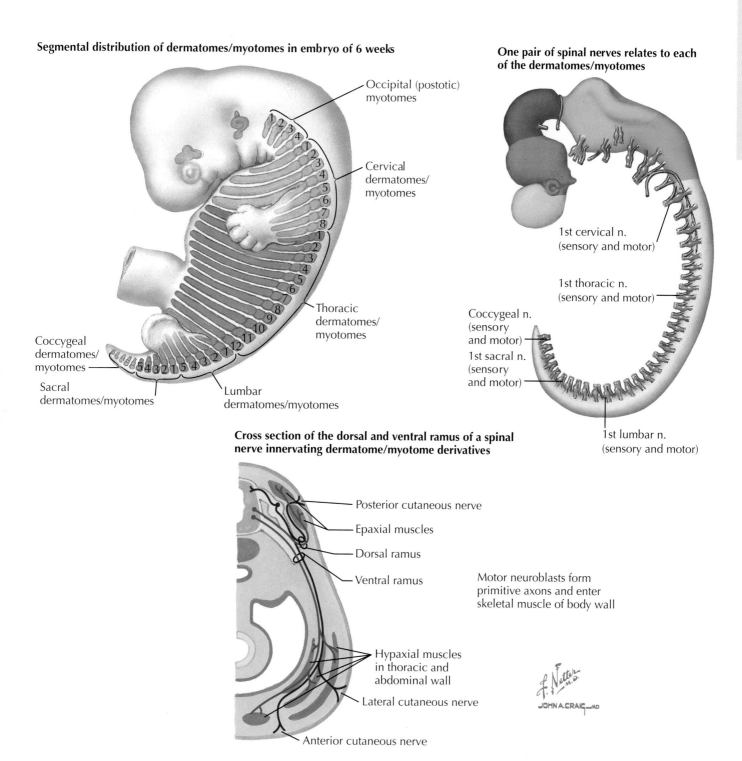

Segmental distribution of dermatomes/myotomes in embryo of 6 weeks

Occipital (postotic) myotomes

Cervical dermatomes/myotomes

Thoracic dermatomes/myotomes

Coccygeal dermatomes/myotomes

Sacral dermatomes/myotomes

Lumbar dermatomes/myotomes

One pair of spinal nerves relates to each of the dermatomes/myotomes

1st cervical n. (sensory and motor)

1st thoracic n. (sensory and motor)

Coccygeal n. (sensory and motor)

1st sacral n. (sensory and motor)

1st lumbar n. (sensory and motor)

Cross section of the dorsal and ventral ramus of a spinal nerve innervating dermatome/myotome derivatives

Posterior cutaneous nerve

Epaxial muscles

Dorsal ramus

Ventral ramus

Motor neuroblasts form primitive axons and enter skeletal muscle of body wall

Hypaxial muscles in thoracic and abdominal wall

Lateral cutaneous nerve

Anterior cutaneous nerve

3.14 EMBRYONIC DERMATOMES

The somites from the paraxial columns of mesoderm in the embryo divide into a sclerotome, myotome, and dermatome. The sclerotome forms bone and cartilage, the myotome differentiates into muscle, and the dermatome contributes to the dermis of the skin. A single spinal nerve relates to each somite, and sensory neuron processes grow into the dermatome to supply its territory of skin via anterior, lateral, and posterior cutaneous nerves. Somatic mesenchyme from the lateral plate is also a source of the dermis and superficial fascia, particularly in the limbs, but the segmental pattern of skin innervation is established by the relationship between the spinal nerves and the dermatomes of the somites.

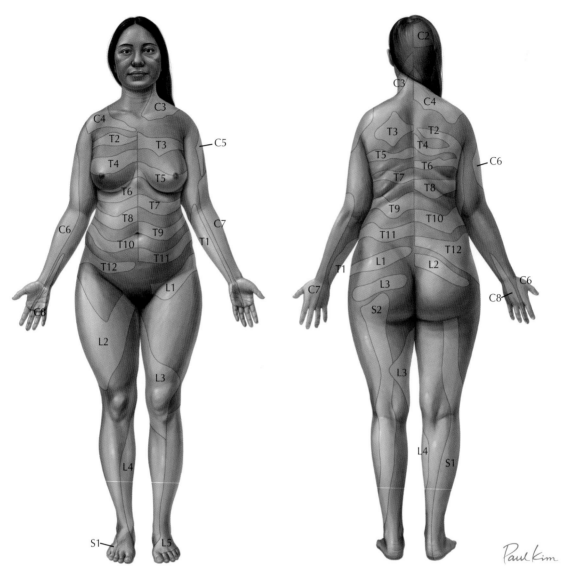

Levels of principal dermatomes

C4	Level of clavicles	**T10**	Level of umbilicus
C5, C6, C7	Lateral surfaces of upper limbs	**L1**	Inguinal region and proximal anterior thigh
C8, T1	Medial surfaces of upper limbs	**L1, L2, L3, L4**	Anteromedial lower limb and gluteal region
C6	Lateral digits	**L4, L5, S1**	Foot
C6, C7, C8	Hand	**L4**	Medial leg
C8	Medial digits	**L5, S1**	Posterolateral lower limb and dorsum of foot
T4	Level of nipples	**S1**	Lateral foot

Schematic based on Lee MW, McPhee RW, Stringer MD. An evidence-based approach to human dermatomes. Clin Anat. 2008; 21(5):363–373. doi: 10.1002/ca.20636. PMID: 18470936. Please note that these areas are not absolute and vary from person to person. S3, S4, S5, and Co supply the perineum but are not shown for reasons of clarity. Of note, the dermatomes are larger than illustrated as the figure is based on best evidence; gaps represent areas in which the data are inconclusive.

3.15 ADULT DERMATOMES

A dermatome in the adult is defined as the area of skin supplied by a single pair of spinal nerves. As the limbs elongate and rotate, some dermatomes lose their continuity with the trunk, and the dermatomes of the lower extremity assume a spiral arrangement. Dermatomes in the limbs also differ from those in the trunk because spinal nerve segments are intermixed in the nerve plexuses that supply the extremities. As a result, one dermatome may be supplied by more than one nerve, and one nerve can contribute to more than one dermatome. Despite these complications, the craniocaudal relationship between dermatomes in the embryo is maintained in the adult. See Chapter 8 for more details on the effect of limb rotation on dermatomes.

CLINICAL POINT

Referred pain. Lesions or other sources of pain originating in visceral sensory spinal segments of internal organs will be projected or "referred" (felt) in the spinal nerve dermatomes of the same spinal segments. The location of pain in the skin or body wall is extremely important for diagnosis of the origin of the pain internally.

Central nervous system at 28 days

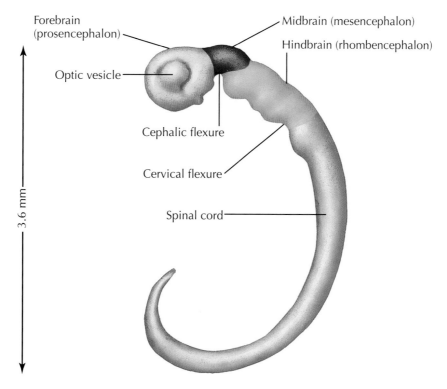

Forebrain
(prosencephalon)

Optic vesicle

Midbrain (mesencephalon)

Hindbrain (rhombencephalon)

Cephalic flexure

Cervical flexure

Spinal cord

3.6 mm

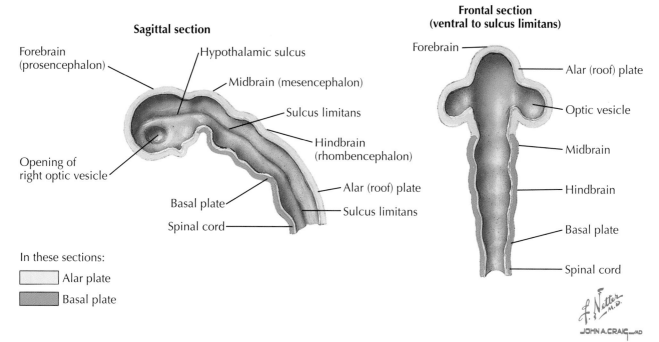

Sagittal section

Forebrain
(prosencephalon)

Hypothalamic sulcus

Midbrain (mesencephalon)

Sulcus limitans

Hindbrain
(rhombencephalon)

Opening of
right optic vesicle

Basal plate

Alar (roof) plate

Sulcus limitans

Spinal cord

In these sections:

Alar plate

Basal plate

**Frontal section
(ventral to sulcus limitans)**

Forebrain

Alar (roof) plate

Optic vesicle

Midbrain

Hindbrain

Basal plate

Spinal cord

3.16 EARLY BRAIN DEVELOPMENT

The brain begins to develop from the neural tube near the end of the first month. Flexures and swellings distinguish the forebrain (**prosencephalon**), midbrain (**mesencephalon**), and hindbrain (**rhombencephalon**). Large **optic vesicles** extend from the forebrain and are the most prominent external features of the primitive brain. They will become the optic nerves and retina of the eyes. As in the spinal cord, the **sulcus limitans** divides the brain into a dorsal **alar plate** that is sensory and ventral **basal plate** that is motor. The exception is the forebrain, which has no basal plate. The only two cranial nerves that connect to the forebrain (olfactory and optic) are special sensory with no motor components.

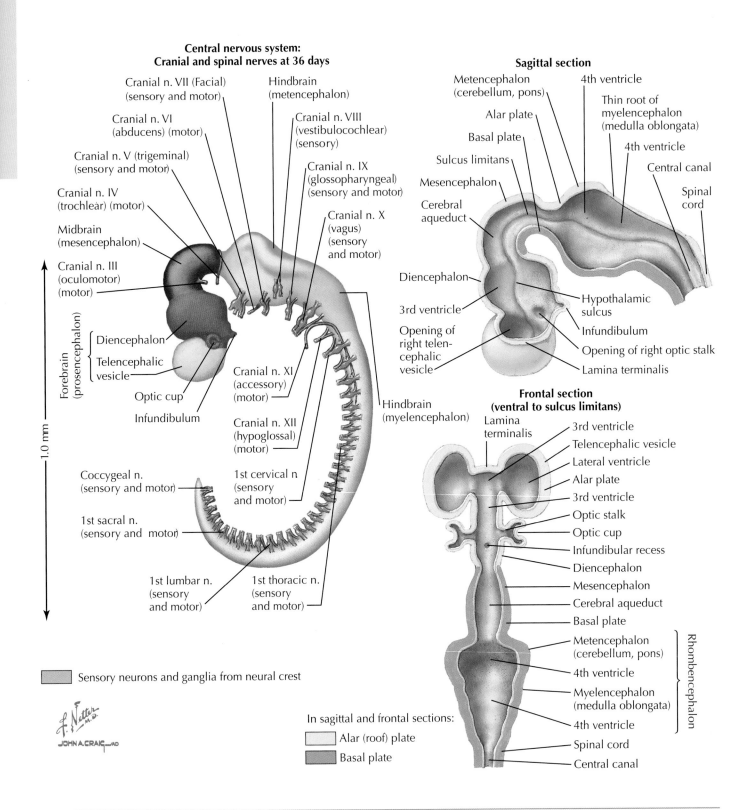

**Central nervous system:
Cranial and spinal nerves at 36 days**

Cranial n. VII (Facial)
(sensory and motor)

Cranial n. VI
(abducens) (motor)

Cranial n. V (trigeminal)
(sensory and motor)

Cranial n. IV
(trochlear) (motor)

Midbrain
(mesencephalon)

Cranial n. III
(oculomotor)
(motor)

Diencephalon

Telencephalic
vesicle

Optic cup

Infundibulum

1.0 mm

Forebrain (prosencephalon)

Hindbrain
(metencephalon)

Cranial n. VIII
(vestibulocochlear)
(sensory)

Cranial n. IX
(glossopharyngeal)
(sensory and motor)

Cranial n. X
(vagus)
(sensory
and motor)

Cranial n. XI
(accessory)
(motor)

Cranial n. XII
(hypoglossal)
(motor)

Hindbrain
(myelencephalon)

Coccygeal n.
(sensory and motor)

1st sacral n.
(sensory and motor)

1st lumbar n.
(sensory
and motor)

1st thoracic n.
(sensory
and motor)

1st cervical n
(sensory
and motor)

Sagittal section

Metencephalon
(cerebellum, pons)

Alar plate

Basal plate

Sulcus limitans

Mesencephalon

Cerebral
aqueduct

4th ventricle

Thin root of
myelencephalon
(medulla oblongata)

4th ventricle

Central canal

Spinal
cord

Diencephalon

3rd ventricle

Opening of
right telen-
cephalic
vesicle

Hypothalamic
sulcus

Infundibulum

Opening of right optic stalk

Lamina terminalis

**Frontal section
(ventral to sulcus limitans)**

Lamina
terminalis

3rd ventricle

Telencephalic vesicle

Lateral ventricle

Alar plate

3rd ventricle

Optic stalk

Optic cup

Infundibular recess

Diencephalon

Mesencephalon

Cerebral aqueduct

Basal plate

Metencephalon
(cerebellum, pons)

4th ventricle

Myelencephalon
(medulla oblongata)

4th ventricle

Spinal cord

Central canal

Rhombencephalon

Sensory neurons and ganglia from neural crest

In sagittal and frontal sections:

Alar (roof) plate

Basal plate

JOHN A.CRAIG—MD

3.17 FURTHER DEVELOPMENT OF FOREBRAIN, MIDBRAIN, AND HINDBRAIN

By 5 weeks, the forebrain has two subdivisions, the **telencephalon** and **diencephalon**, and the hindbrain has two parts, the **metencephalon** and **myelencephalon**. Each optic vesicle forms an **optic cup and stalk** extending from the diencephalon. The telencephalon is the future cerebral cortex. It consists of bilateral vesicles that

grow rapidly to surpass the optic structures as the dominant features of the forebrain. The **infundibulum** (posterior lobe of the pituitary gland and connecting structures) extends from the floor of the diencephalon. The **hypothalamic sulcus** separates the thalamus from hypothalamus and is not a continuation of the sulcus limitans. The cavity of the neural tube develops into the ventricular system, which contains CSF.

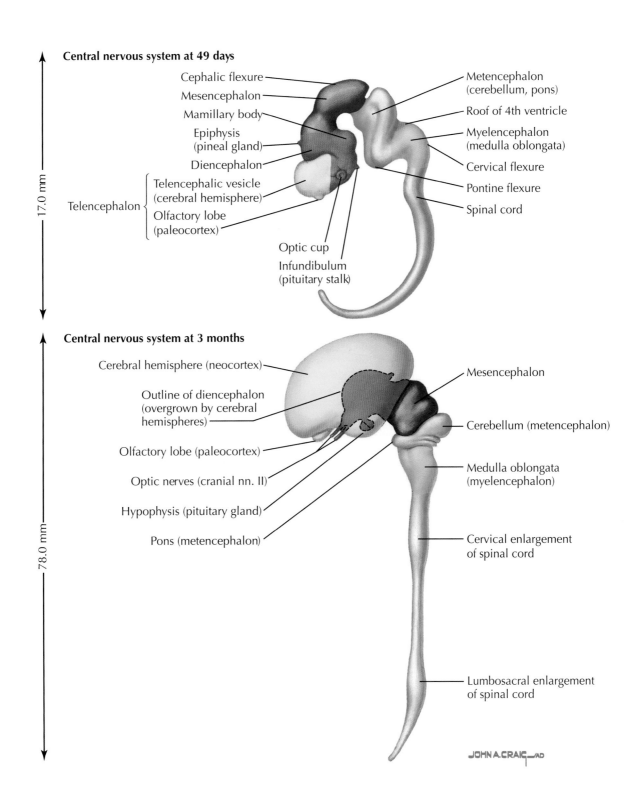

Central nervous system at 49 days

17.0 mm

Cephalic flexure
Mesencephalon
Mamillary body
Epiphysis (pineal gland)
Diencephalon
Telencephalon { Telencephalic vesicle (cerebral hemisphere)
Olfactory lobe (paleocortex)
Optic cup
Infundibulum (pituitary stalk)

Metencephalon (cerebellum, pons)
Roof of 4th ventricle
Myelencephalon (medulla oblongata)
Cervical flexure
Pontine flexure
Spinal cord

Central nervous system at 3 months

78.0 mm

Cerebral hemisphere (neocortex)
Outline of diencephalon (overgrown by cerebral hemispheres)
Olfactory lobe (paleocortex)
Optic nerves (cranial nn. II)
Hypophysis (pituitary gland)
Pons (metencephalon)

Mesencephalon
Cerebellum (metencephalon)
Medulla oblongata (myelencephalon)
Cervical enlargement of spinal cord
Lumbosacral enlargement of spinal cord

JOHN A.CRAIG⎯AD

3.18 DEVELOPMENT OF MAJOR BRAIN STRUCTURES

By 3 months, the major regions, structures, and features of the brain are recognizable. The **cerebral hemispheres** from the telencephalon overgrow the diencephalon. The **cerebellum** and **pons** differentiate from the metencephalon, and the myelencephalon is now the **medulla oblongata**. The **olfactory** lobes are prominent in the brains of lower animals, but in humans they become a restricted area of **"paleo" cortex**, and their proximal portions have evolved more complex structures of the **limbic system** (lobe) involved with emotions, memory, and learning. The cervical and lumbosacral enlargements of the spinal cord contain extra neurons required for the innervation of the limbs.

Brain at 6 months

←——————— 8.0 mm ———————→

Frontal lobe of left
cerebral hemisphere

Insula (island of Reil) in
lateral (sylvian) sulcus

Olfactory bulb

Temporal lobe

Pons

Pyramid

Central (rolandic) sulcus

Parietal lobe

Parietooccipital sulcus

Occipital lobe

Cerebellum

Medulla oblongata

Spinal cord

Brain at 9 months (birth)

←——————— 10.5 mm ———————→

Precentral (motor) gyrus

Precentral sulcus

Frontal lobe

Left cerebral hemisphere

Lateral (sylvian) sulcus

Insula (island of Reil)

Olfactory bulb

Temporal lobe

Pons

Pyramid

Olive

Central (rolandic) sulcus

Postcentral (sensory) gyrus

Postcentral sulcus

Parietooccipital sulcus

Parietal lobe

Occipital lobe

Cerebellum

Medulla oblongata

Spinal cord

JOHN A.CRAIG—AD

3.19 GROWTH OF THE CEREBRAL HEMISPHERES

The appearance of the brain changes dramatically from 3 months to birth with the rapid enlargement of the cerebral hemispheres and the elaboration of their **frontal, parietal, temporal,** and **occipital lobes**. The surface of the hemispheres becomes convoluted with primary, secondary, and tertiary **sulci** separating several irregular folded **gyri**. This greatly increases the surface area of the cerebral cortex. Cortical enlargement is an evolutionary novelty related to higher mental function in mammals and birds, and most of this cortex is called **neocortex**. The human brain at birth is 25% of its adult weight (nearly 50% at 6 months, 75% at 2.5 years, 90% at 5 years, and 95% at 10 years).

Adult derivatives of brain primordia

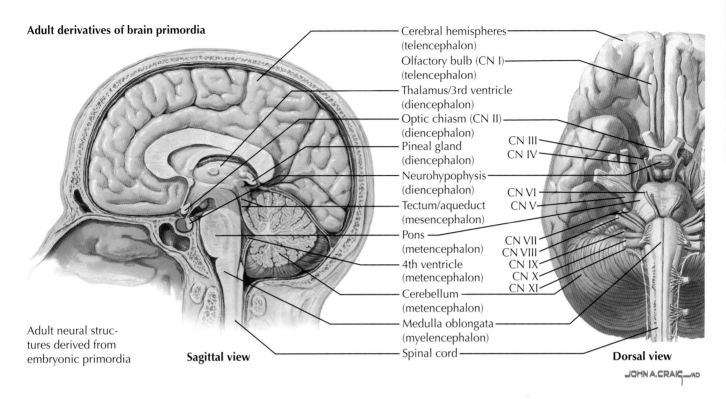

Cerebral hemispheres
(telencephalon)
Olfactory bulb (CN I)
(telencephalon)
Thalamus/3rd ventricle
(diencephalon)
Optic chiasm (CN II)
(diencephalon)
Pineal gland
(diencephalon)
Neurohypophysis
(diencephalon)
Tectum/aqueduct
(mesencephalon)
Pons
(metencephalon)
4th ventricle
(metencephalon)
Cerebellum
(metencephalon)
Medulla oblongata
(myelencephalon)
Spinal cord

CN III
CN IV
CN VI
CN V
CN VII
CN VIII
CN IX
CN X
CN XI

Adult neural structures derived from embryonic primordia

Sagittal view

Dorsal view

JOHN A. CRAIG—AD

ADULT DERIVATIVES OF THE FOREBRAIN, MIDBRAIN, AND HINDBRAIN

Forebrain	Telencephalon	Cerebral hemispheres (neocortex) Olfactory cortex (paleocortex) Hippocampus (archicortex) Basal ganglia/corpus striatum Lateral and 3rd ventricles	Nerves: Olfactory (I)
	Diencephalon	Optic cup/nerves Thalamus Hypothalamus Mammillary bodies Part of 3rd ventricle	Optic (II)
Midbrain	Mesencephalon	Tectum (superior, inferior colliculi) Cerebral aqueduct Red nucleus Substantia nigra Crus cerebri	Oculomotor (III) Trochlear (IV)
Hindbrain	Metencephalon	Pons Cerebellum	Trigeminal (V) Abducens(VI)
	Myelencephalon	Medulla oblongata	Facial (VII) Vestibulocochlear (VIII) Glossopharyngeal (IX) Vagus (X) Hypoglossal (XII)

3.20 DERIVATIVES OF THE FOREBRAIN, MIDBRAIN, AND HINDBRAIN

The telencephalon has three major components: the large **cerebral hemispheres**, **olfactory cortex** (including the hippocampus and limbic system), and **basal ganglia**. The latter two are intimately connected to the thalamus, epithalamus, and hypothalamus of the diencephalon for a number of integrative, autonomic, and endocrine control functions relating to a variety of mental processes. The midbrain **tectum** has visual and auditory integrative functions, and the ventral part has motor interconnections. The relatively large **cerebellum** functions in equilibrium, locomotion, and posture. The **medulla oblongata** and **pons** are sensory and motor relays between the spinal cord and brain and between the cerebrum and cerebellum; they also contain the motor nuclei of cranial nerves.

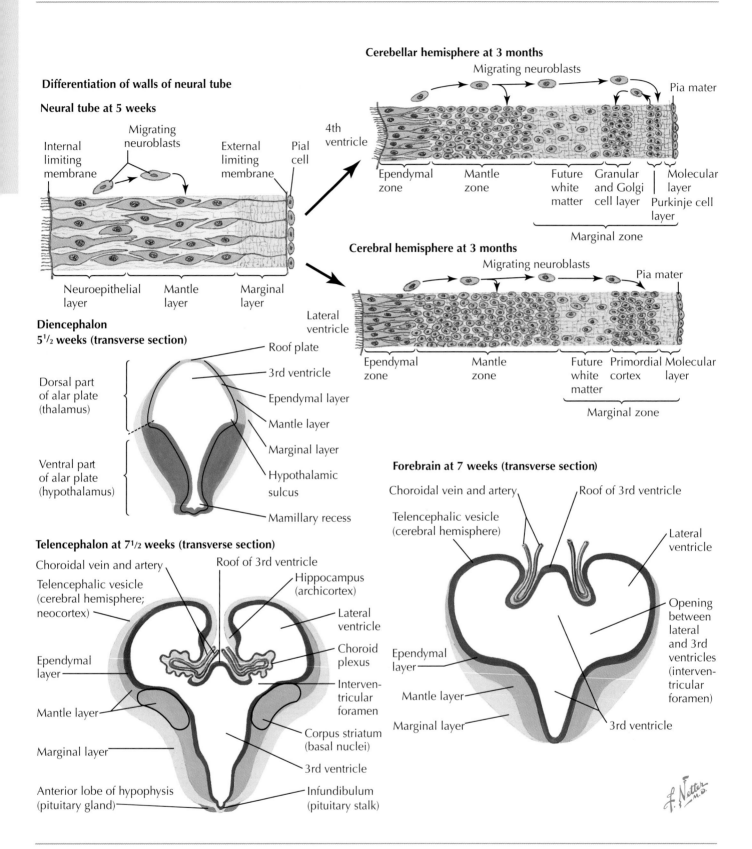

Differentiation of walls of neural tube

Neural tube at 5 weeks

Internal limiting membrane
Migrating neuroblasts
External limiting membrane
Pial cell

Neuroepithelial layer
Mantle layer
Marginal layer

Cerebellar hemisphere at 3 months

Migrating neuroblasts
Pia mater

Ependymal zone
Mantle zone
Future white matter
Granular and Golgi cell layer
Molecular layer
Purkinje cell layer
Marginal zone

Cerebral hemisphere at 3 months

Migrating neuroblasts
Pia mater

Ependymal zone
Mantle zone
Future white matter
Primordial cortex
Molecular layer
Marginal zone

Diencephalon
5½ weeks (transverse section)

Dorsal part of alar plate (thalamus)
Ventral part of alar plate (hypothalamus)

Roof plate
3rd ventricle
Ependymal layer
Mantle layer
Marginal layer
Hypothalamic sulcus
Mamillary recess

4th ventricle

Lateral ventricle

Telencephalon at 7½ weeks (transverse section)

Choroidal vein and artery
Telencephalic vesicle (cerebral hemisphere; neocortex)
Ependymal layer
Mantle layer
Marginal layer
Anterior lobe of hypophysis (pituitary gland)

Roof of 3rd ventricle
Hippocampus (archicortex)
Lateral ventricle
Choroid plexus
Interventricular foramen
Corpus striatum (basal nuclei)
3rd ventricle
Infundibulum (pituitary stalk)

Forebrain at 7 weeks (transverse section)

Choroidal vein and artery
Telencephalic vesicle (cerebral hemisphere)
Ependymal layer
Mantle layer
Marginal layer

Roof of 3rd ventricle
Lateral ventricle
Opening between lateral and 3rd ventricles (interventricular foramen)
3rd ventricle

3.21 FOREBRAIN WALL AND VENTRICLES

Because of the evolutionary enlargement of the telencephalon of the forebrain, the cerebrum (neocortex) is the largest part of the brain and dominates its appearance in humans. It also differs from the organization of the CNS in the histological composition of the marginal zone and in the absence of the basal plate—the ventral, motor component of the neural tube. Neuroblasts in the embryonic walls of the cerebral hemispheres (and cerebellum) migrate beyond the intermediate mantle zone to form gray matter layers in the outer marginal zone near the surface of the cortex. The cavity of the neural tube enlarges to form **lateral ventricles** in the cerebral hemispheres and the **third ventricle** in the diencephalon.

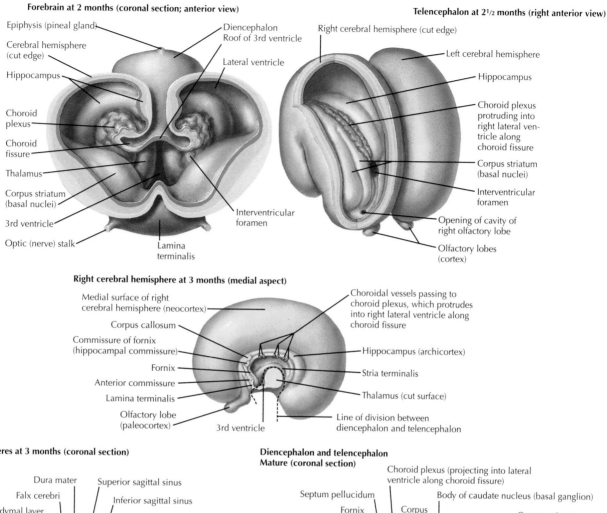

Forebrain at 2 months (coronal section; anterior view)

Epiphysis (pineal gland)
Cerebral hemisphere (cut edge)
Hippocampus
Choroid plexus
Choroid fissure
Thalamus
Corpus striatum (basal nuclei)
3rd ventricle
Optic (nerve) stalk
Diencephalon
Roof of 3rd ventricle
Lateral ventricle
Interventricular foramen
Lamina terminalis

Telencephalon at 2½ months (right anterior view)

Right cerebral hemisphere (cut edge)
Left cerebral hemisphere
Hippocampus
Choroid plexus protruding into right lateral ventricle along choroid fissure
Corpus striatum (basal nuclei)
Interventricular foramen
Opening of cavity of right olfactory lobe
Olfactory lobes (cortex)

Right cerebral hemisphere at 3 months (medial aspect)

Medial surface of right cerebral hemisphere (neocortex)
Corpus callosum
Commissure of fornix (hippocampal commissure)
Fornix
Anterior commissure
Lamina terminalis
Olfactory lobe (paleocortex)
3rd ventricle
Choroidal vessels passing to choroid plexus, which protrudes into right lateral ventricle along choroid fissure
Hippocampus (archicortex)
Stria terminalis
Thalamus (cut surface)
Line of division between diencephalon and telencephalon

Cerebral hemispheres at 3 months (coronal section)

Dura mater
Falx cerebri
Ependymal layer
Mantle layer
Marginal layer
Neocortex
Hippocampal cortex
Corpus striatum (basal nuclei) { Caudate nucleus / Lenticular nucleus }
Optic recess of 3rd ventricle
Superior sagittal sinus
Inferior sagittal sinus
Lateral ventricle
Ependymal-pial covering of choroid plexus
Choroidal vein and artery
Internal capsule
Interventricular foramen
Anterior commissure
Choroid plexus of roof of 3rd ventricle

Diencephalon and telencephalon Mature (coronal section)

Septum pellucidum
Fornix
Choroid plexus in roof of 3rd ventricle
Interthalamic adhesion (bridging 3rd ventricle)
Thalamus
Hypothalamus
Mamillary bodies
Choroid plexus (projecting into lateral ventricle along choroid fissure)
Corpus callosum
Body of caudate nucleus (basal ganglion)
Internal capsule
Corpus striatum (basal nuclei)
Claustrum
Insula
Lateral sulcus
Temporal lobe of cerebral hemisphere (from alar plate)
Cerebral cortex (gray matter)
Tracts (white matter)
Amygdala
Line of fusion between diencephalon and telencephalon

3.22 RELATIONSHIP BETWEEN TELENCEPHALON AND DIENCEPHALON

The diencephalon gives rise to the epithalamus, thalamus, and hypothalamus. The epithalamus forms the pineal body and tela choroidea extending into the roof of the third ventricle. The telencephalon overgrows the diencephalon, and the basal ganglia and internal capsule of the telencephalon flank the thalamus and hypothalamus. The internal capsule is white matter connecting the cerebral cortex to the brain stem. Anterior to the diencephalon is the limbic system. Limbus is Latin for "border"; this proximal part of the olfactory cortex is at the structural and functional interface between the telencephalon and diencephalon. The choroid plexus protrudes into the lateral ventricles to become the most extensive source of CSF.

Spinal cord

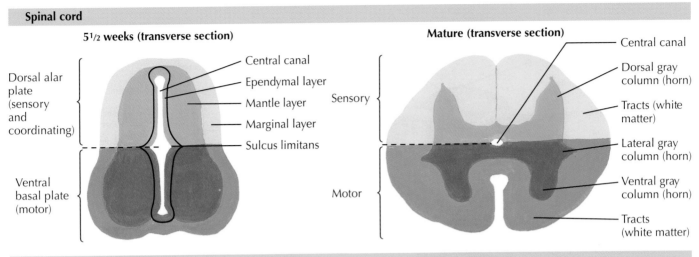

5½ weeks (transverse section)

Dorsal alar plate (sensory and coordinating)

Ventral basal plate (motor)

- Central canal
- Ependymal layer
- Mantle layer
- Marginal layer
- Sulcus limitans

Mature (transverse section)

Sensory

Motor

- Central canal
- Dorsal gray column (horn)
- Tracts (white matter)
- Lateral gray column (horn)
- Ventral gray column (horn)
- Tracts (white matter)

Medulla oblongata

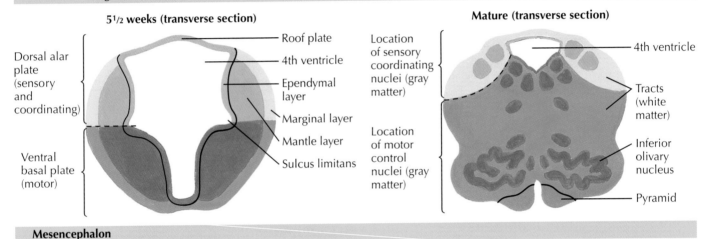

5½ weeks (transverse section)

Dorsal alar plate (sensory and coordinating)

Ventral basal plate (motor)

- Roof plate
- 4th ventricle
- Ependymal layer
- Marginal layer
- Mantle layer
- Sulcus limitans

Mature (transverse section)

Location of sensory coordinating nuclei (gray matter)

Location of motor control nuclei (gray matter)

- 4th ventricle
- Tracts (white matter)
- Inferior olivary nucleus
- Pyramid

Mesencephalon

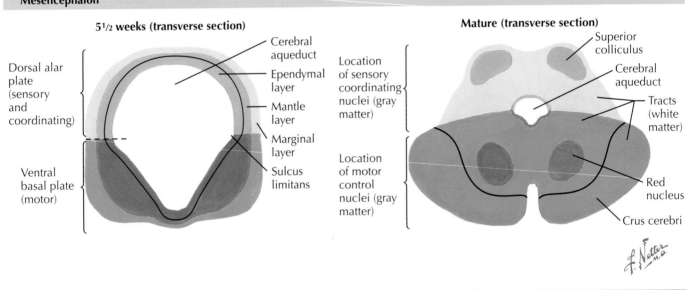

5½ weeks (transverse section)

Dorsal alar plate (sensory and coordinating)

Ventral basal plate (motor)

- Cerebral aqueduct
- Ependymal layer
- Mantle layer
- Marginal layer
- Sulcus limitans

Mature (transverse section)

Location of sensory coordinating nuclei (gray matter)

Location of motor control nuclei (gray matter)

- Superior colliculus
- Cerebral aqueduct
- Tracts (white matter)
- Red nucleus
- Crus cerebri

3.23 CROSS SECTIONS OF THE MIDBRAIN AND HINDBRAIN

The brain or brain stem and spinal cord have more similarities than may be apparent by casual inspection. Dorsal is sensory; ventral is motor. The sensory and motor gray matter columns of the spinal cord extend into the brain stem. Cranial and spinal nerves provide sensory and motor innervation to the body tissues in segmental fashion. These similarities are obscured by the loss of dorsal/ventral symmetry in the brain. Sensory areas are displaced laterally by the dorsal location of the ventricles. Other differences include the organization of brain stem gray matter into nuclei instead of columns and the greater variety of nuclei for new types of neurons in cranial nerves.

Medulla oblongata at 3½ months (transverse section)

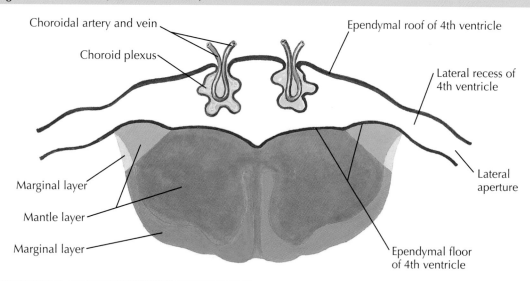

Choroidal artery and vein

Choroid plexus

Ependymal roof of 4th ventricle

Lateral recess of 4th ventricle

Lateral aperture

Marginal layer

Mantle layer

Marginal layer

Ependymal floor of 4th ventricle

Medulla oblongata, mature (transverse section)

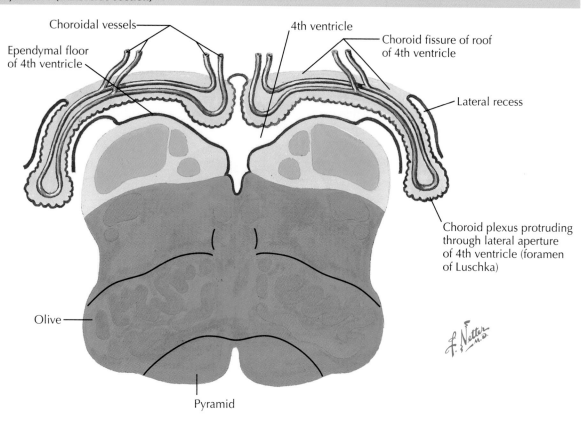

Choroidal vessels

Ependymal floor of 4th ventricle

4th ventricle

Choroid fissure of roof of 4th ventricle

Lateral recess

Choroid plexus protruding through lateral aperture of 4th ventricle (foramen of Luschka)

Olive

Pyramid

3.24 PRODUCTION OF CEREBROSPINAL FLUID

The ependyma, pia mater, and a rich plexus of blood vessels extend into the ventricles within the brain. This elaborate vascular membrane is the **tela choroidea** with its **choroid plexus** of capillaries, the site of production of **CSF** that surrounds and protects the brain and spinal cord in the subarachnoid space. CSF is an ultrafiltrate of arterial blood, and the tight junctions between the epithelial cells of the ependyma form a selective barrier in the passage of CSF from the choroid capillaries into the ventricles. Shown in Fig. 3.24 schematically is the development of the choroid plexus in the roof of the **fourth ventricle** in the medulla oblongata. The **foramina of Luschka** in the fourth ventricle are sites of passage of CSF into the subarachnoid space.

Frontal section (ventral to sulcus limitans) at 36 days

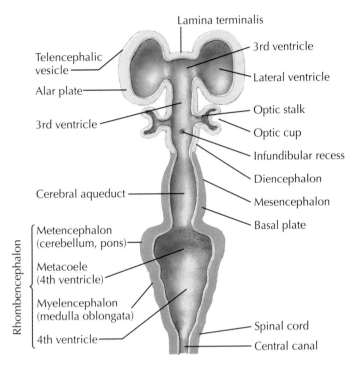

Ependymal lining of cavities of brain at 3 months

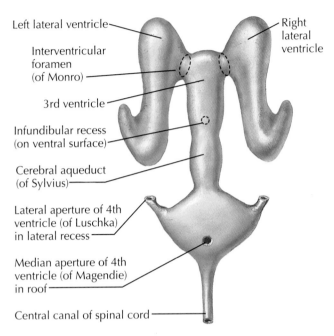

Ependymal lining of cavities of brain at 9 months (birth)

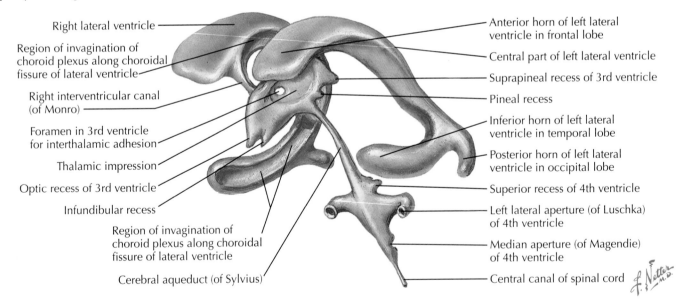

3.25 DEVELOPMENT OF THE VENTRICLES

The lumen of the neural tube enlarges in the brain to form the **ventricles**, a series of interconnected chambers where **CSF** is produced. CSF exits the fourth ventricle from paired lateral apertures (**foramina of Luschka**) and a median aperture (**foramen of Magendie**) to surround the brain and spinal cord in the subarachnoid space. CSF reenters the bloodstream through arachnoid granulations that protrude into the superior sagittal sinus, a venous channel within the dura mater at the top of the falx cerebri, and through capillaries of the CNS and pia mater.

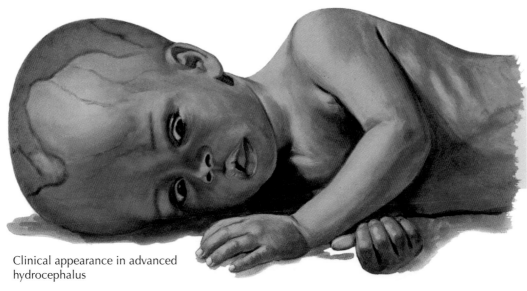

Clinical appearance in advanced hydrocephalus

Potential lesion sites in obstructive hydrocephalus

1. Interventricular foramen (of Monro)
2. Cerebral aqueduct (of Sylvius)
3. Lateral apertures (of Luschka)
4. Median aperture (of Magendie)

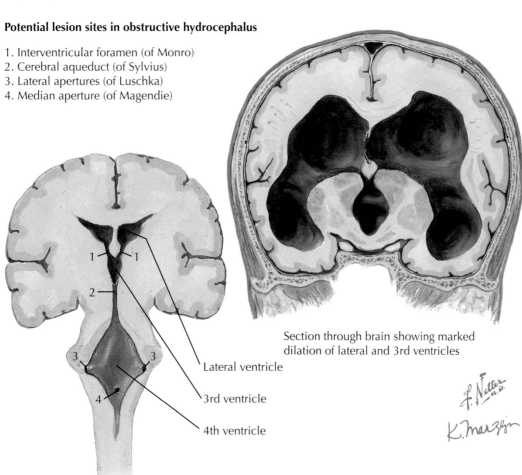

Lateral ventricle

3rd ventricle

4th ventricle

Section through brain showing marked dilation of lateral and 3rd ventricles

3.26 CONGENITAL VENTRICULAR DEFECTS

Obstructive hydrocephalus is a congenital type of "water in the head." CSF accumulates within the ventricles because of a blockage of flow from one ventricle to another or from exiting the fourth ventricle into the subarachnoid space. The enlarging ventricles compress the brain against the neurocranium, which, in response to the increased pressure, grows at an abnormally fast rate compared with the viscerocranium. Postnatal hydrocephalus is more often caused by the interruption of CSF passing back into the bloodstream through the arachnoid granulations. Fluid accumulates in the subarachnoid space surrounding the brain instead of the ventricles, and the brain is compressed externally instead of internally.

CLINICAL POINT

Hydrocephalus. Symptoms and findings include headache associated with nausea or vomiting and aggravated by physical activity, cranial nerve VI palsy, depressed mental status, gait instability, and increased head circumference.

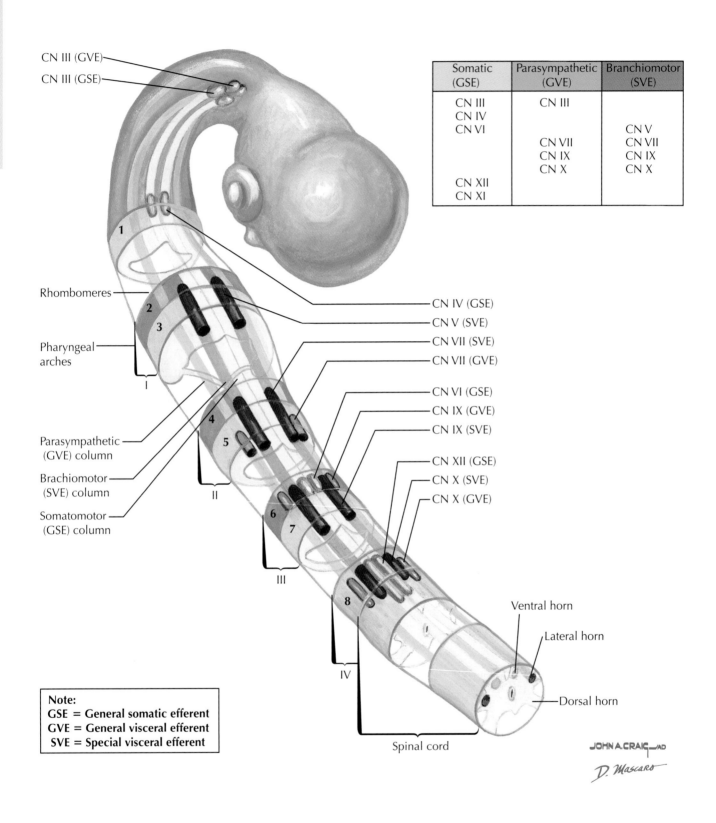

	Somatic (GSE)	Parasympathetic (GVE)	Branchiomotor (SVE)
	CN III	CN III	
	CN IV		
	CN VI		CN V
		CN VII	CN VII
		CN IX	CN IX
		CN X	CN X
	CN XII		
	CN XI		

CN III (GVE)
CN III (GSE)

Rhombomeres

Pharyngeal arches

Parasympathetic (GVE) column

Brachiomotor (SVE) column

Somatomotor (GSE) column

CN IV (GSE)
CN V (SVE)
CN VII (SVE)
CN VII (GVE)
CN VI (GSE)
CN IX (GVE)
CN IX (SVE)
CN XII (GSE)
CN X (SVE)
CN X (GVE)

Ventral horn
Lateral horn
Dorsal horn

Spinal cord

Note:
GSE = General somatic efferent
GVE = General visceral efferent
SVE = Special visceral efferent

JOHN A. CRAIG—AD
D. Mascaro

3.27 DEVELOPMENT OF MOTOR NUCLEI IN THE BRAIN STEM

The gray matter columns for somatomotor cell bodies (ventral horn) and presynaptic autonomic neurons (lateral horn) in the spinal cord extend into the brain stem. They maintain the same positional relationship to each other but are organized into a series of separate but aligned nuclei. A third series of nuclei is present in the hindbrain for motor neurons (branchiomotor) supplying the pharyngeal arch muscles.

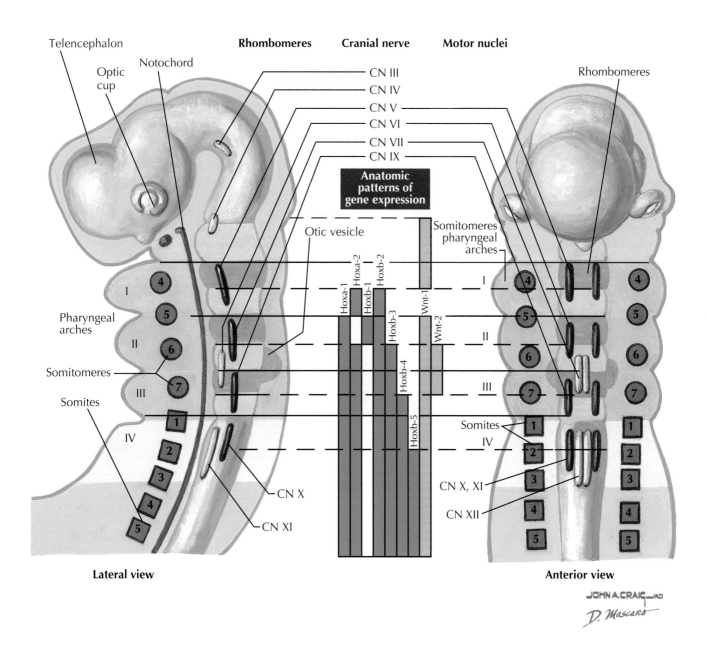

Telencephalon

Optic cup

Notochord

Rhombomeres   **Cranial nerve**   **Motor nuclei**

CN III
CN IV
CN V
CN VI
CN VII
CN IX

Anatomic patterns of gene expression

Otic vesicle

Somitomeres pharyngeal arches

Hoxa-1   Hoxa-2   Hoxb-1   Hoxb-2   Hoxb-3   Hoxb-4   Hoxb-5   Wnt-1   Wnt-2

Pharyngeal arches

Somitomeres

Somites

CN X

CN XI

Lateral view

Rhombomeres

Somites

CN X, XI

CN XII

Anterior view

JOHN A. CRAIG—AD

D. Mascaro

3.28 SEGMENTATION OF THE HINDBRAIN

Segmentation is evident in the hindbrain as a series of swellings and in the pattern of blood supply. This segmentation pattern is extended into the pharyngeal arches, somitomeres, and their nerves, which are all in register with the rhombomeres. Segmentation in these structures is related to the pattern of homeotic and segmentation gene expression (mainly of the *Hox* gene family). The segmental nature of the spinal nerves is obvious, but the developing spinal cord has no visible equivalent of rhombomeres, and the process that determines the path of peripheral neuron growth appears to be different in the hindbrain compared with the spinal cord.

Midsagittal sections of the development of the anterior and posterior lobes of the pituitary gland. Anterior is to the right.

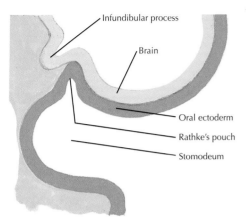

Infundibular process

Brain

Oral ectoderm

Rathke's pouch

Stomodeum

1. Beginning formation of Rathke's pouch and infundibular process

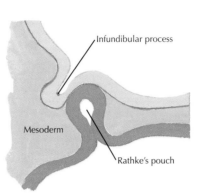

Infundibular process

Mesoderm

Rathke's pouch

2. Neck of Rathke's pouch constricted by growth of mesoderm

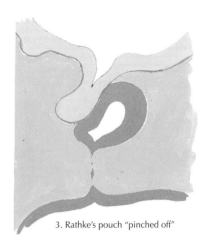

3. Rathke's pouch "pinched off"

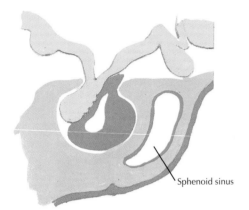

Sphenoid sinus

4. "Pinched off" segment conforms to neural process, forming pars distalis, pars intermedia and pars tuberalis

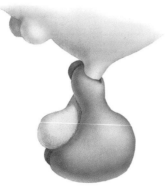

5. Pars tuberalis encircles infundibular stalk (lateral surface view)

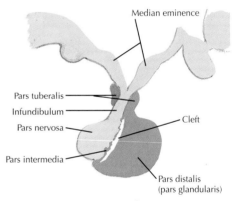

Median eminence

Pars tuberalis

Infundibulum

Pars nervosa

Pars intermedia

Cleft

Pars distalis (pars glandularis)

6. Mature form

PITUITARY HORMONES

From the Anterior Lobe (Pars Distalis)		From the Posterior Lobe (Pars Nervosa)
Follicle-stimulating hormone (FSH)	Thyroid-stimulating hormone (TSH)	Vasopressin
Luteinizing hormone (LH)	Adrenocorticotropic hormone (ACTH)	Oxytocin
Prolactin	Growth hormone (GH)	

3.29 DEVELOPMENT OF THE PITUITARY GLAND

The pituitary gland is unusual in that it develops from the fusion of outgrowths from two embryonic primordia that are separate from each other in structure and function. The **anterior lobe** (**adenohypophysis** or **pars distalis**) is an outgrowth of the roof of the stomodeum. It encircles the base of the **posterior lobe** or **neurohypophysis**, which is an extension of the brain. The anterior lobe is glandular endocrine tissue that secretes its hormones in response to hypothalamic neuroendocrine products transmitted in the hypophyseal portal system of veins. The posterior lobe consists of specialized hypothalamic nerve terminations that store and release hormones.

Terminology

Auerbach's plexus	Part of the enteric nervous system, it is an autonomic plexus with ganglia in the smooth muscle wall of the gastrointestinal tract.
Central canal	Cavity within the neural tube. It diminishes within the spinal cord, but, in the brain, it forms the system of interconnected ventricles that produce cerebrospinal fluid.
Central nervous system	Brain and spinal cord.
Cortex	(L., "bark" or "shell") The outer, stratified, gray matter covering of the brain.
Dermatome	Area of skin innervated by one spinal nerve pair; or the part of a somite that gives rise to the dermis of skin supplied by one spinal nerve.
Enteric nervous system	Autonomic nerve plexus in the walls of the gastrointestinal tract.
Ganglion	(G., "swelling" or "knot") A collection of somatic (sensory) or autonomic nerve cell bodies in the peripheral nervous system.
Glia	(G., "glue") Supporting cells of the central nervous system, including astrocytes, oligodendrocytes, microglia, and ependymal cells.
Gray matter	Tissue in the central nervous system where cell bodies predominate in contrast to white matter consisting of nerve cell processes.
Meissner's plexus	Part of the enteric nervous system, it is an autonomic plexus with ganglia in the submucosa of the gastrointestinal tract wall.
Nerve	Collections of neuron cell processes enveloped by a connective tissue sheath of epineurium in the peripheral nervous system.
Nerve fiber	The long process of a single neuron enveloped by the connective tissue sheath of endoneurium.
Neural crest	Part of the folding neural tube that pinches off to form the cell bodies of all neurons and supporting cells outside the central nervous system. Also gives rise to pia, arachnoid, and mesenchyme in the head that will form bone, muscle, and connective tissue.
Neural plate	Thickening of ectoderm in the bilaminar embryonic disc that gives rise to all of the nervous system.
Neural tube	Tube derived from the neural plate of surface ectoderm that gives rise to the brain and spinal cord (central nervous system) and all of the nerve cell bodies within them.
Neurotransmitter	Chemical that relays an electrical impulse from one neuron to another at the synapse, the narrow gap between neurons. Also secreted at the end of a nerve for its effect on muscle, glandular tissue, and so forth.
Node of Ranvier	Gaps between Schwann cells along myelinated nerve fibers.
Nucleus	Discreet aggregation of gray matter cell bodies in the brainstem. The term is morphologically equivalent to ganglia in the peripheral nervous system or the gray matter horns of the spinal cord.
Perineurium	Sheath around bundles of nerve cell processes in peripheral nerves that has epithelial, contractile, and connective tissue properties.
Peripheral nervous system	All cranial, spinal, and autonomic nerves that are in the body tissues outside the brain and spinal cord (central nervous system).
Plexus	(L., "braid") Interconnecting networks of peripheral nerves (or vessels).
Rhombomeres	Segmentation of the hindbrain related to the pattern of segmentation/homeotic gene expression (mainly *Hox* genes).
Somatopleure	Lateral plate mesoderm with surface ectoderm that is the basis for the body wall bone, striated muscle, skin, and connective tissue.
Somites	Epithelial blocks of mesoderm flanking the notochord that develop from the paraxial columns of mesoderm. They will form bone, muscle, and connective tissue.

Terminology—cont'd

Somitomeres	The first evidence of segmentation of the paraxial columns in the process of somite formation. In the head, they never fully separate into distinct somite blocks and retain the term, somitomeres.
Splanchnopleure	Lateral plate mesoderm with endoderm that forms the wall of visceral organs and their suspending mesenteries.
Sulcus limitans	Bilateral groove in the central canal dividing the neural tube into dorsal alar plates (sensory) and ventral basal plates (motor).
Tela choroidea	(G., "weblike membrane") Vascular layers of pia mater and ependyma in the walls of the ventricles that produce cerebrospinal fluid.
Tethered cord syndrome	A low positioning of the termination of the spinal cord below L1 by the filum terminale that may result from abnormal secondary neurulation. May be associated with sensory and motor symptoms in pelvic organs and the lower extremities.
White matter	Tissue in the central nervous system consisting largely of nerve cell processes extending from cell bodies in the gray matter.

4

THE CARDIOVASCULAR SYSTEM

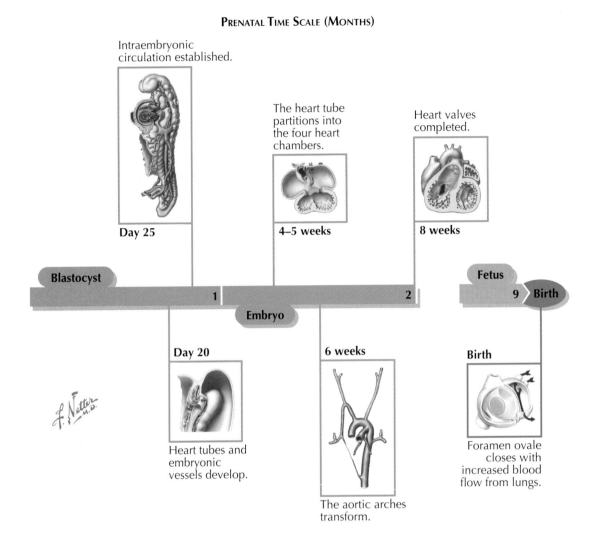

PRENATAL TIME SCALE (MONTHS)

Intraembryonic circulation established.

Day 25

The heart tube partitions into the four heart chambers.

4–5 weeks

Heart valves completed.

8 weeks

Blastocyst

Fetus

9 Birth

Embryo

Day 20

Heart tubes and embryonic vessels develop.

6 weeks

The aortic arches transform.

Birth

Foramen ovale closes with increased blood flow from lungs.

4.1 TIMELINE

HEART PRIMORDIUM

Cardiogenic mesoderm at the cranial end of the embryonic disc. Most is splanchnic mesoderm from the primitive streak. Mesoderm in the outflow portions of the heart is cranial mesoderm from the neural crest and paraxial columns.

PLAN

The cardiovascular system is the first functioning system. The heart begins as a primitive tube with peristaltic waves of contraction starting by day 22. Blood circulates within the embryo and to the placenta and yolk sac. The single heart tube is partitioned into four chambers, with a systemic outflow on the left and pulmonary outflow on the right. Pulmonary circulation is minimal because gas exchange occurs in the placenta and the airway is filled with amniotic fluid. Blood bypasses the nonfunctioning lungs in two temporary "shunts," one between the atria (foramen ovale) and one between the pulmonary trunk and aortic arch (ductus arteriosus). The fetal circulatory system is designed to be capable of converting to the adult pattern with the first breath.

INCLUSION AND BIAS CONSIDERATION: SKIN TONE REPRESENTATION FOR BETTER CLINICAL ASSESSMENT

This chapter focuses on introducing some major clinical correlations as they relate to the development of the cardiovascular system. Frequently, there is reference to the presentation of conditions related to vascular supply, such as the pallor, erythema, or cyanosis. In these types of visual patient assessments, it is critically important to be aware of how such conditions present on a variety of skin tones. Historically, the images that have often been used in medical texts and guides lack diversity, particularly for people with darker skin tones. However, this can lead to large gaps in understanding the breadth of patient assessment, ultimately perpetuating health disparities and outcomes, particularly for people with dark skin tones. Educating oneself on the variety of presentations, in addition to increasing the representation of presentations, is key for inclusive clinical practice. Fig. 4.24 of this chapter provides more details for this as it relates to the condition of cyanosis.

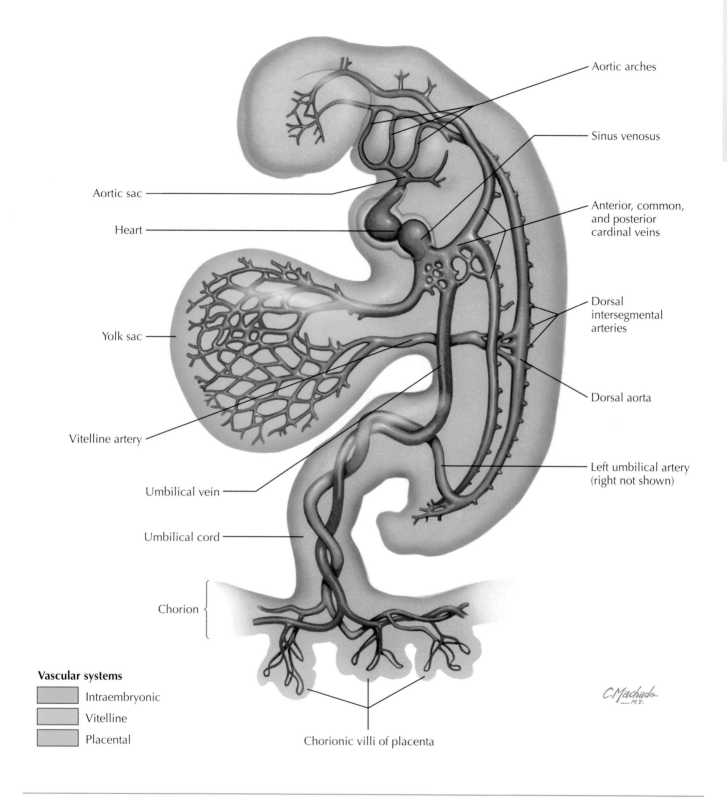

Aortic arches

Sinus venosus

Aortic sac

Anterior, common, and posterior cardinal veins

Heart

Dorsal intersegmental arteries

Yolk sac

Dorsal aorta

Vitelline artery

Left umbilical artery (right not shown)

Umbilical vein

Umbilical cord

Chorion

Vascular systems

Intraembryonic

Vitelline

Placental

Chorionic villi of placenta

C. Machado
M.D.

4.2 **EARLY VASCULAR SYSTEMS**

By the end of the third week, blood flow is established within the embryo and to the placenta and yolk sac. Oxygen and nutrients derived from maternal blood in the placenta enter the embryo in the umbilical vein. The primary intraembryonic arteries are the dorsal aorta, the intersegmental arteries between somites, and the aortic arch arteries within the pharyngeal arches in the head and neck region of the embryo. The cardinal system of veins brings embryonic venous blood back to the heart, where it mixes with blood from the umbilical vein. The yolk sac is not a primary source of nutrition as in egg-laying animals, but it is important as the first source of blood cells that enter the embryonic circulation via the vitelline veins.

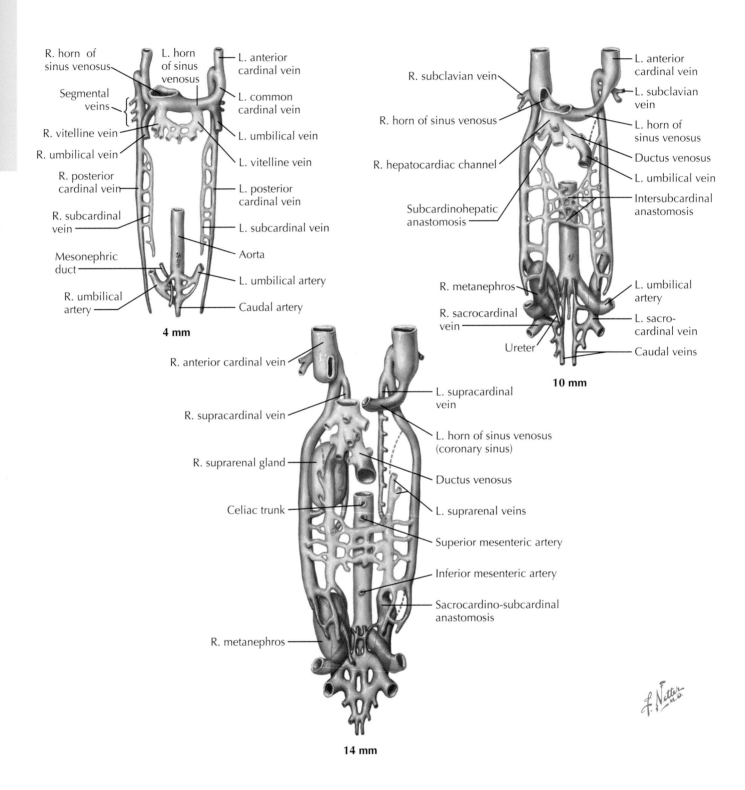

R. horn of sinus venosus

L. horn of sinus venosus

L. anterior cardinal vein

Segmental veins

L. common cardinal vein

R. vitelline vein

L. umbilical vein

R. umbilical vein

L. vitelline vein

R. posterior cardinal vein

L. posterior cardinal vein

R. subcardinal vein

L. subcardinal vein

Mesonephric duct

Aorta

L. umbilical artery

R. umbilical artery

Caudal artery

4 mm

R. subclavian vein

L. anterior cardinal vein

L. subclavian vein

R. horn of sinus venosus

L. horn of sinus venosus

R. hepatocardiac channel

Ductus venosus

L. umbilical vein

Subcardinohepatic anastomosis

Intersubcardinal anastomosis

R. metanephros

L. umbilical artery

R. sacrocardinal vein

L. sacro-cardinal vein

Ureter

Caudal veins

10 mm

R. anterior cardinal vein

L. supracardinal vein

R. supracardinal vein

L. horn of sinus venosus (coronary sinus)

R. suprarenal gland

Ductus venosus

Celiac trunk

L. suprarenal veins

Superior mesenteric artery

Inferior mesenteric artery

Sacrocardino-subcardinal anastomosis

R. metanephros

14 mm

4.3 EARLY DEVELOPMENT OF THE CARDINAL SYSTEM OF VEINS

The cardinal, subcardinal, and supracardinal veins develop and interconnect in temporal sequence, forming the **intraembryonic cardinal system of veins**. Anterior cardinal veins become the veins cranial to the heart. Supracardinal veins relate to the late-growing thoracic wall. The major events occur in the abdomen, where the left and right posterior cardinal veins disappear, and blood from the lower half of the embryo shifts to the subcardinal veins. The right subcardinal vein will connect to the heart via the most proximal segment of the right vitelline vein that is forming the intrahepatic segment of the inferior vena cava, the hepatic veins, and the hepatic portal vein.

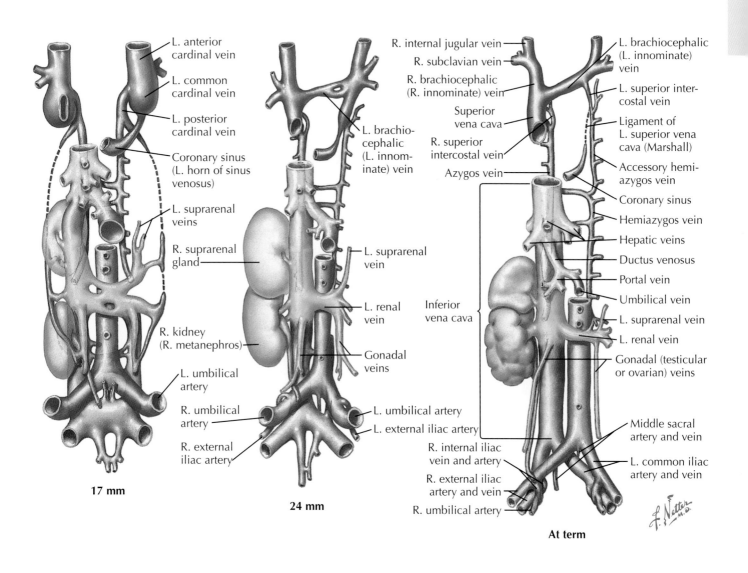

17 mm

24 mm

At term

4.4 TRANSFORMATION TO THE POSTNATAL PATTERN

Blood from the pelvis and lower extremity converges on the developing common iliac veins. As the posterior cardinal veins diminish in size, the **subcardinal veins** connect to the common iliac veins and greatly enlarge on the right side of the body to form the **lower inferior vena cava**. They also form the **renal and gonadal veins**. The vitelline veins give rise to the upper, intrahepatic portion of the inferior vena cava. The veins of the abdominal viscera are related to the proximal vitelline veins because of the endodermal continuity of the yolk sac and midgut. The subcardinal portion of the inferior vena cava joins the portal and hepatic circulation by anastomosis with the vitelline veins on the right.

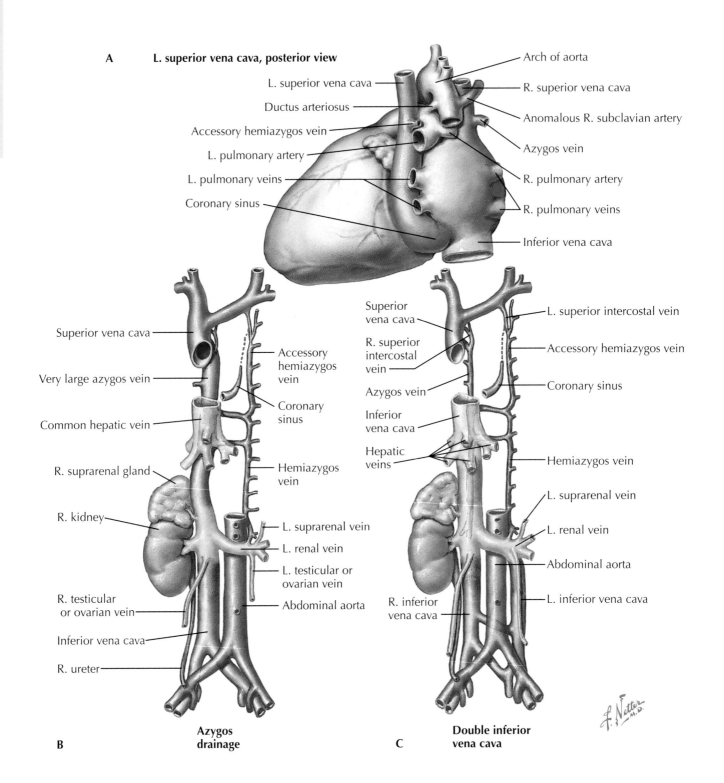

A   **L. superior vena cava, posterior view**

Arch of aorta

L. superior vena cava

Ductus arteriosus

Accessory hemiazygos vein

L. pulmonary artery

L. pulmonary veins

Coronary sinus

R. superior vena cava

Anomalous R. subclavian artery

Azygos vein

R. pulmonary artery

R. pulmonary veins

Inferior vena cava

Superior vena cava

Very large azygos vein

Common hepatic vein

R. suprarenal gland

R. kidney

R. testicular
or ovarian vein

Inferior vena cava

R. ureter

Accessory
hemiazygos
vein

Coronary
sinus

Hemiazygos
vein

L. suprarenal vein

L. renal vein

L. testicular or
ovarian vein

Abdominal aorta

B   **Azygos
drainage**

Superior
vena cava

R. superior
intercostal
vein

Azygos vein

Inferior
vena cava

Hepatic
veins

R. inferior
vena cava

L. superior intercostal vein

Accessory hemiazygos vein

Coronary sinus

Hemiazygos vein

L. suprarenal vein

L. renal vein

Abdominal aorta

L. inferior vena cava

C   **Double inferior
vena cava**

4.5 VEIN ANOMALIES

All three cardinal systems begin as paired veins of similar size. Later in fetal development veins in the right side of the body predominates as the superior and inferior vena cavae and related veins. The bilateral nature of the veins may persist as a double superior vena cava (Fig. 4.5A), inferior vena cava (Fig, 4.5C), or both. The persistent left superior vena cava will drain into the heart via a greatly enlarged coronary sinus, a remnant of the left horn of the sinus venosus (Fig. 4.5A). The complicated sequences of venous development may result in abnormal connections. For example, if the anastomoses between the subcardinal and vitelline veins fail to develop, the lower inferior vena cava continues as the azygous vein, and the inferior vena cava entering the right atrium drains blood only from the gut via the hepatic veins and hepatic portal vein (Fig. 4.5B).

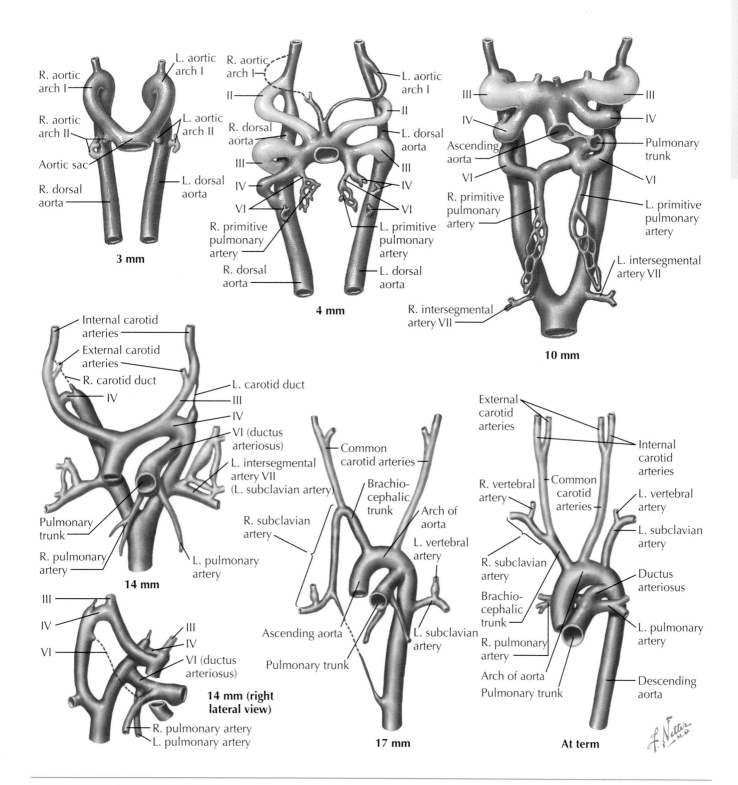

R. aortic arch I
R. aortic arch II
Aortic sac
R. dorsal aorta
L. aortic arch I
L. aortic arch II
L. dorsal aorta

3 mm

R. aortic arch I
II
R. dorsal aorta
III
IV
VI
R. primitive pulmonary artery
R. dorsal aorta
L. aortic arch I
II
L. dorsal aorta
III
IV
VI
L. primitive pulmonary artery
L. dorsal aorta

4 mm

III
IV
Ascending aorta
VI
R. primitive pulmonary artery
III
IV
Pulmonary trunk
VI
L. primitive pulmonary artery
L. intersegmental artery VII
R. intersegmental artery VII

10 mm

Internal carotid arteries
External carotid arteries
R. carotid duct
IV
L. carotid duct
III
IV
VI (ductus arteriosus)
L. intersegmental artery VII (L. subclavian artery)
Pulmonary trunk
R. pulmonary artery
L. pulmonary artery

14 mm

III
IV
VI
III
IV
VI (ductus arteriosus)
R. pulmonary artery
L. pulmonary artery

14 mm (right lateral view)

Common carotid arteries
Brachiocephalic trunk
Arch of aorta
L. vertebral artery
R. subclavian artery
Ascending aorta
Pulmonary trunk
L. subclavian artery

17 mm

External carotid arteries
Internal carotid arteries
R. vertebral artery
Common carotid arteries
L. vertebral artery
L. subclavian artery
R. subclavian artery
Brachiocephalic trunk
Ductus arteriosus
R. pulmonary artery
L. pulmonary artery
Arch of aorta
Pulmonary trunk
Descending aorta

At term

4.6 AORTIC ARCH ARTERIES

At the end of week 4, blood flows from the primitive heart to the tissues through a series of paired arteries that pass through the pharyngeal arches of mesoderm flanking the foregut. They connect to a left and right dorsal aorta that fuse into a single aorta caudal to the pharyngeal arches. The right dorsal aorta disappears as the aortic arches transform into the adult pattern during the sixth week.

Major Aortic Arch Derivatives

- **Arch 1:** Mostly disappear but contribute to the maxillary arteries
- **Arch 2:** Mostly disappear
- **Arch 3:** Common and internal carotid arteries
- **Arch 4:** Right subclavian artery and part of the arch of the aorta
- **Arch 6:** Ductus arteriosus and proximal parts of the pulmonary arteries

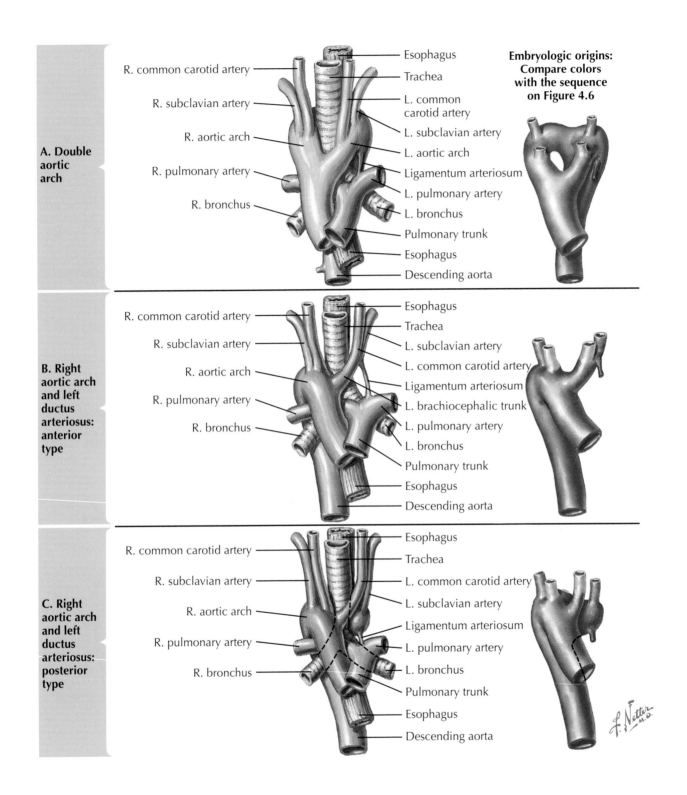

A. Double aortic arch

- R. common carotid artery
- R. subclavian artery
- R. aortic arch
- R. pulmonary artery
- R. bronchus
- Esophagus
- Trachea
- L. common carotid artery
- L. subclavian artery
- L. aortic arch
- Ligamentum arteriosum
- L. pulmonary artery
- L. bronchus
- Pulmonary trunk
- Esophagus
- Descending aorta

Embryologic origins: Compare colors with the sequence on Figure 4.6

B. Right aortic arch and left ductus arteriosus: anterior type

- R. common carotid artery
- R. subclavian artery
- R. aortic arch
- R. pulmonary artery
- R. bronchus
- Esophagus
- Trachea
- L. subclavian artery
- L. common carotid artery
- Ligamentum arteriosum
- L. brachiocephalic trunk
- L. pulmonary artery
- L. bronchus
- Pulmonary trunk
- Esophagus
- Descending aorta

C. Right aortic arch and left ductus arteriosus: posterior type

- R. common carotid artery
- R. subclavian artery
- R. aortic arch
- R. pulmonary artery
- R. bronchus
- Esophagus
- Trachea
- L. common carotid artery
- L. subclavian artery
- Ligamentum arteriosum
- L. pulmonary artery
- L. bronchus
- Pulmonary trunk
- Esophagus
- Descending aorta

4.7 AORTIC ARCH ANOMALIES

A double aortic arch results when the initial connection between the aortic sac and the aortic arches on the right remains (Fig. 4.7A). A right aortic arch forms when this connection persists while the one on the left that forms the ascending aorta degenerates. Two variations of a right aortic arch are shown: one with the left subclavian artery passing in front of the trachea (Fig. 4.7B) and one with it passing behind (Fig. 4.7C).

CLINICAL POINT

Vascular sling. If a component of an aortic arch passes behind the trachea (Figs. 4.7A and 4.7C), difficulty in swallowing may occur because it will compress the esophagus behind it.

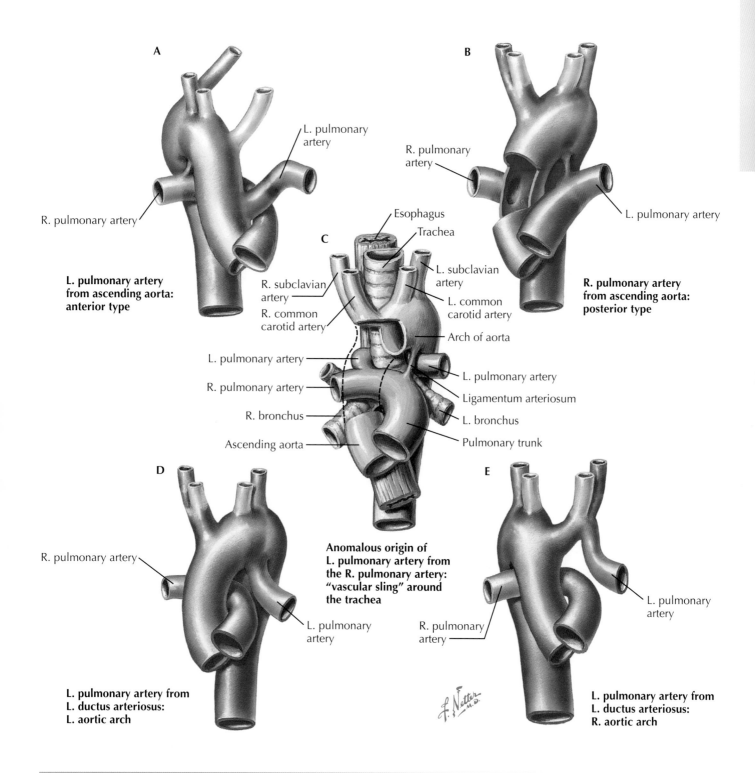

A

L. pulmonary artery

R. pulmonary artery

**L. pulmonary artery
from ascending aorta:
anterior type**

B

R. pulmonary artery

L. pulmonary artery

**R. pulmonary artery
from ascending aorta:
posterior type**

C

Esophagus

Trachea

R. subclavian artery

L. subclavian artery

R. common carotid artery

L. common carotid artery

Arch of aorta

L. pulmonary artery

L. pulmonary artery

R. pulmonary artery

Ligamentum arteriosum

R. bronchus

L. bronchus

Ascending aorta

Pulmonary trunk

**Anomalous origin of
L. pulmonary artery from
the R. pulmonary artery:
"vascular sling" around
the trachea**

D

R. pulmonary artery

L. pulmonary artery

**L. pulmonary artery from
L. ductus arteriosus:
L. aortic arch**

E

R. pulmonary artery

L. pulmonary artery

**L. pulmonary artery from
L. ductus arteriosus:
R. aortic arch**

4.8 ANOMALOUS ORIGINS OF THE PULMONARY ARTERIES

The sequence of events in the transformation of the aortic arches is complex, and there are many opportunities for disruptions in the process. The pulmonary arteries and the ductus arteriosus develop from the most caudal pair of aortic arches (sixth), so the division of the truncus arteriosus into the ascending aorta and pulmonary trunk can affect their connections. Pulmonary arteries can originate from the ascending aorta (Fig. 4.8A and 4.8B), from a right aortic arch (Fig. 4.8E), from the inferior end of the ductus arteriosus (Figs. 4.8D and 4.8E), or from the opposite pulmonary artery (Fig. 4.8C). Like the anomalous left subclavian artery in Fig. 4.7C, the origin of the left pulmonary artery from the right pulmonary artery (Fig. 4.8C) also creates a vascular sling around the trachea that results in difficulty swallowing caused by anterior compression of the esophagus by the anomalous pulmonary artery.

Coarctation of the aorta

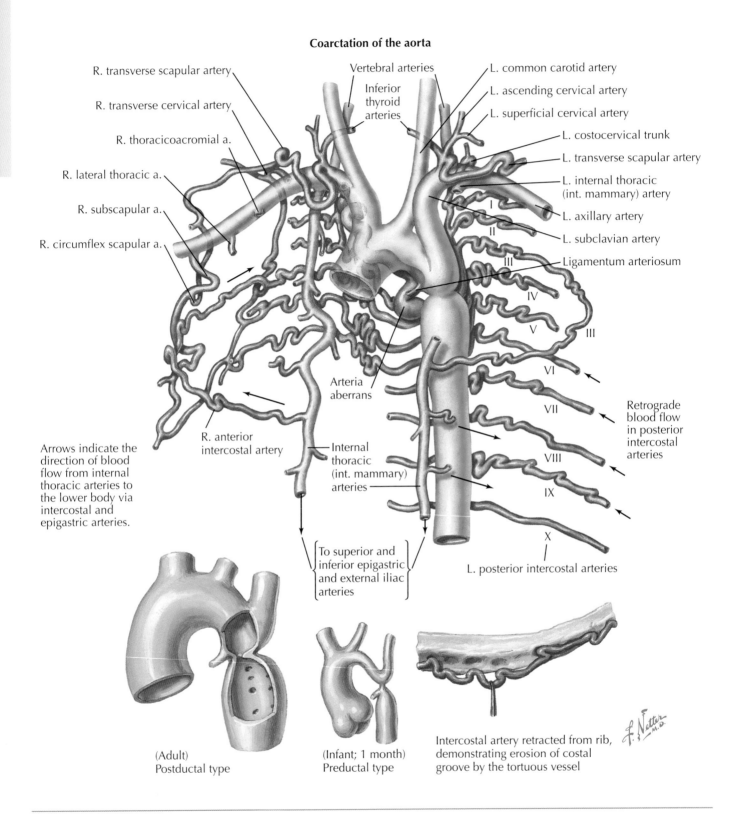

R. transverse scapular artery

R. transverse cervical artery

R. thoracicoacromial a.

R. lateral thoracic a.

R. subscapular a.

R. circumflex scapular a.

Vertebral arteries

Inferior thyroid arteries

L. common carotid artery

L. ascending cervical artery

L. superficial cervical artery

L. costocervical trunk

L. transverse scapular artery

L. internal thoracic (int. mammary) artery

L. axillary artery

L. subclavian artery

Ligamentum arteriosum

Arteria aberrans

Arrows indicate the direction of blood flow from internal thoracic arteries to the lower body via intercostal and epigastric arteries.

R. anterior intercostal artery

Internal thoracic (int. mammary) arteries

To superior and inferior epigastric and external iliac arteries

Retrograde blood flow in posterior intercostal arteries

L. posterior intercostal arteries

(Adult) Postductal type

(Infant; 1 month) Preductal type

Intercostal artery retracted from rib, demonstrating erosion of costal groove by the tortuous vessel

4.9 INTERSEGMENTAL ARTERIES AND COARCTATION OF THE AORTA

Coarctation of the aorta is a congenital narrowing that occurs near the entrance of the ductus arteriosus. Blood flows through two collateral routes via the internal thoracic arteries to get to the lower body: (1) the deep superior and inferior epigastric arteries into the external iliac; and (2) intercostal arteries with retrograde flow into the thoracic aorta inferior to the coarctation. The intercostal arteries are dilated and tortuous from the increase in blood pressure and flow. They develop from embryonic **intersegmental arteries** that pass between each of the somites from the dorsal aorta. They also contribute to the vertebral, subclavian, lumbar, common iliac, and lateral sacral arteries.

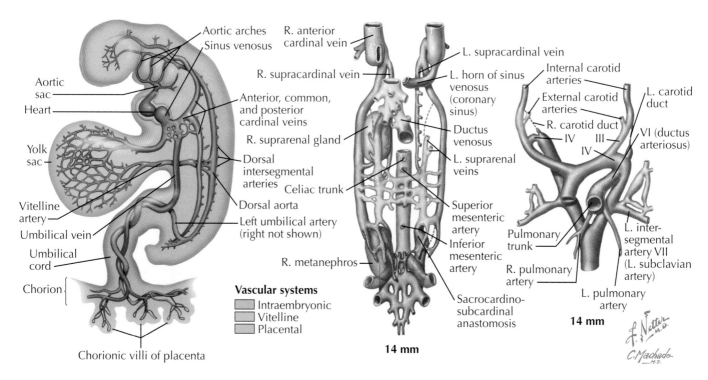

EMBRYONIC BLOOD VESSEL DERIVATIVES

Embryonic Vessels	Major Derivatives
Aortic arch artery 1	Part of maxillary arteries
Aortic arch artery 3	Common and internal carotid arteries
Aortic arch artery 4	Right subclavian artery; part of aortic arch
Aortic arch artery 6	Ductus arteriosus; proximal pulmonary arteries
Intersegmental arteries	Intercostal arteries Lumbar arteries Common iliac arteries Parts of vertebral, subclavian, and lateral sacral arteries
Umbilical arteries	Medial umbilical ligaments on the internal aspect of the abdominal wall
Umbilical vein	Round ligament of the liver (ligamentum teres)
Vitelline arteries	Celiac trunk Superior mesenteric artery Inferior mesenteric artery
Vitelline veins	Hepatic portal system Hepatic veins Intrahepatic segment of the inferior vena cava
Anterior cardinal veins	Superior vena cava Brachiocephalic (innominate) veins Internal jugular veins
Subcardinal veins (and anastomoses between the systems)	Lower inferior vena cava Renal and suprarenal veins Gonadal veins
Supracardinal veins	Azygous system of veins Segment of the inferior vena cava between the kidneys and liver

4.10 SUMMARY OF EMBRYONIC BLOOD VESSEL DERIVATIVES

The umbilical vessels become fibrous ligaments. The development of gastrointestinal vessels from the vitelline circulation reflects the close relationship between the endodermal yolk sac and gut tube. Veins cranial to the heart come from the anterior cardinal veins. Veins below the liver (lower inferior vena cava, renal, gonadal) develop from the subcardinal system, and veins of the thoracic wall arise from the supracardinal veins. The aortic arch arteries form the arteries between the maxillary artery (arch 1) in the head and pulmonary arteries/ductus arteriosus in the mediastinum (arch 6). Halfway in between are the common carotid arteries that develop from the middle (arch 3).

Presomite stage (1.5-mm embryo) at approximately 20 days

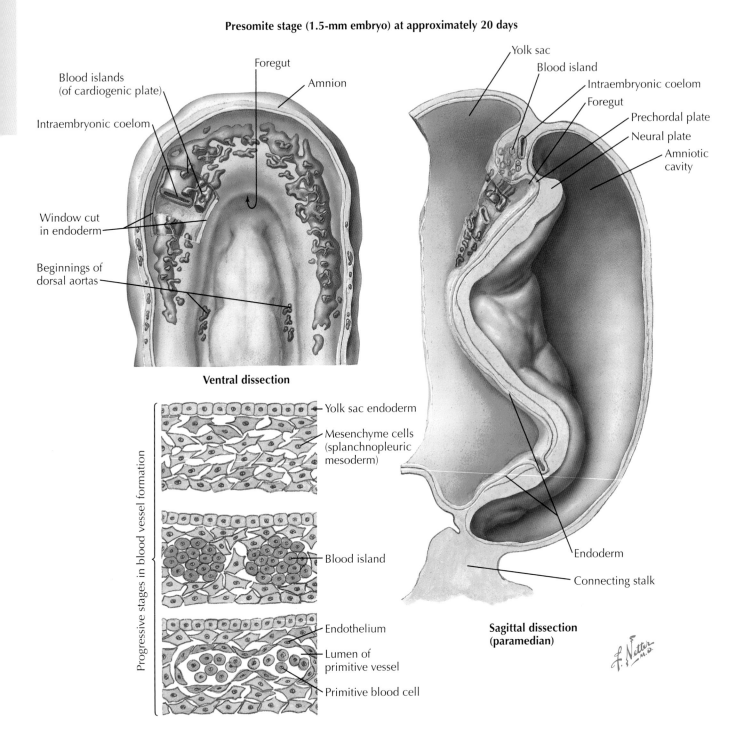

Blood islands
(of cardiogenic plate)

Intraembryonic coelom

Window cut
in endoderm

Beginnings of
dorsal aortas

Foregut

Amnion

Ventral dissection

Yolk sac

Blood island

Intraembryonic coelom

Foregut

Prechordal plate

Neural plate

Amniotic
cavity

Endoderm

Connecting stalk

**Sagittal dissection
(paramedian)**

Progressive stages in blood vessel formation

Yolk sac endoderm

Mesenchyme cells
(splanchnopleuric
mesoderm)

Blood island

Endothelium

Lumen of
primitive vessel

Primitive blood cell

4.11 FORMATION OF BLOOD VESSELS

Blood vessels first appear next to the intraembryonic coelom in the lateral plate and cardiogenic mesoderm and in the extraembryonic mesoderm of the yolk sac and connecting stalk. Mesenchyme condenses into interconnecting cords of cells that cavitate to form the vascular lumen. Some mesenchymal cells remain within the lumen to differentiate into primitive blood cells near the end of week 3. The yolk sac and allantois are the first sources of embryonic blood cells. The fetal liver and spleen take over this function, with postnatal hemopoiesis occurring primarily in the bone marrow.

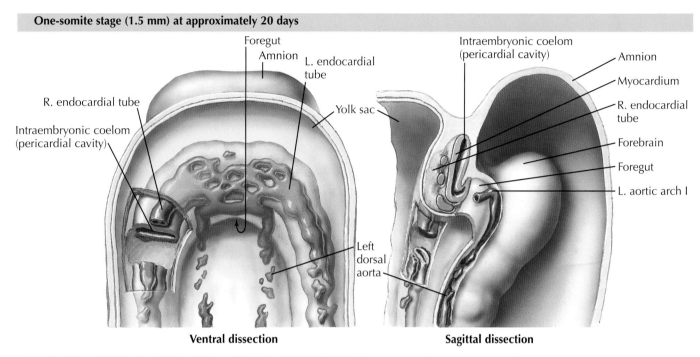

One-somite stage (1.5 mm) at approximately 20 days

Foregut
Amnion
L. endocardial tube
R. endocardial tube
Intraembryonic coelom (pericardial cavity)
Yolk sac
Left dorsal aorta

Ventral dissection

Intraembryonic coelom (pericardial cavity)
Amnion
Myocardium
R. endocardial tube
Forebrain
Foregut
L. aortic arch I

Sagittal dissection

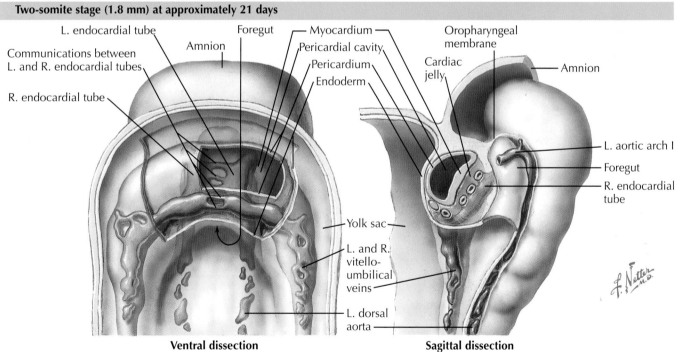

Two-somite stage (1.8 mm) at approximately 21 days

L. endocardial tube
Communications between L. and R. endocardial tubes
R. endocardial tube
Amnion
Foregut
Myocardium
Pericardial cavity
Pericardium
Endoderm
Yolk sac
L. and R. vitello-umbilical veins
L. dorsal aorta

Ventral dissection

Oropharyngeal membrane
Cardiac jelly
Amnion
L. aortic arch I
Foregut
R. endocardial tube

Sagittal dissection

4.12 FORMATION OF THE LEFT AND RIGHT HEART TUBES

Vascular spaces coalesce into left and right heart tubes that begin to communicate with each other in the midline. Cardiogenic mesoderm adjacent to the heart tubes differentiates into a jelly-like layer of connective tissue surrounded by a layer of muscle cells (myocardium). Ventral to the heart tubes, the cardiogenic mesoderm forms a cavity that is continuous with the intraembryonic coelom in the lateral plate mesoderm on both sides. By the beginning of the fourth week, peristaltic waves of contraction move blood through the embryonic tissues via aortic arch arteries surrounding the foregut, a left and right dorsal aorta, and the developing embryonic vasculature.

Four-somite stage (2.0 mm) at approximately 22 days

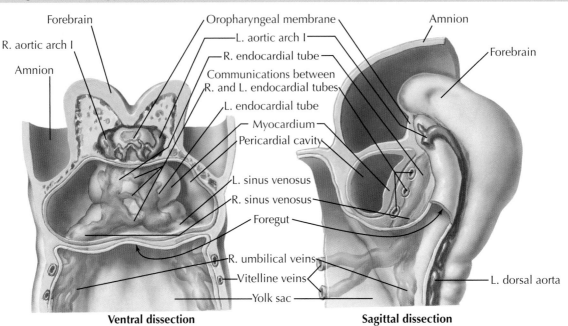

Ventral dissection   Sagittal dissection

Seven-somite stage (2.2 mm) at approximately 23 days

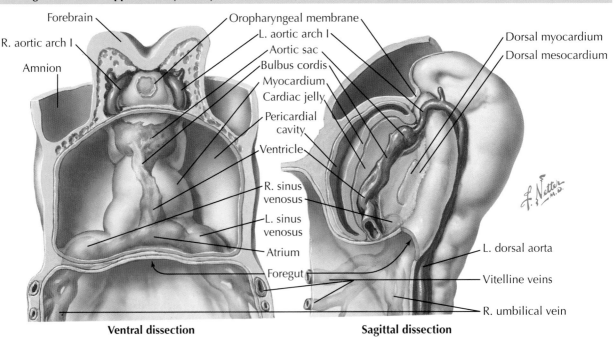

Ventral dissection   Sagittal dissection

4.13 FORMATION OF A SINGLE HEART TUBE

The left and right heart tubes fuse into a single epithelial tube surrounded by an acellular layer of **cardiac jelly** and **mantle layer** that forms the heart muscle (**myocardium**). The enlarging tube sinks into the primitive pericardial coelom (cavity) and is suspended by a mesentery, the **dorsal mesocardium**. Epithelial cells from the cardiac mesoderm on the sinus venosus migrate over the myocardium to form the epicardium (visceral pericardium).

Ten-somite stage (2.5 mm) at approximately 23 days

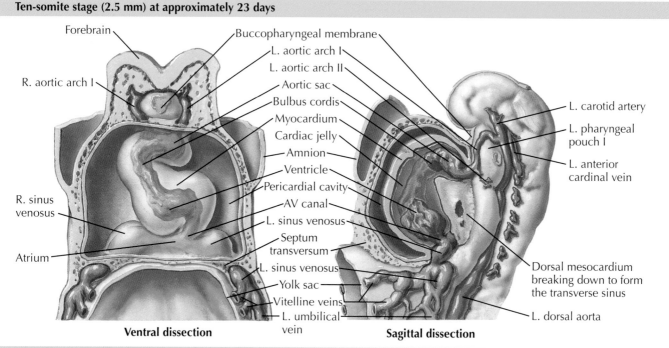

Forebrain

Buccopharyngeal membrane

L. aortic arch I

L. aortic arch II

R. aortic arch I

Aortic sac

Bulbus cordis

Myocardium

Cardiac jelly

Amnion

Ventricle

Pericardial cavity

R. sinus venosus

AV canal

L. sinus venosus

Septum transversum

Atrium

L. sinus venosus

Yolk sac

Vitelline veins

L. umbilical vein

L. carotid artery

L. pharyngeal pouch I

L. anterior cardinal vein

Dorsal mesocardium breaking down to form the transverse sinus

L. dorsal aorta

Ventral dissection

Sagittal dissection

Fourteen-somite stage (3.0 mm) at approximately 24 days

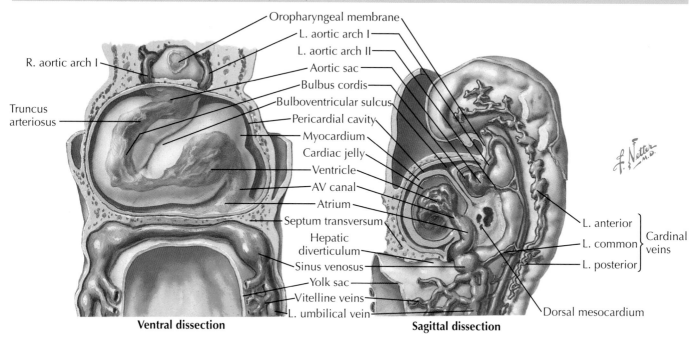

Oropharyngeal membrane

L. aortic arch I

L. aortic arch II

R. aortic arch I

Aortic sac

Bulbus cordis

Bulboventricular sulcus

Truncus arteriosus

Pericardial cavity

Myocardium

Cardiac jelly

Ventricle

AV canal

Atrium

Septum transversum

Hepatic diverticulum

Sinus venosus

Yolk sac

Vitelline veins

L. umbilical vein

L. anterior

L. common ⎫ Cardinal

L. posterior ⎭ veins

Dorsal mesocardium

Ventral dissection

Sagittal dissection

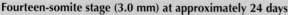

4.14 CHAMBERS OF THE HEART TUBE

Blood flows through a sequence of chambers in the single heart tube. From the venous end to the arterial end, they consist of the **sinus venosus, atrium, ventricle, bulbus cordis, truncus arteriosus**, and **aortic sac** that gives rise to the and **aortic sac** that gives rise to the aortic arch arteries. The heart tube bends between the ventricle and bulbus cordis, and the venous end of the heart moves cranially behind the arterial part of the tube. The **dorsal mesentery** breaks down to form the **transverse sinus**, the space at the top of the heart between the great arteries and veins. The single atrium and single ventricle begin to form left and right chambers.

CLINICAL POINT

Transverse sinus: The transverse sinus behind the ascending aorta and pulmonary trunk in adults gives easier access to these arteries in heart surgery (e.g., in clamping or suturing).

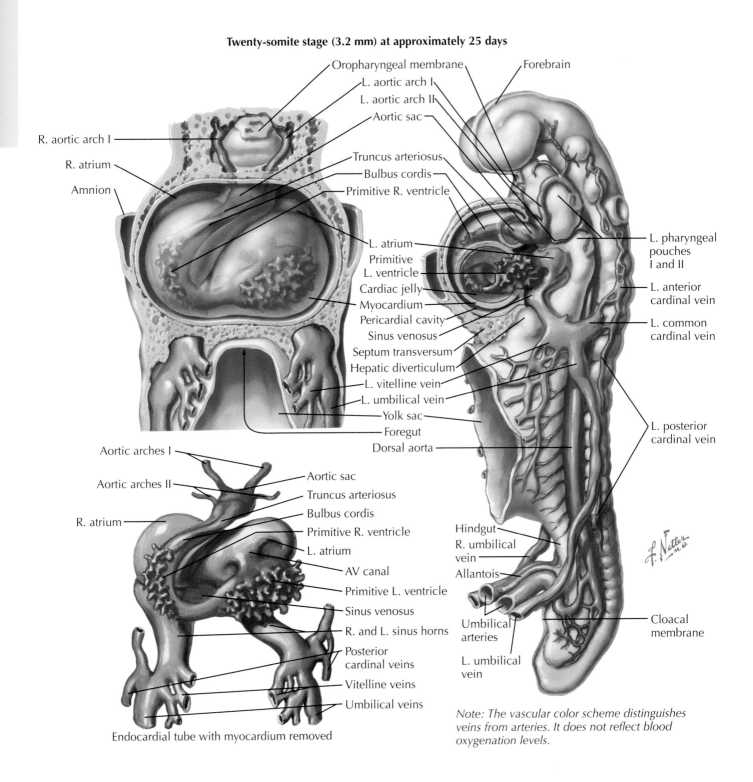

Twenty-somite stage (3.2 mm) at approximately 25 days

Oropharyngeal membrane
L. aortic arch I
L. aortic arch II
Aortic sac
Forebrain
R. aortic arch I
R. atrium
Truncus arteriosus
Bulbus cordis
Primitive R. ventricle
Amnion
L. atrium
Primitive L. ventricle
Cardiac jelly
Myocardium
Pericardial cavity
Sinus venosus
Septum transversum
Hepatic diverticulum
L. vitelline vein
L. umbilical vein
Yolk sac
Foregut
Dorsal aorta
L. pharyngeal pouches I and II
L. anterior cardinal vein
L. common cardinal vein
L. posterior cardinal vein

Aortic arches I
Aortic arches II
R. atrium
Aortic sac
Truncus arteriosus
Bulbus cordis
Primitive R. ventricle
L. atrium
AV canal
Primitive L. ventricle
Sinus venosus
R. and L. sinus horns
Posterior cardinal veins
Vitelline veins
Umbilical veins

Hindgut
R. umbilical vein
Allantois
Umbilical arteries
L. umbilical vein
Cloacal membrane

Endocardial tube with myocardium removed

Note: The vascular color scheme distinguishes veins from arteries. It does not reflect blood oxygenation levels.

4.15 OVERVIEW NEAR THE END OF THE FOURTH WEEK

Blood flow is still in a single path through the primitive heart. The venous and arterial ends of the tube assume the dorsal and superior positions they occupy in adults. Partitions begin to divide the single atrium and ventricle into left and right chambers. The three systems of veins converge on the sinus venosus leading into the heart tube: the common cardinal veins from embryonic tissues, the vitelline veins from the yolk sac, and the umbilical veins (soon to become one) from the placenta.

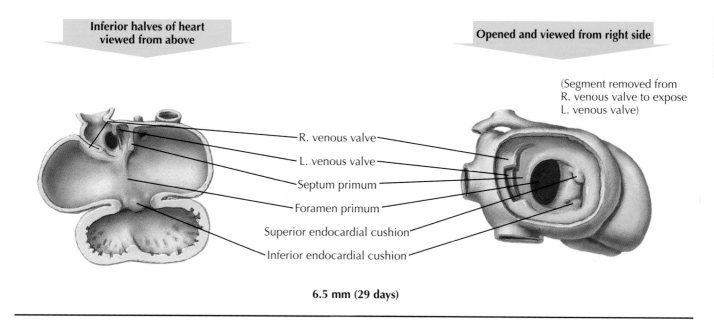

Inferior halves of heart viewed from above

Opened and viewed from right side

(Segment removed from R. venous valve to expose L. venous valve)

R. venous valve

L. venous valve

Septum primum

Foramen primum

Superior endocardial cushion

Inferior endocardial cushion

6.5 mm (29 days)

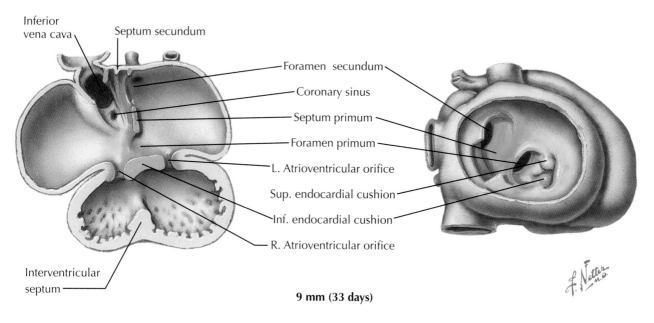

Inferior vena cava

Septum secundum

Foramen secundum

Coronary sinus

Septum primum

Foramen primum

L. Atrioventricular orifice

Sup. endocardial cushion

Inf. endocardial cushion

R. Atrioventricular orifice

Interventricular septum

9 mm (33 days)

4.16 PARTITIONING OF THE HEART TUBE

Dorsal (superior) and ventral (inferior) **endocardial cushions** divide the atrioventricular canal (and blood flow) into left and right sides. An **interventricular septum** and a primary interatrial septum (**septum primum**) grow toward the endocardial cushions.

The canal connecting the two atria is the **foramen primum**. As it diminishes in size with growth of the septum primum toward the endocardial cushions, the **foramen secundum** appears high up on the septum primum. A second interatrial septum, the **septum secundum**, develops on the right side of the septum primum.

After fusion of the endocardial cushions and the establishment of a left and right flow of blood, the heart still has one primary site of entry for blood (right atrium) and one primary site of exit (right ventricle). Blood must be able to pass between the atria and between the ventricles.

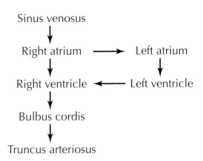

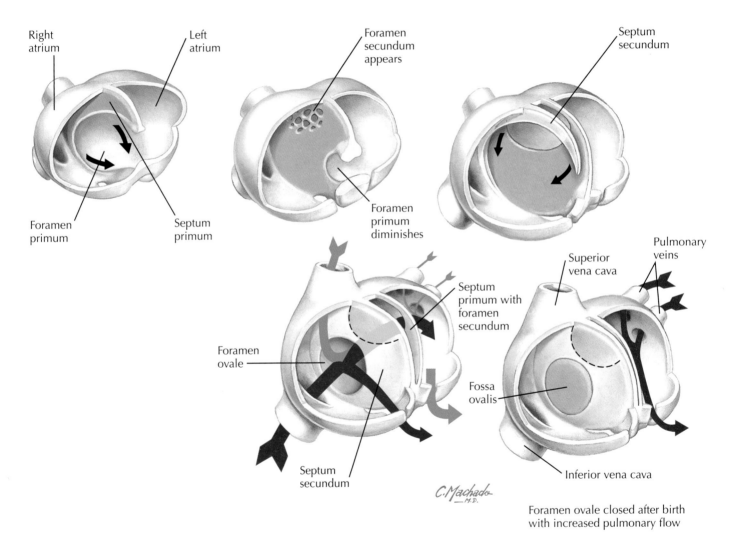

Foramen ovale closed after birth with increased pulmonary flow

4.17 ATRIAL SEPARATION

The atria are divided by two septa: a **septum primum** with a **foramen secundum**, and **septum secundum** with a **foramen ovale**. The foramen primum disappears as the septum primum grows toward and fuses to the endocardial cushions. The two foramina (secundum and ovale) are not aligned, and the two septa act as a simple valve permitting blood flow from right to left as blood from the inferior vena cava is directed toward the septum primum in the foramen ovale. When left atrial pressure rises at birth with the establishment of pulmonary blood flow, the septa are pushed together, and the interatrial lung shunt is effectively closed.

4 to 5 mm (approximately 27 days)

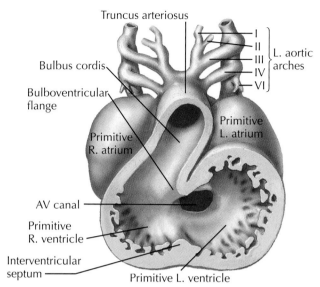

Truncus arteriosus

Bulbus cordis

Bulboventricular flange

L. aortic arches
I
II
III
IV
VI

Primitive R. atrium

Primitive L. atrium

AV canal

Primitive R. ventricle

Interventricular septum

Primitive L. ventricle

6 to 7 mm (approximately 29 days)

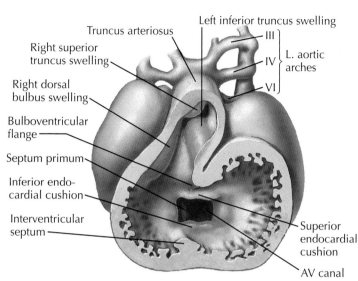

Truncus arteriosus

Right superior truncus swelling

Right dorsal bulbus swelling

Bulboventricular flange

Septum primum

Inferior endo-cardial cushion

Interventricular septum

Left inferior truncus swelling

L. aortic arches
III
IV
VI

Superior endocardial cushion

AV canal

8 to 9 mm (approximately 31 days)

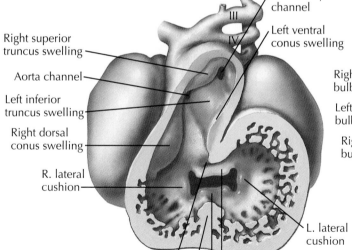

Right superior truncus swelling

Aorta channel

Left inferior truncus swelling

Right dorsal conus swelling

R. lateral cushion

Bulboventricular flange

Interventricular septum

Pulmonary channel

III

IV

Left ventral conus swelling

L. lateral cushion

Superior
Inferior
Endocardial cushions

9 to 10 mm (approximately 33 days)

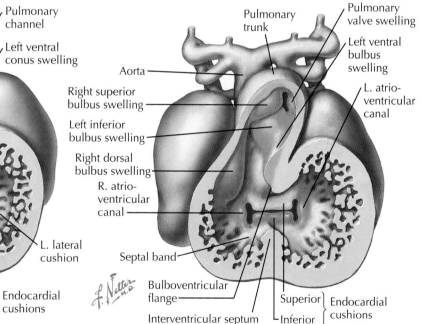

Pulmonary trunk

Aorta

Right superior bulbus swelling

Left inferior bulbus swelling

Right dorsal bulbus swelling

R. atrio-ventricular canal

Septal band

Bulboventricular flange

Interventricular septum

Pulmonary valve swelling

Left ventral bulbus swelling

L. atrio-ventricular canal

Superior
Inferior
Endocardial cushions

4.18 SPIRAL (AORTICOPULMONARY) SEPTUM

Division of the left and right ventricles is intimately related to division of the bulbus cordis and truncus arteriosus. The single ventricle begins to form left and right chambers with the appearance of the interventricular (IV) septum and the formation of the left and right atrioventricular canals by the superior and inferior (or dorsal/ventral) endocardial cushions. The division of the ventricles by the IV septum is not complete, and all blood exits the heart via the right ventricle, bulbus cordis, and truncus arteriosus. The blood takes a spiral path through these chambers, and ridges form a spiral septum between the streams. The septum is also called the aorticopulmonary septum because of the two arteries it forms from the truncus arteriosus.

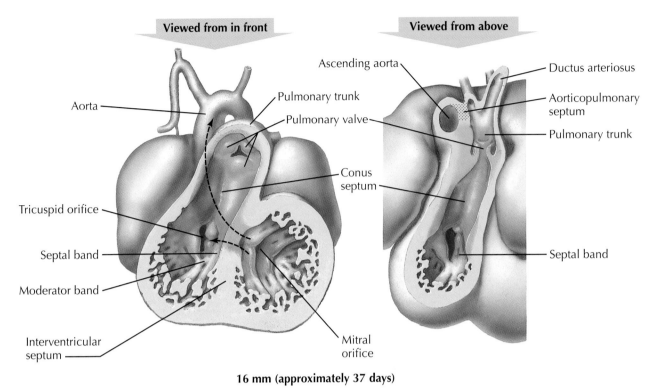

Viewed from in front

Aorta

Ascending aorta

Pulmonary trunk

Pulmonary valve

Tricuspid orifice

Septal band

Moderator band

Interventricular septum

Conus septum

Mitral orifice

16 mm (approximately 37 days)

Viewed from above

Ductus arteriosus

Aorticopulmonary septum

Pulmonary trunk

Septal band

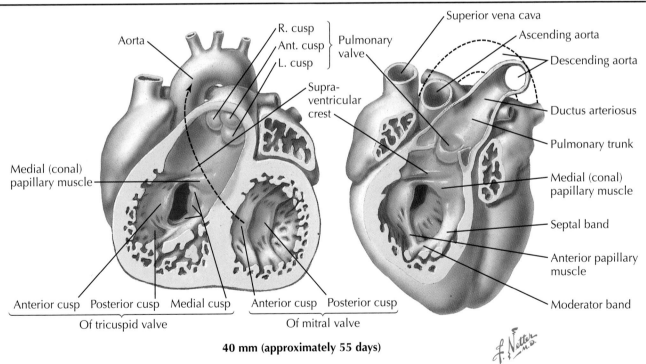

Aorta

R. cusp
Ant. cusp
L. cusp
} Pulmonary valve

Supra-ventricular crest

Medial (conal) papillary muscle

Anterior cusp Posterior cusp Medial cusp
Of tricuspid valve

Anterior cusp Posterior cusp
Of mitral valve

Superior vena cava

Ascending aorta

Descending aorta

Ductus arteriosus

Pulmonary trunk

Medial (conal) papillary muscle

Septal band

Anterior papillary muscle

Moderator band

40 mm (approximately 55 days)

f. Netter M.D.

4.19 COMPLETION OF THE SPIRAL (AORTICOPULMONARY) SEPTUM

The longitudinal swellings in the outflow portion of the heart tube grow together to complete the spiral septum that divides the bulbus cordis and truncus arteriosus. The spiral septum fuses with the IV septum and endocardial cushions inferiorly to complete the division of the left and right ventricles. The **bulbus cordis** forms the smooth upper portion of each ventricle below the semilunar valves (**aortic vestibule** in left ventricle, **conus arteriosus** in the right). The **truncus arteriosus** divides into the **ascending aorta** and **pulmonary trunk**. The latter connects to the aortic arch via the **ductus arteriosus**, the second shunt where blood bypasses the fetal lungs. Valve development is completed by 8 weeks.

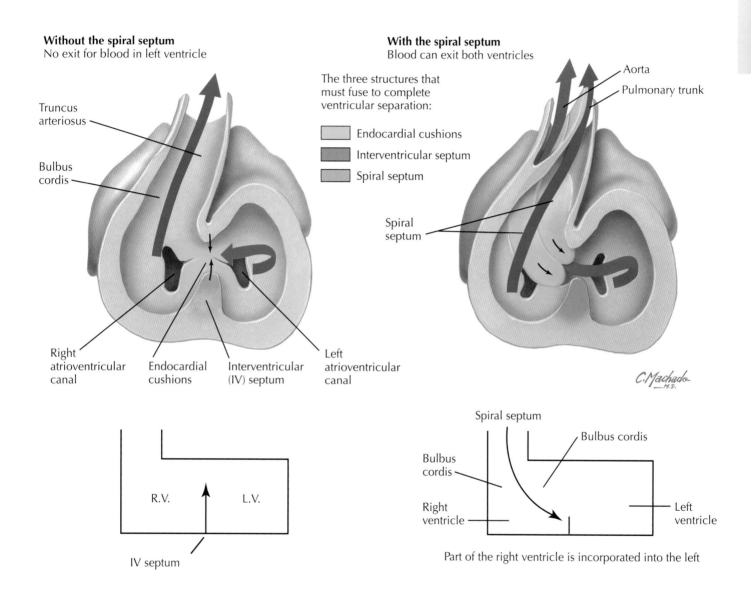

Without the spiral septum
No exit for blood in left ventricle

Truncus arteriosus

Bulbus cordis

Right atrioventricular canal

Endocardial cushions

Interventricular (IV) septum

Left atrioventricular canal

R.V.   L.V.

IV septum

With the spiral septum
Blood can exit both ventricles

The three structures that must fuse to complete ventricular separation:

Endocardial cushions

Interventricular septum

Spiral septum

Aorta

Pulmonary trunk

Spiral septum

C. Machado
—M.D.

Spiral septum

Bulbus cordis

Bulbus cordis

Right ventricle

Left ventricle

Part of the right ventricle is incorporated into the left

4.20 VENTRICULAR SEPARATION AND BULBUS CORDIS

The bulbus cordis and truncus arteriosus are continuations of the right ventricle. If the IV septum grew to the endocardial cushions to separate the ventricles, there would be no exit of blood from the left ventricle. Three primordia must fuse with each other to complete ventricular separation: the spiral septum, the IV septum, and the endocardial cushions. These structures form the upper membranous part of the IV septum, the most common site of ventricular septal defects. The primary IV septum forms the lower muscular part. Because the spiral septum extends obliquely to the IV septum, part of the right ventricle gets incorporated into the left ventricle, and the bulbus cordis contributes to both chambers.

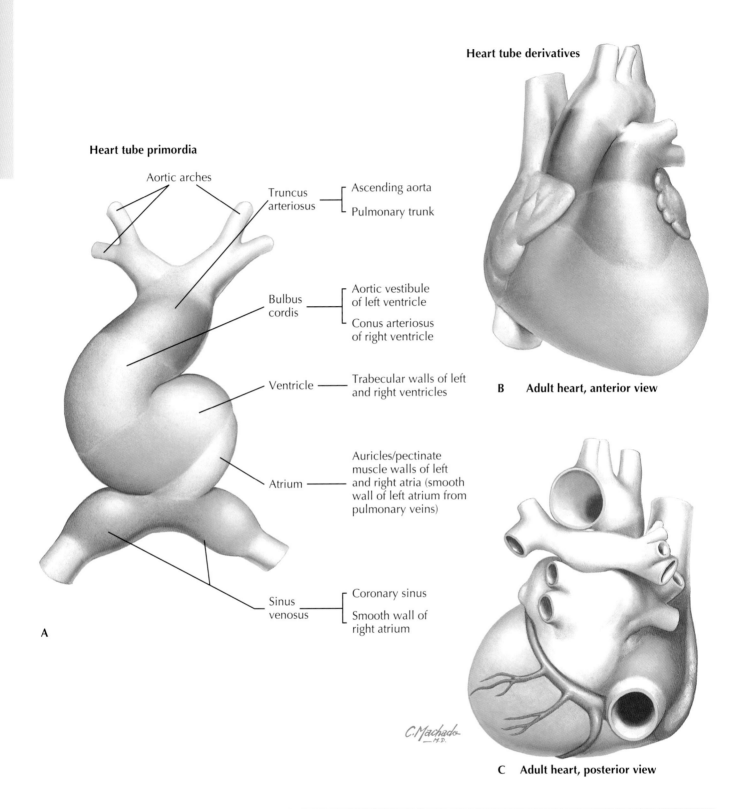

Heart tube primordia

Aortic arches

Truncus arteriosus
- Ascending aorta
- Pulmonary trunk

Bulbus cordis
- Aortic vestibule of left ventricle
- Conus arteriosus of right ventricle

Ventricle — Trabecular walls of left and right ventricles

Atrium — Auricles/pectinate muscle walls of left and right atria (smooth wall of left atrium from pulmonary veins)

Sinus venosus
- Coronary sinus
- Smooth wall of right atrium

A

Heart tube derivatives

B   Adult heart, anterior view

C   Adult heart, posterior view

4.21 ADULT DERIVATIVES OF THE HEART TUBE CHAMBERS

The primitive heart tube (Fig. 4.21A) is color-coded according to the derivatives in the adult heart (Figs. 4.21B and C). The chambers of the heart are mostly lined with ridges of cardiac muscle, but the walls are smooth in both the inflow parts of the atria and outflow parts of the ventricles. The **primitive atrium** and **primitive ventricle** in the embryo give rise to the walls of the heart with ridged muscle, the **pectinate muscle** in the auricles of the atria, and the **trabeculae carneae** in the ventricles. The smooth posterior wall of the right atrium comes from the right horn of the sinus venosus. The smooth outflow portion of both ventricles derives from the bulbous cordis. The smooth wall of the left atrium forms from a merging of the proximal portions of the pulmonary veins.

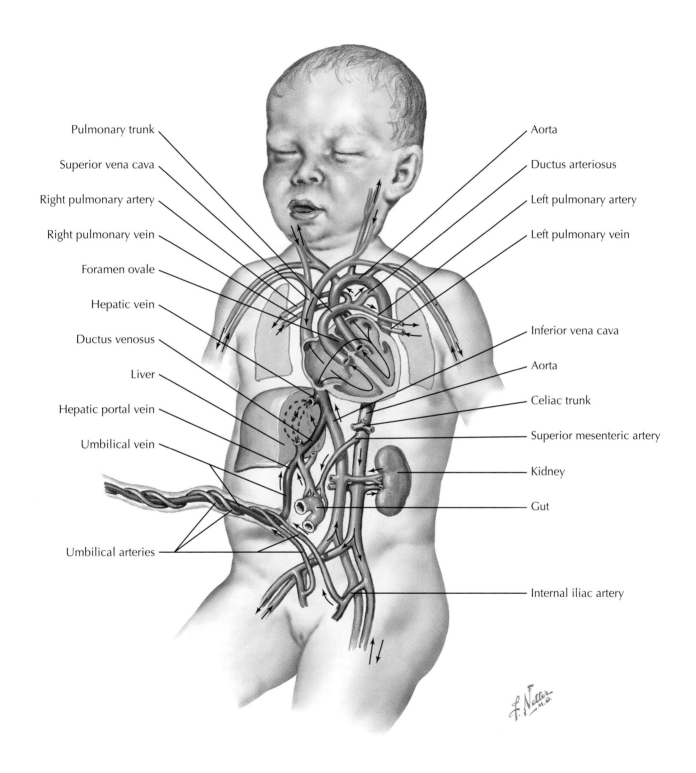

Pulmonary trunk

Superior vena cava

Right pulmonary artery

Right pulmonary vein

Foramen ovale

Hepatic vein

Ductus venosus

Liver

Hepatic portal vein

Umbilical vein

Umbilical arteries

Aorta

Ductus arteriosus

Left pulmonary artery

Left pulmonary vein

Inferior vena cava

Aorta

Celiac trunk

Superior mesenteric artery

Kidney

Gut

Internal iliac artery

4.22 FETAL CIRCULATION

In prenatal circulation, oxygenated blood in the umbilical vein bypasses the liver via the **ductus venosus** and the lungs via two routes. Most blood from the inferior vena cava is directed toward the **foramen ovale** in the interatrial septum to flow to the left systemic side of the heart. Most blood from the superior vena cava flows into the right ventricle and pulmonary trunk, where it is diverted from the pulmonary arteries into the lower-pressure aorta through the **ductus arteriosus**.

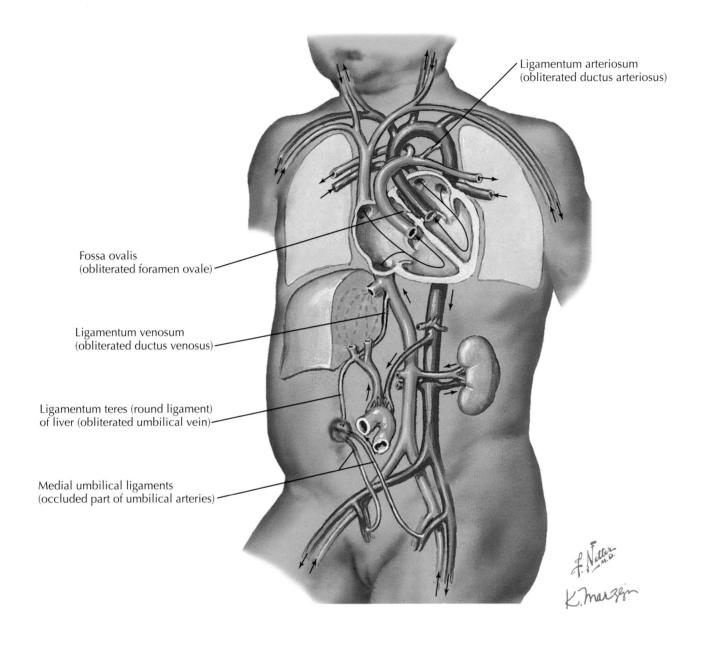

Ligamentum arteriosum
(obliterated ductus arteriosus)

Fossa ovalis
(obliterated foramen ovale)

Ligamentum venosum
(obliterated ductus venosus)

Ligamentum teres (round ligament)
of liver (obliterated umbilical vein)

Medial umbilical ligaments
(occluded part of umbilical arteries)

4.23 TRANSITION TO POSTNATAL CIRCULATION

Transition from fetal to postnatal circulation:

1. The first breath clears the airway of amniotic fluid, greatly reducing the pressure within the pulmonary vascular beds.
2. Lower pulmonary pressure causes blood to enter the lungs instead of passing through the ductus arteriosus to the aortic arch.
3. Blood rushes from the lungs into the left atrium, where the septum primum is pressed against the septum secundum to effectively close the foramen ovale.
4. Higher oxygen levels in the umbilical arteries cause them to spasm.

5. The uterus contracts, forcing most of the placental blood into the fetus. The umbilical vein collapses from lack of blood.

CLINICAL POINT

Umbilical Line. In newborns and especially premature infants in neonatal intensive care units, the umbilical vein and/or an umbilical artery can be used for catheter access (an **umbilical line**) to the internal circulation for a variety of functions, including transfusions or fluid infusion, drug administration, blood gas monitoring, and drawing blood samples. An umbilical catheter can also be used to access the heart for repair of congenital heart defects.

Clinical characteristics of too little pulmonary flow

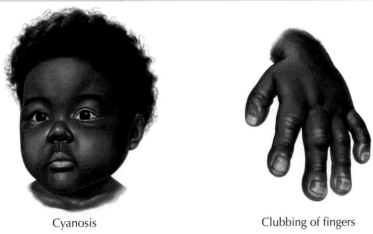

Cyanosis   Clubbing of fingers

Clinical characteristics of too much pulmonary flow (pulmonary volume overload)

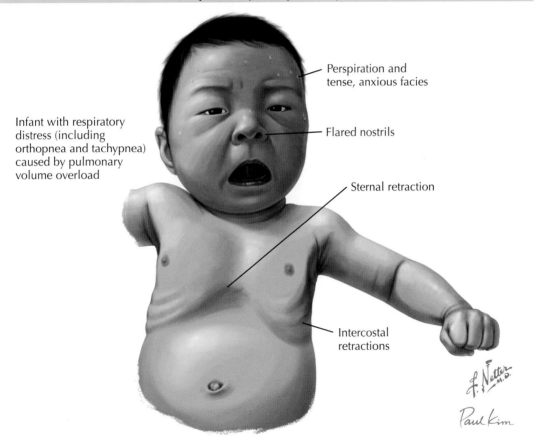

Perspiration and tense, anxious facies

Flared nostrils

Infant with respiratory distress (including orthopnea and tachypnea) caused by pulmonary volume overload

Sternal retraction

Intercostal retractions

4.24 CONGENITAL HEART DEFECT CONCEPTS

Congenital heart defects result in problems if the lungs get too much or too little blood. Too little blood in the lungs may be caused by pulmonary stenosis or right ventricular outflow obstruction, in which case not enough blood is oxygenated to meet the metabolic demands of the body. Clinical presentation includes cyanosis and clubbing of the fingers. It is important to note that for individuals with dark skin, cyanosis may be easier to see in the mucous membranes of the lips, mouth or eyes, or fingernails. It can also present as more of a peripheral gray-green in dark skin tones, rather than the frequently described blue/purple of light skin tones. Too much blood to the lungs results in excessive pulmonary return to the heart, which may overload the left atrium, left ventricle, and mitral valve. Blood backs up in the lungs, and fluid accumulates. This type of congestive heart failure is usually caused by abnormal communication between the two ventricles or between the ascending aorta and pulmonary trunk. See next few sections for more details on the embryonic basis of congestive heart failure.

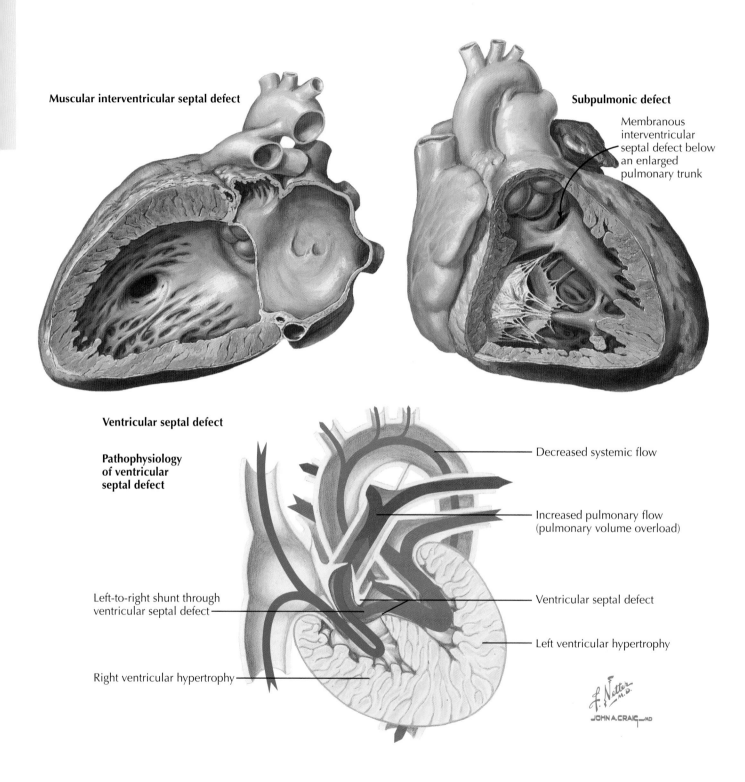

Muscular interventricular septal defect

Subpulmonic defect

Membranous
interventricular
septal defect below
an enlarged
pulmonary trunk

Ventricular septal defect

**Pathophysiology
of ventricular
septal defect**

Decreased systemic flow

Increased pulmonary flow
(pulmonary volume overload)

Left-to-right shunt through
ventricular septal defect

Ventricular septal defect

Left ventricular hypertrophy

Right ventricular hypertrophy

4.25 VENTRICULAR SEPTAL DEFECTS

Ventricular septal defects (VSDs) are detected in about 1 in 1000 infants and are the most common congenital heart defects (about 25%). Holes can develop anywhere in the muscular IV septum, but the most common VSDs occur in the upper membranous part of the septum. The embryonic basis is the failure of the spiral septum to properly fuse with the IV septum and endocardial cushions. Blood is diverted from the left ventricle to the right through the VSD as the systemic blood pressure increases relative to the pulmonary with growth of the infant and maturation of the airway. The lungs and left side of the heart get too much blood, and congestive heart failure and pulmonary edema can result.

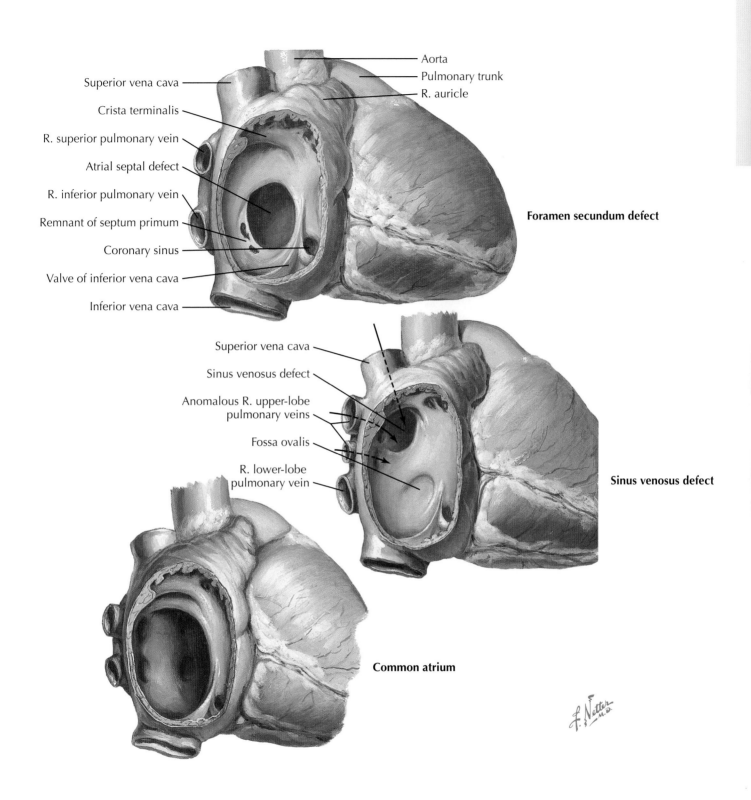

Aorta
Pulmonary trunk
R. auricle

Superior vena cava
Crista terminalis
R. superior pulmonary vein
Atrial septal defect
R. inferior pulmonary vein
Remnant of septum primum
Coronary sinus
Valve of inferior vena cava
Inferior vena cava

Foramen secundum defect

Superior vena cava
Sinus venosus defect
Anomalous R. upper-lobe pulmonary veins
Fossa ovalis
R. lower-lobe pulmonary vein

Sinus venosus defect

Common atrium

4.26 ATRIAL SEPTAL DEFECTS

Atrial septal defects (ASDs) usually occur when the **foramen ovale** or **foramen secundum** is too large, resulting in overlap with each other. A very small opening of this type is a "probe patent" foramen ovale found in 25% of the population, which is typically asymptomatic. Other ASDs result when the septum primum fails to fuse with the endocardial cushions, when the sinus venosus is not properly incorporated into the right atrium, or when perforations develop anywhere in the interatrial septum. With the low blood pressure in the atria, most ASDs are not clinically significant unless other heart defects cause a shunting of blood between the atria.

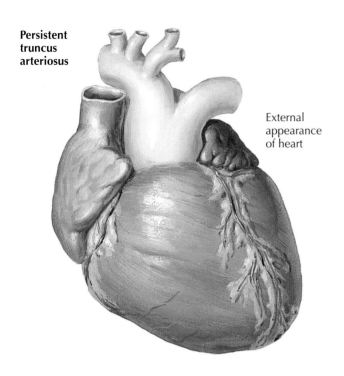

Persistent truncus arteriosus

External appearance of heart

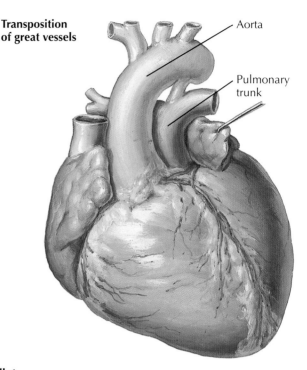

Transposition of great vessels

Aorta

Pulmonary trunk

Tetralogy of Fallot

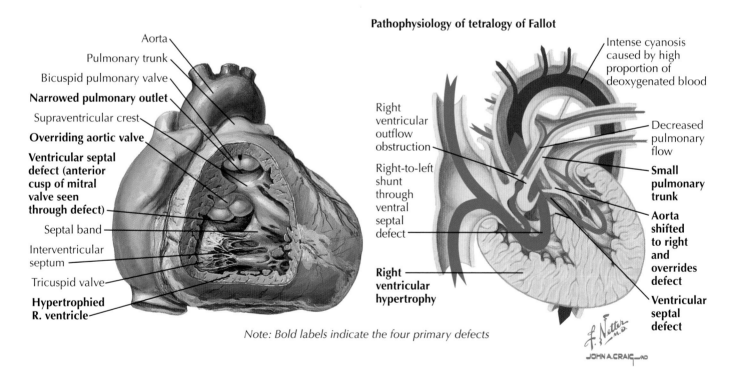

Aorta

Pulmonary trunk

Bicuspid pulmonary valve

Narrowed pulmonary outlet

Supraventricular crest

Overriding aortic valve

Ventricular septal defect (anterior cusp of mitral valve seen through defect)

Septal band

Interventricular septum

Tricuspid valve

Hypertrophied R. ventricle

Note: Bold labels indicate the four primary defects

Pathophysiology of tetralogy of Fallot

Intense cyanosis caused by high proportion of deoxygenated blood

Right ventricular outflow obstruction

Right-to-left shunt through ventral septal defect

Right ventricular hypertrophy

Decreased pulmonary flow

Small pulmonary trunk

Aorta shifted to right and overrides defect

Ventricular septal defect

4.27 SPIRAL SEPTUM DEFECTS

The spiral septum may not develop (**persistent truncus arteriosus**), may not take a spiral course (**transposition of the great vessels**), or may divide the truncus arteriosus unequally, leading to the four primary defects in **tetralogy of Fallot**, shown in Fig. 4.27. Any communication between the ascending aorta and pulmonary trunk has a physiological result similar to VSD—blood is diverted from the systemic to the lower-pressure pulmonary circulation. Transposition results in death at birth unless there is mixing of blood between the two systems (e.g., through a VSD). A patent ductus arteriosus is often present in tetralogy of Fallot. If it is large, it is a significant route for blood to get to the lungs from the systemic circulation in the aortic arch.

Patent ductus arteriosus

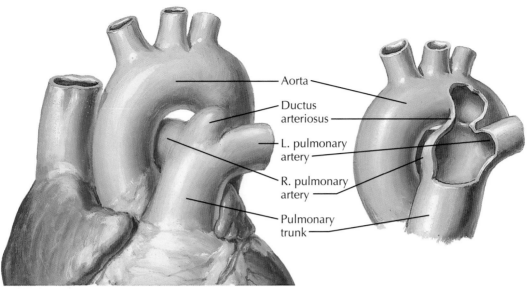

- Aorta
- Ductus arteriosus
- L. pulmonary artery
- R. pulmonary artery
- Pulmonary trunk

Pathophysiology of patent ductus arteriosus

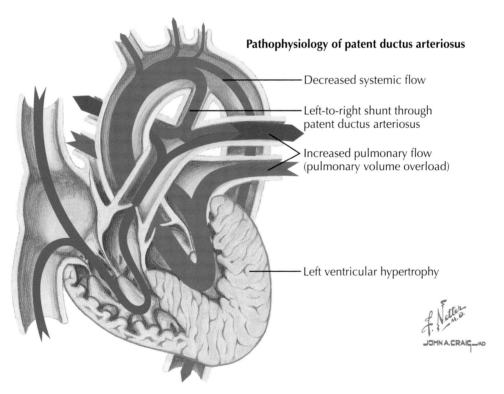

- Decreased systemic flow
- Left-to-right shunt through patent ductus arteriosus
- Increased pulmonary flow (pulmonary volume overload)
- Left ventricular hypertrophy

4.28 PATENT DUCTUS ARTERIOSUS

Large, patent ductus arteriosus results in pulmonary overload if it persists. Any communication between the left and right outflow tracts is subject to the pressure differential that develops as the pulmonary blood pressure becomes lower than the systemic pressure.

CLINICAL POINT

Neonatal cyanosis with patent ductus arteriosus. A normal-sized ductus arteriosus remains patent for 2 weeks after birth. Although pulmonary vascular resistance begins to fall during this time, it is possible for blood to be diverted from the pulmonary trunk into the aorta if intrapleural pressure rises. This accounts for cyanosis in infants with prolonged crying spells.

Terminology

Angiogenesis	Blood vessel development.
Aortic arch arteries	Arteries within the pharyngeal (branchial) arches flanking the foregut that connect the aortic sac with the paired dorsal aortae and give rise to most of the arteries of the neck.
Aortic sac	Arterial chamber at the distal end of the outflow tract of the primitive heart tube ventral to the foregut. It directs blood from the truncus arteriosus into the aortic arch arteries.
Bulbus cordis	A chamber in the primitive heart tube that develops into the upper, smooth, outflow portion of each ventricle.
Cardinal veins	Cardinal, subcardinal, and supracardinal veins are embryonic systems of veins that develop in temporal sequence and form most of the major somatic, renal, and gonadal veins.
Cardiac jelly	A gelatinous connective tissue layer between the endothelial heart tube and the myocardial mantle layer. Its significance is unknown.
Cardiogenic mesoderm	Mesoderm from the primitive streak that migrates around the oropharyngeal (oral) membrane to a midline position at the cranial end of the embryo. It is continuous with the lateral plate mesoderm on either side. All structures of the heart and pericardial sac develop from cardiogenic mesoderm.
Coarctation	An abnormal constriction.
Cyanosis	(G., "blue") Bluish coloration of the body tissues due to lower oxygen levels in the blood. It is seen best in thin skin and mucous membranes.
Ductus arteriosus	A lung shunt connecting the pulmonary trunk to the arch of the aorta. After birth it remains patent for a few weeks before forming the fibrous ligamentum arteriosum.
Ductus venosus	Liver bypass shunting blood from the umbilical vein into the inferior vena cava. It becomes the ligamentum venosum.
Endocardial cushions	Dorsal and ventral (or superior/inferior) partitions of the heart tube that fuse to first separate blood flow into left and right sides.
Epicardium	Visceral pericardium on the surface of the heart. Cells from the cardiogenic mesoderm on the sinus venosus migrate over the myocardial mantle layer to form the epicardium.
Foramen ovale	A lung shunt where blood passes from the right atrium to the left atrium. In common usage it refers to the entire atrial bypass that includes the foramen secundum.
Sinus venosus	The first part of the venous end of the heat tube receiving blood from the umbilical vein, common cardinal veins, and vitelline veins.
Stenosis	(G., "narrowing") The narrowing of a vessel, duct, or canal.
Tetralogy of Fallot	"Four" secondary heart defects resulting from a primary spiral septum defect that divides the truncus arteriosus unequally: (1) pulmonary stenosis, (2) ventricular septal defect, (3) aorta overriding and draining both ventricles, and (4) right ventricular hypertrophy.
Transverse sinus	The space between the great arteries and the superior vena cava occupied by the dorsal mesentery of the heart. The heart tube sinks into the pericardial coelom and becomes suspended by a mesentery, the dorsal mesocardium. As the arterial and venous ends of the heart tube approach each other, the mesocardium breaks down to form the transverse sinus.
Vitelline vessels	Circulation to the yolk sac, which is the first source of blood cell production. The proximal, intraembryonic portions persist as the major midgut and hindgut arteries, liver veins, and hepatic portal system.

5

THE RESPIRATORY SYSTEM

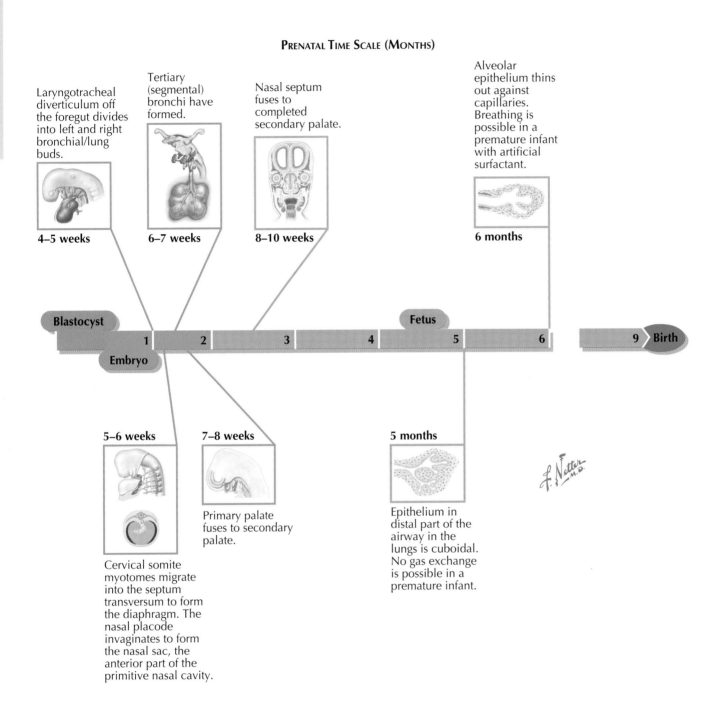

PRENATAL TIME SCALE (MONTHS)

Laryngotracheal diverticulum off the foregut divides into left and right bronchial/lung buds.

4–5 weeks

Tertiary (segmental) bronchi have formed.

6–7 weeks

Nasal septum fuses to completed secondary palate.

8–10 weeks

Alveolar epithelium thins out against capillaries. Breathing is possible in a premature infant with artificial surfactant.

6 months

Blastocyst

Embryo

Fetus

1   2   3   4   5   6   9 Birth

5–6 weeks

7–8 weeks

Primary palate fuses to secondary palate.

Cervical somite myotomes migrate into the septum transversum to form the diaphragm. The nasal placode invaginates to form the nasal sac, the anterior part of the primitive nasal cavity.

5 months

Epithelium in distal part of the airway in the lungs is cuboidal. No gas exchange is possible in a premature infant.

5.1 TIMELINE

PRIMORDIA FOR THE UPPER AIRWAY
Nasal sac (from nasal placode), stomodeum, and foregut.

PRIMORDIA FOR THE LOWER AIRWAY
Laryngotracheal diverticulum (lung bud) of foregut splanchnopleure.

PLAN
The main developmental event in the upper airway is the division of the stomodeum by the palate into separate respiratory (nasal) and gastrointestinal (oral) components so that respiration can occur during mastication. The development of the lower airway is characterized by the creation of the pleural cavity and the extensive branching of the airway within it. The continuous intraembryonic coelom is partitioned into separate pleural, pericardial, and peritoneal components, each lined by mesothelium. A bud from the laryngotracheal diverticulum pushes into each pleural sac and continues to branch for more than 22 generations to produce a surface area of 85 m² for gas exchange between alveoli and the bloodstream.

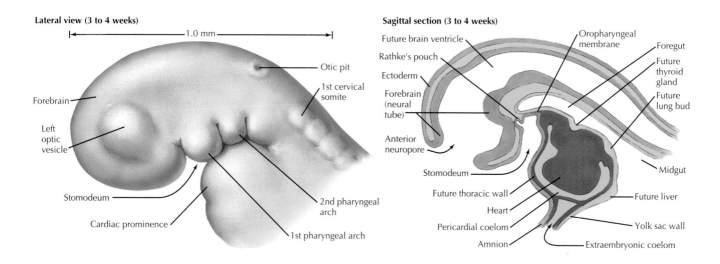

Lateral view (3 to 4 weeks)

1.0 mm

Otic pit

1st cervical somite

Forebrain

Left optic vesicle

Stomodeum

Cardiac prominence

2nd pharyngeal arch

1st pharyngeal arch

Sagittal section (3 to 4 weeks)

Future brain ventricle

Rathke's pouch

Ectoderm

Forebrain (neural tube)

Anterior neuropore

Stomodeum

Future thoracic wall

Heart

Pericardial coelom

Amnion

Oropharyngeal membrane

Foregut

Future thyroid gland

Future lung bud

Midgut

Future liver

Yolk sac wall

Extraembryonic coelom

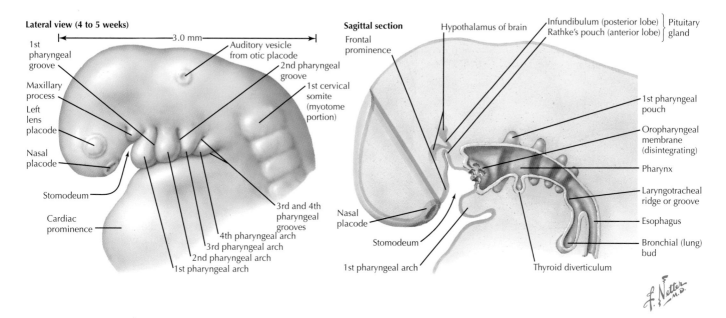

Lateral view (4 to 5 weeks)

3.0 mm

1st pharyngeal groove

Maxillary process

Left lens placode

Nasal placode

Stomodeum

Cardiac prominence

Auditory vesicle from otic placode

2nd pharyngeal groove

1st cervical somite (myotome portion)

3rd and 4th pharyngeal grooves

4th pharyngeal arch

3rd pharyngeal arch

2nd pharyngeal arch

1st pharyngeal arch

Sagittal section

Frontal prominence

Hypothalamus of brain

Infundibulum (posterior lobe) ⎫ Pituitary
Rathke's pouch (anterior lobe) ⎬ gland

Nasal placode

Stomodeum

1st pharyngeal arch

Thyroid diverticulum

1st pharyngeal pouch

Oropharyngeal membrane (disintegrating)

Pharynx

Laryngotracheal ridge or groove

Esophagus

Bronchial (lung) bud

f. Netter m.d.

5.2 EARLY PRIMORDIA
The early primordia of the upper (left) and lower (right) airways:

Stomodeum	Laryngotracheal diverticulum (lung bud)
Nasal placode	Septum transversum
Foregut	Intraembryonic coelom

A. Cross section of embryo

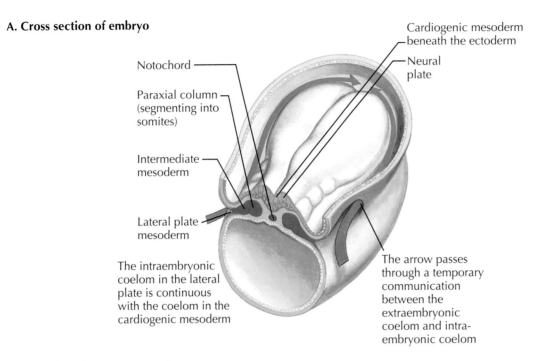

Notochord

Paraxial column (segmenting into somites)

Intermediate mesoderm

Lateral plate mesoderm

Cardiogenic mesoderm beneath the ectoderm

Neural plate

The intraembryonic coelom in the lateral plate is continuous with the coelom in the cardiogenic mesoderm

The arrow passes through a temporary communication between the extraembryonic coelom and intra-embryonic coelom

B. Sagittal section at 5 to 6 weeks

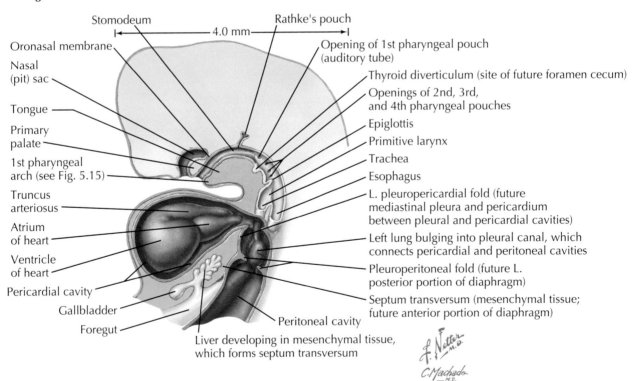

Stomodeum

4.0 mm

Rathke's pouch

Oronasal membrane

Nasal (pit) sac

Tongue

Primary palate

1st pharyngeal arch (see Fig. 5.15)

Truncus arteriosus

Atrium of heart

Ventricle of heart

Pericardial cavity

Gallbladder

Foregut

Opening of 1st pharyngeal pouch (auditory tube)

Thyroid diverticulum (site of future foramen cecum)

Openings of 2nd, 3rd, and 4th pharyngeal pouches

Epiglottis

Primitive larynx

Trachea

Esophagus

L. pleuropericardial fold (future mediastinal pleura and pericardium between pleural and pericardial cavities)

Left lung bulging into pleural canal, which connects pericardial and peritoneal cavities

Pleuroperitoneal fold (future L. posterior portion of diaphragm)

Septum transversum (mesenchymal tissue; future anterior portion of diaphragm)

Peritoneal cavity

Liver developing in mesenchymal tissue, which forms septum transversum

5.3 FORMATION OF THE PLEURAL CAVITIES

The **intraembryonic coelom** begins as cavities form in the lateral plate mesoderm on each side and in the midline cardiogenic mesoderm (see Fig. 5.3A). Shown in Fig. 5.3B is the interior of the coelom on the left extending from the abdominal region through the left pleural canal into the pericardial cavity. From there it continues under the heart and back down the other side of the midline gastrointestinal tract and its supporting dorsal and ventral mesenteries. The U-shaped coelomic tube is partitioned into separate peritoneal, pleural, and pericardial cavities by **pleuroperitoneal membranes** and pleuropericardial folds, where the common cardinal veins (not shown) pinch the coelom to separate the pleural cavity from the pericardial cavity.

Sagittal section at 6 to 7 weeks

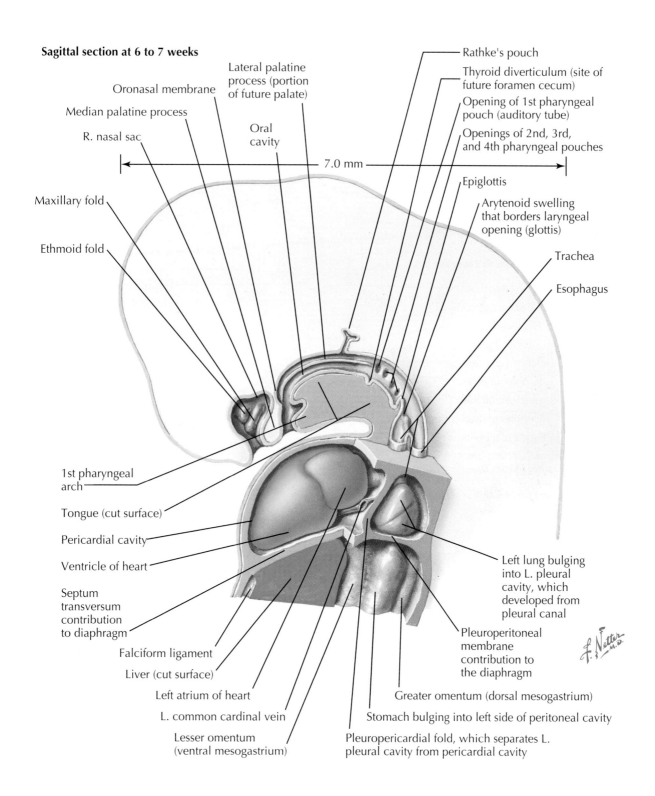

Rathke's pouch

Thyroid diverticulum (site of future foramen cecum)

Opening of 1st pharyngeal pouch (auditory tube)

Openings of 2nd, 3rd, and 4th pharyngeal pouches

Epiglottis

Arytenoid swelling that borders laryngeal opening (glottis)

Trachea

Esophagus

Lateral palatine process (portion of future palate)

Oronasal membrane

Median palatine process

R. nasal sac

Oral cavity

7.0 mm

Maxillary fold

Ethmoid fold

1st pharyngeal arch

Tongue (cut surface)

Pericardial cavity

Ventricle of heart

Septum transversum contribution to diaphragm

Falciform ligament

Liver (cut surface)

Left atrium of heart

L. common cardinal vein

Lesser omentum (ventral mesogastrium)

Left lung bulging into L. pleural cavity, which developed from pleural canal

Pleuroperitoneal membrane contribution to the diaphragm

Greater omentum (dorsal mesogastrium)

Stomach bulging into left side of peritoneal cavity

Pleuropericardial fold, which separates L. pleural cavity from pericardial cavity

5.4 THE RELATIONSHIP BETWEEN LUNGS AND PLEURAL CAVITIES

The **septum transversum** and **pleuroperitoneal membranes** of the developing diaphragm separate the peritoneal cavity from the pleural and pericardial cavities in the thorax. The pleural and pericardial cavities are also separate from each other. The mesenchyme lining the three cavities differentiates into the simple squamous epithelium (**mesothelium**) of pleura, peritoneum, and pericardium. The lungs grow into the pleural sac of mesothelium much like a fist pushing into a balloon. The mesothelium on the surface of the lung is **visceral pleura**. **Parietal pleura** lines the thoracic wall, diaphragm, and mediastinum.

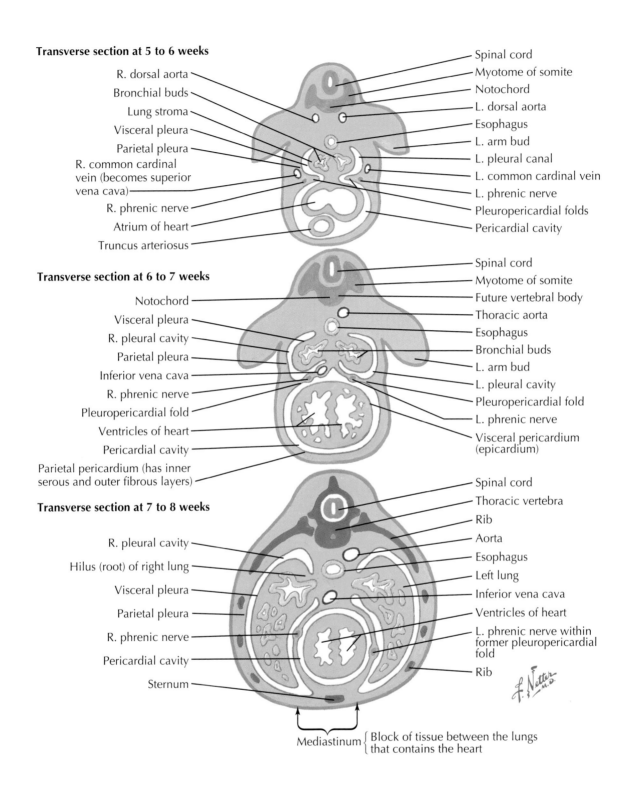

Transverse section at 5 to 6 weeks

- R. dorsal aorta
- Bronchial buds
- Lung stroma
- Visceral pleura
- Parietal pleura
- R. common cardinal vein (becomes superior vena cava)
- R. phrenic nerve
- Atrium of heart
- Truncus arteriosus

- Spinal cord
- Myotome of somite
- Notochord
- L. dorsal aorta
- Esophagus
- L. arm bud
- L. pleural canal
- L. common cardinal vein
- L. phrenic nerve
- Pleuropericardial folds
- Pericardial cavity

Transverse section at 6 to 7 weeks

- Notochord
- Visceral pleura
- R. pleural cavity
- Parietal pleura
- Inferior vena cava
- R. phrenic nerve
- Pleuropericardial fold
- Ventricles of heart
- Pericardial cavity
- Parietal pericardium (has inner serous and outer fibrous layers)

- Spinal cord
- Myotome of somite
- Future vertebral body
- Thoracic aorta
- Esophagus
- Bronchial buds
- L. arm bud
- L. pleural cavity
- Pleuropericardial fold
- L. phrenic nerve
- Visceral pericardium (epicardium)

Transverse section at 7 to 8 weeks

- R. pleural cavity
- Hilus (root) of right lung
- Visceral pleura
- Parietal pleura
- R. phrenic nerve
- Pericardial cavity
- Sternum

- Spinal cord
- Thoracic vertebra
- Rib
- Aorta
- Esophagus
- Left lung
- Inferior vena cava
- Ventricles of heart
- L. phrenic nerve within former pleuropericardial fold
- Rib

Mediastinum { Block of tissue between the lungs that contains the heart

5.5 VISCERAL AND PARIETAL PLEURA

The division of pleural and pericardial cavities is complete by 7 weeks. Visceral and parietal pleura are continuous with each other at the root of the lung. As the lungs enlarge, the pleural cavity becomes a potential space with a little serous fluid to reduce friction as visceral and parietal pleura slide against each other during respiration.

CLINICAL POINT

Pneumothorax. Visceral and parietal pleura are attached to each other only by surface tension involving a thin film of serous fluid. If the seal is broken from a puncture wound through the thoracic wall or rupture of a bleb of air near the surface of the lung, air will accumulate in the pleural cavity with the negative pressure of inhalation, and the lung may collapse. If not treated, it is a medical emergency because of pressure ultimately compressing the heart and great vessels.

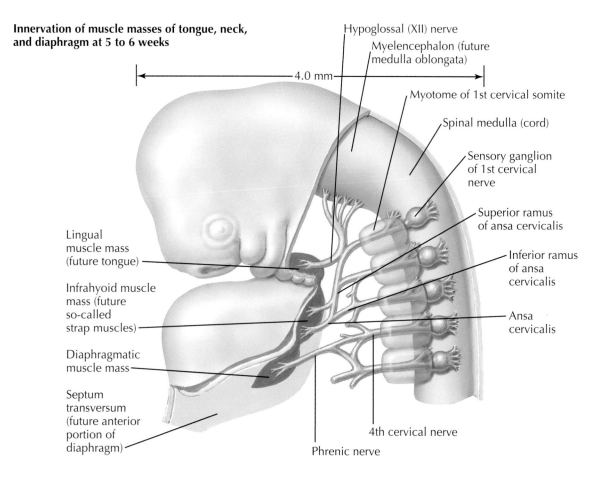

Innervation of muscle masses of tongue, neck, and diaphragm at 5 to 6 weeks

Hypoglossal (XII) nerve

Myelencephalon (future medulla oblongata)

4.0 mm

Myotome of 1st cervical somite

Spinal medulla (cord)

Sensory ganglion of 1st cervical nerve

Superior ramus of ansa cervicalis

Inferior ramus of ansa cervicalis

Ansa cervicalis

Lingual muscle mass (future tongue)

Infrahyoid muscle mass (future so-called strap muscles)

Diaphragmatic muscle mass

Septum transversum (future anterior portion of diaphragm)

4th cervical nerve

Phrenic nerve

Embryological origins of diaphragm

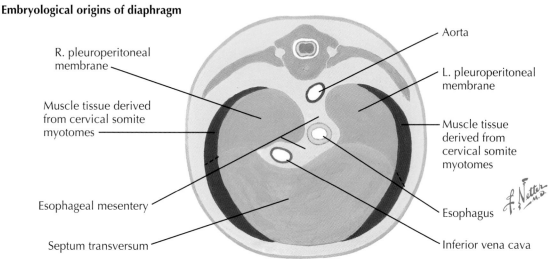

R. pleuroperitoneal membrane

Aorta

L. pleuroperitoneal membrane

Muscle tissue derived from cervical somite myotomes

Muscle tissue derived from cervical somite myotomes

Esophageal mesentery

Esophagus

Septum transversum

Inferior vena cava

5.6 DEVELOPMENT OF THE DIAPHRAGM

The diaphragm develops from four primordia:

- **Septum transversum**, a mesenchyme partition between the embryonic thorax and abdomen
- **Pleuroperitoneal membranes**
- **Mesentery of the esophagus**
- **Cervical somite myotomes** (for muscle cells of the diaphragm)

The septum transversum develops adjacent to the cervical region; it then "descends" relative to the growth of the embryonic trunk. It carries with it the **phrenic nerve** consisting of the ventral rami of spinal nerve segments C3, C4, and C5.

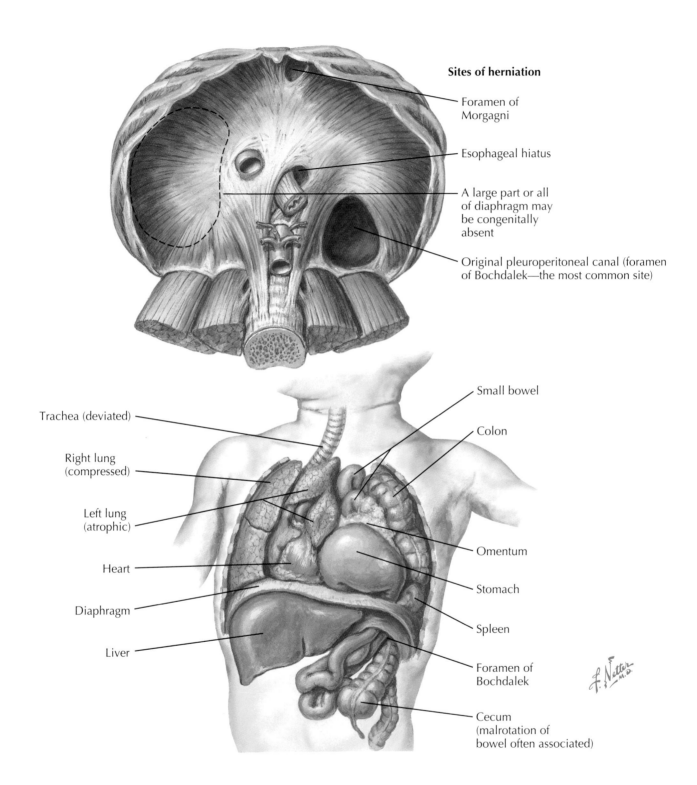

Sites of herniation

Foramen of Morgagni

Esophageal hiatus

A large part or all of diaphragm may be congenitally absent

Original pleuroperitoneal canal (foramen of Bochdalek—the most common site)

Trachea (deviated)

Right lung (compressed)

Left lung (atrophic)

Heart

Diaphragm

Liver

Small bowel

Colon

Omentum

Stomach

Spleen

Foramen of Bochdalek

Cecum (malrotation of bowel often associated)

5.7 CONGENITAL DIAPHRAGMATIC HERNIA

This is the most common diaphragmatic hernia. It results from a failure of the pleuroperitoneal membranes to grow across the intraembryonic coelom. Abdominal organs may extend into the thoracic cavity, resulting in an abnormally distended thorax and flat stomach region. Other diaphragmatic hernias are septum transversum defects or result from natural openings that are unusually large.

CLINICAL POINT

Congenital vs. sliding hernias. A sliding diaphragmatic hernia is where part of the stomach extends through the esophageal opening of the diaphragm. A symptom or consequence of this is gastroesophageal reflux disease, where stomach acid has retrograde passage into the esophagus to cause "heartburn" and damage to the esophagus. It usually develops postnatally.

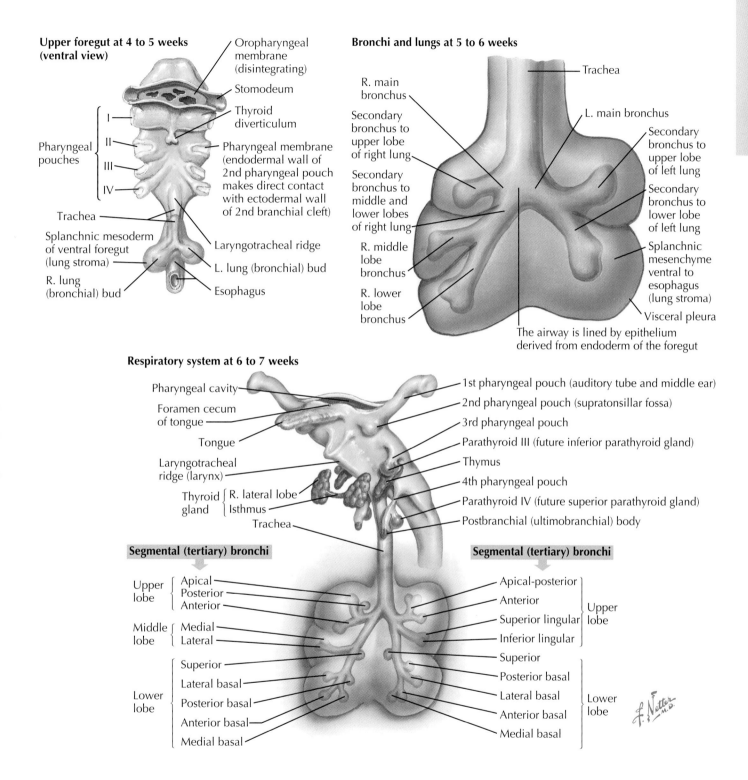

Upper foregut at 4 to 5 weeks (ventral view)

- Oropharyngeal membrane (disintegrating)
- Stomodeum
- Thyroid diverticulum
- I, II, III, IV — Pharyngeal pouches
- Pharyngeal membrane (endodermal wall of 2nd pharyngeal pouch makes direct contact with ectodermal wall of 2nd branchial cleft)
- Trachea
- Splanchnic mesoderm of ventral foregut (lung stroma)
- R. lung (bronchial) bud
- Laryngotracheal ridge
- L. lung (bronchial) bud
- Esophagus

Bronchi and lungs at 5 to 6 weeks

- Trachea
- R. main bronchus
- L. main bronchus
- Secondary bronchus to upper lobe of right lung
- Secondary bronchus to upper lobe of left lung
- Secondary bronchus to middle and lower lobes of right lung
- Secondary bronchus to lower lobe of left lung
- R. middle lobe bronchus
- Splanchnic mesenchyme ventral to esophagus (lung stroma)
- R. lower lobe bronchus
- Visceral pleura

The airway is lined by epithelium derived from endoderm of the foregut

Respiratory system at 6 to 7 weeks

- Pharyngeal cavity
- Foramen cecum of tongue
- Tongue
- Laryngotracheal ridge (larynx)
- Thyroid gland { R. lateral lobe / Isthmus }
- Trachea
- 1st pharyngeal pouch (auditory tube and middle ear)
- 2nd pharyngeal pouch (supratonsillar fossa)
- 3rd pharyngeal pouch
- Parathyroid III (future inferior parathyroid gland)
- Thymus
- 4th pharyngeal pouch
- Parathyroid IV (future superior parathyroid gland)
- Postbranchial (ultimobranchial) body

Segmental (tertiary) bronchi

Upper lobe { Apical / Posterior / Anterior }
Middle lobe { Medial / Lateral }
Lower lobe { Superior / Lateral basal / Posterior basal / Anterior basal / Medial basal }

Segmental (tertiary) bronchi

Apical-posterior / Anterior / Superior lingular / Inferior lingular } Upper lobe
Superior / Posterior basal / Lateral basal / Anterior basal / Medial basal } Lower lobe

5.8 **THE AIRWAY AT 4 TO 7 WEEKS**

The **laryngotracheal diverticulum** grows ventrally off the foregut and begins an extensive series of branching in the fourth week. It is composed of splanchnopleure, with the endoderm forming the epithelial **parenchyma** of the future airway and the mesoderm forming the connective tissue **stroma**. The diverticulum first branches into a left and right lung bud with **primary bronchi.** The next division forms the lobes of the lung with their **secondary (lobar) bronchi**. Secondary bronchi divide into **tertiary (segmental)** bronchi that supply the **bronchopulmonary segments** of the lungs.

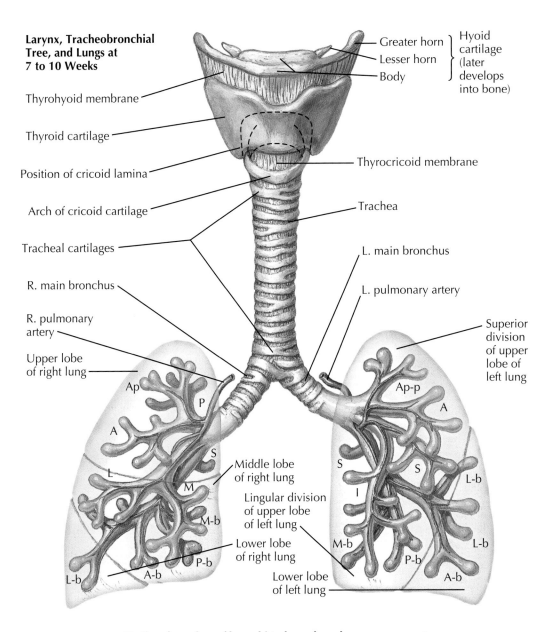

Larynx, Tracheobronchial Tree, and Lungs at 7 to 10 Weeks

Thyrohyoid membrane

Thyroid cartilage

Position of cricoid lamina

Arch of cricoid cartilage

Tracheal cartilages

R. main bronchus

R. pulmonary artery

Upper lobe of right lung

Greater horn
Lesser horn
Body
} Hyoid cartilage (later develops into bone)

Thyrocricoid membrane

Trachea

L. main bronchus

L. pulmonary artery

Superior division of upper lobe of left lung

Middle lobe of right lung

Lingular division of upper lobe of left lung

Lower lobe of right lung

Lower lobe of left lung

Tertiary branches of bronchi to bronchopulmonary segments

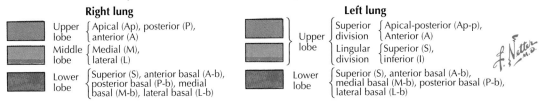

Right lung		Left lung		
Upper lobe	Apical (Ap), posterior (P), anterior (A)	Upper lobe	Superior division	Apical-posterior (Ap-p), Anterior (A)
Middle lobe	Medial (M), lateral (L)		Lingular division	Superior (S), inferior (I)
Lower lobe	Superior (S), anterior basal (A-b), posterior basal (P-b), medial basal (M-b), lateral basal (L-b)	Lower lobe		Superior (S), anterior basal (A-b), medial basal (M-b), posterior basal (P-b), lateral basal (L-b)

5.9 THE AIRWAY AT 7 TO 10 WEEKS

By 10 weeks, the cartilages of the larynx and cartilage rings of the trachea and larger bronchi have formed. The bronchi continue their generations of branching. There are 10 bronchopulmonary segments in the right lung and 9 in the left. The left lung has only two lobes (and two secondary bronchi) instead of three. The lingula of the left lung is equivalent to the middle lobe of the right. The pulmonary arteries branch with the bronchi, and the veins run between the segments.

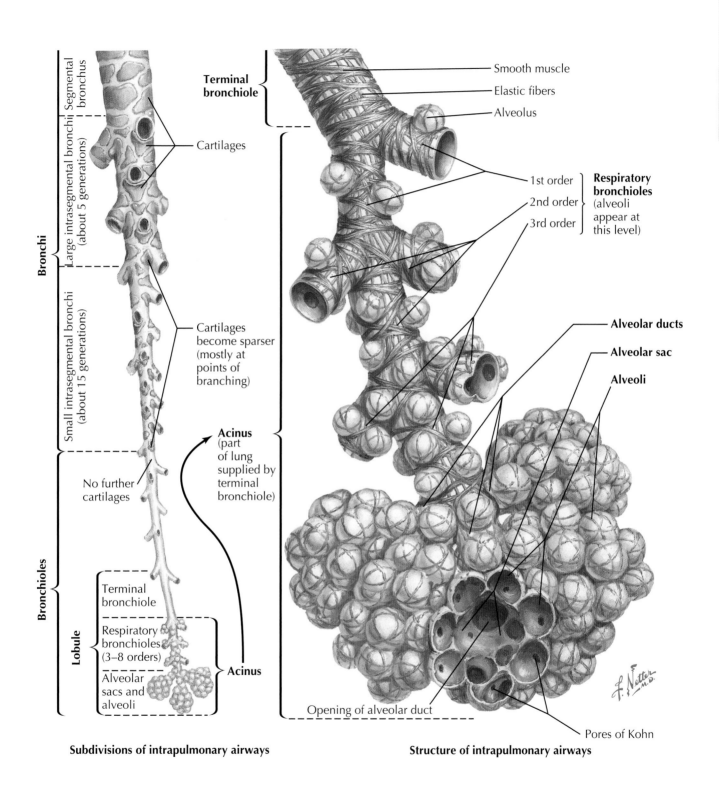

Subdivisions of intrapulmonary airways

Structure of intrapulmonary airways

(Labels in illustration:)

Segmental bronchus

Large intrasegmental bronchi (about 5 generations)

Bronchi

Small intrasegmental bronchi (about 15 generations)

Bronchioles

Lobule

Cartilages

Cartilages become sparser (mostly at points of branching)

No further cartilages

Acinus (part of lung supplied by terminal bronchiole)

Terminal bronchiole

Respiratory bronchioles (3–8 orders)

Alveolar sacs and alveoli

Acinus

Terminal bronchiole

Smooth muscle

Elastic fibers

Alveolus

1st order

2nd order

3rd order

Respiratory bronchioles (alveoli appear at this level)

Alveolar ducts

Alveolar sac

Alveoli

Opening of alveolar duct

Pores of Kohn

5.10 DEVELOPMENT OF BRONCHIOLES AND ALVEOLI

The tertiary bronchi continue to divide for many generations; the total ranges from 23 to 30, depending on the region of the lung. Bronchi become bronchioles when hyaline cartilage is no longer present in the walls. The bronchial tree eventually terminates in **alveoli**, the saclike structures where gas exchange occurs.

Terminal air tube at 20 weeks

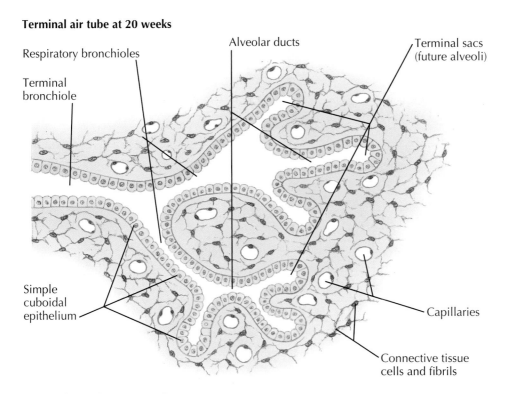

Respiratory bronchioles

Terminal bronchiole

Alveolar ducts

Terminal sacs (future alveoli)

Simple cuboidal epithelium

Capillaries

Connective tissue cells and fibrils

Terminal air tube at 24 weeks

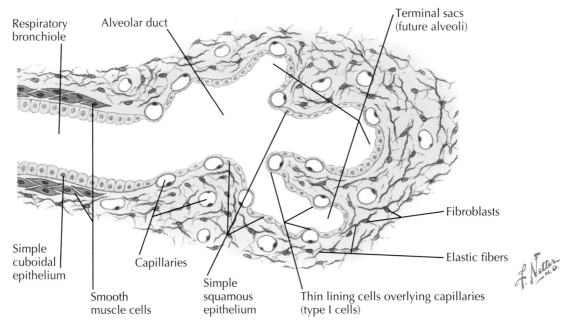

Respiratory bronchiole

Alveolar duct

Terminal sacs (future alveoli)

Simple cuboidal epithelium

Smooth muscle cells

Capillaries

Simple squamous epithelium

Thin lining cells overlying capillaries (type I cells)

Fibroblasts

Elastic fibers

5.11 BRONCHIAL EPITHELIUM MATURATION

The trachea and larger bronchi are lined by **pseudostratified columnar (respiratory) epithelium** with cilia and mucus-producing goblet cells. The epithelium becomes simple cuboidal in the smaller bronchi and simple squamous in mature alveoli. At 20 weeks, all epithelium is simple cuboidal in the distal airway and not closely applied to the capillaries. No gas exchange is possible in a premature infant of this age.

CLINICAL POINT

Earliest airway functioning. At 6 months, the future alveoli are mature enough for gas exchange, but the type II alveolar cells are not yet producing surfactant, which reduces the surface tension that prevents alveoli from collapsing. Life can be sustained only by introducing artificial surfactant or by maintaining positive pressure in the alveoli.

A. Tracheoesophageal fistula

Most common form (90% to 95%) of tracheoesophageal fistula. Upper segment of esophagus ending in blind pouch; lower segment originating from trachea just above bifurcation. The two segments may be connected by a solid cord

B. Variations of tracheoesophageal fistula and rare anomalies of trachea

Upper segment of esophagus ending in trachea; lower segment of variable length

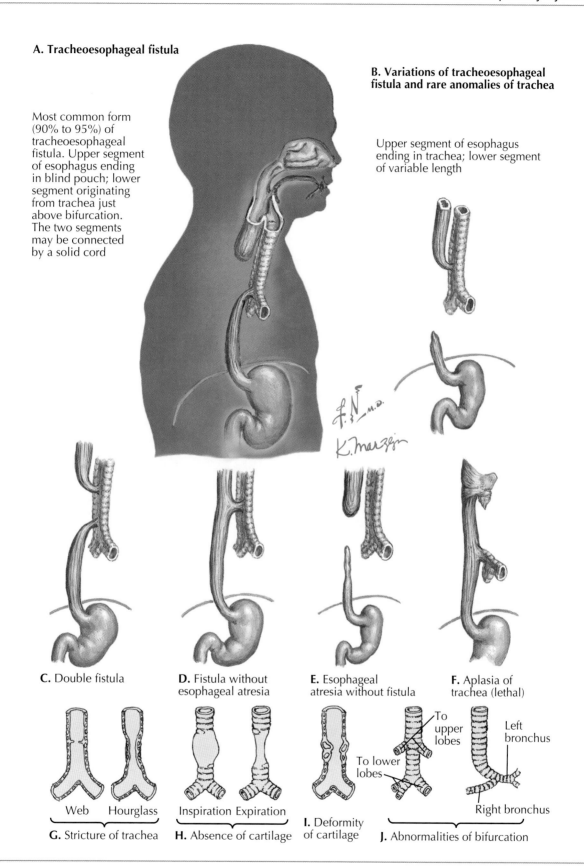

C. Double fistula

D. Fistula without esophageal atresia

E. Esophageal atresia without fistula

F. Aplasia of trachea (lethal)

Web   Hourglass

G. Stricture of trachea

Inspiration Expiration

H. Absence of cartilage

I. Deformity of cartilage

To upper lobes

To lower lobes

Left bronchus

Right bronchus

J. Abnormalities of bifurcation

5.12 CONGENITAL ANOMALIES OF THE LOWER AIRWAY

The laryngotracheal diverticulum is closely applied to the ventral surface of the developing esophagus. The lumen of the esophagus closes from the proliferation of epithelial cells and then reopens.

Disruption of this process can result in **tracheoesophageal fistula** (i.e., abnormal communication between the trachea and esophagus). A variety of possibilities and other types of anomalies of the trachea are illustrated.

Pulmonary agenesis, aplasia, and hypoplasia

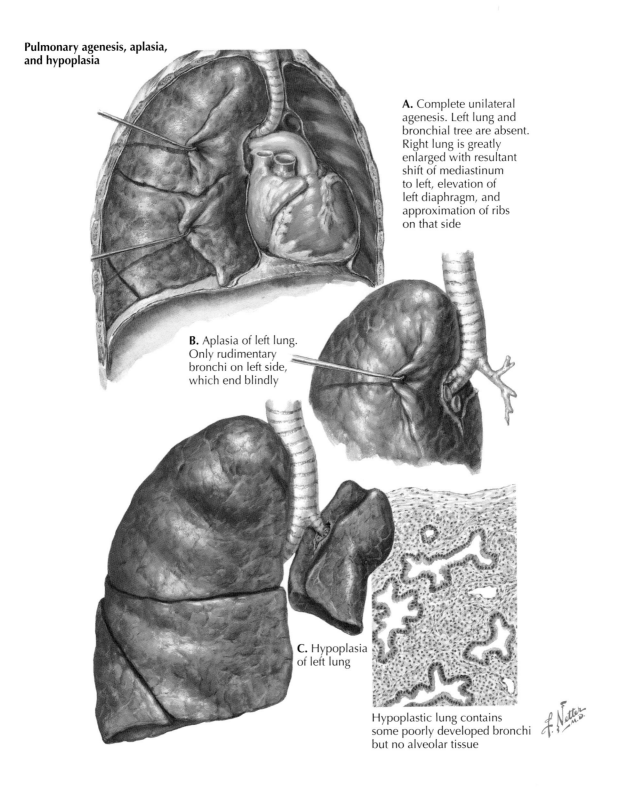

A. Complete unilateral agenesis. Left lung and bronchial tree are absent. Right lung is greatly enlarged with resultant shift of mediastinum to left, elevation of left diaphragm, and approximation of ribs on that side

B. Aplasia of left lung. Only rudimentary bronchi on left side, which end blindly

C. Hypoplasia of left lung

Hypoplastic lung contains some poorly developed bronchi but no alveolar tissue

5.13 AIRWAY BRANCHING ANOMALIES

Like any organ or gland that develops by the sequential branching of its primordium, there are numerous possibilities for asymmetry (and other branching abnormalities, as seen in Fig. 5.12J). Fig. 5.13 shows the result of the lack of a left lung bud or a small left bronchial bud with and without lung tissue.

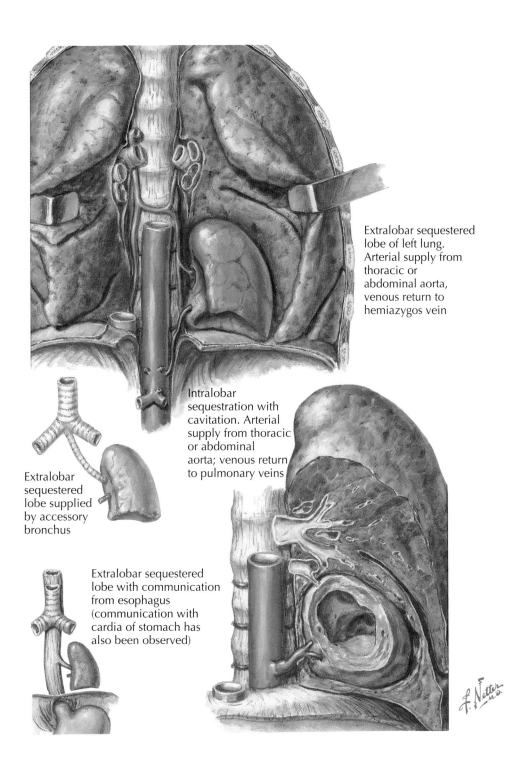

Extralobar sequestered lobe of left lung. Arterial supply from thoracic or abdominal aorta, venous return to hemiazygos vein

Intralobar sequestration with cavitation. Arterial supply from thoracic or abdominal aorta; venous return to pulmonary veins

Extralobar sequestered lobe supplied by accessory bronchus

Extralobar sequestered lobe with communication from esophagus (communication with cardia of stomach has also been observed)

5.14 BRONCHOPULMONARY SEQUESTRATION

More complicated than branching asymmetry is **sequestration**, the separation of a small extra lobe of lung tissue from the normal bronchial tree. It may be inside or outside the lung, but it is typically supplied by the systemic circulation rather than by the pulmonary. It may have abnormal communications with intralobar bronchi or develop from an extra bud off the laryngotracheal diverticulum or even other components of the foregut (e.g., esophagus or stomach).

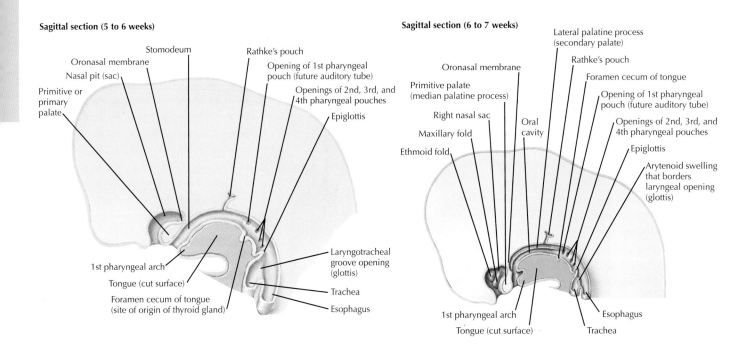

Sagittal section (5 to 6 weeks)

Stomodeum
Oronasal membrane
Nasal pit (sac)
Primitive or primary palate
Rathke's pouch
Opening of 1st pharyngeal pouch (future auditory tube)
Openings of 2nd, 3rd, and 4th pharyngeal pouches
Epiglottis
1st pharyngeal arch
Tongue (cut surface)
Foramen cecum of tongue (site of origin of thyroid gland)
Laryngotracheal groove opening (glottis)
Trachea
Esophagus

Sagittal section (6 to 7 weeks)

Lateral palatine process (secondary palate)
Rathke's pouch
Foramen cecum of tongue
Opening of 1st pharyngeal pouch (future auditory tube)
Openings of 2nd, 3rd, and 4th pharyngeal pouches
Epiglottis
Arytenoid swelling that borders laryngeal opening (glottis)
Oronasal membrane
Primitive palate (median palatine process)
Right nasal sac
Maxillary fold
Ethmoid fold
Oral cavity
1st pharyngeal arch
Tongue (cut surface)
Esophagus
Trachea

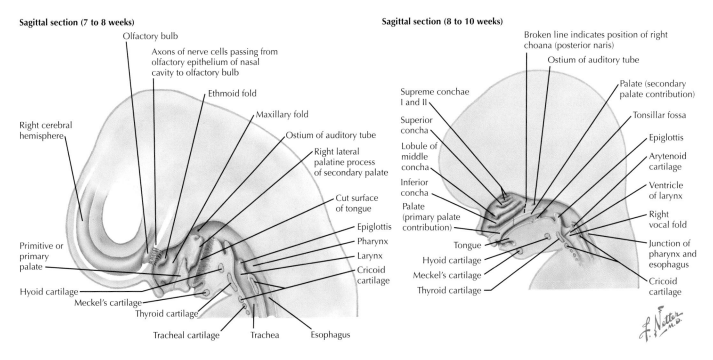

Sagittal section (7 to 8 weeks)

Olfactory bulb
Axons of nerve cells passing from olfactory epithelium of nasal cavity to olfactory bulb
Ethmoid fold
Maxillary fold
Ostium of auditory tube
Right lateral palatine process of secondary palate
Cut surface of tongue
Epiglottis
Pharynx
Larynx
Cricoid cartilage
Right cerebral hemisphere
Primitive or primary palate
Hyoid cartilage
Meckel's cartilage
Thyroid cartilage
Tracheal cartilage
Trachea
Esophagus

Sagittal section (8 to 10 weeks)

Broken line indicates position of right choana (posterior naris)
Ostium of auditory tube
Palate (secondary palate contribution)
Tonsillar fossa
Epiglottis
Arytenoid cartilage
Ventricle of larynx
Right vocal fold
Junction of pharynx and esophagus
Cricoid cartilage
Supreme conchae I and II
Superior concha
Lobule of middle concha
Inferior concha
Palate (primary palate contribution)
Tongue
Hyoid cartilage
Meckel's cartilage
Thyroid cartilage

5.15 PALATE FORMATION IN THE UPPER AIRWAY

The upper airway develops from the **foregut**, the upper half of the **stomodeum**, and the **nasal sacs**, which are invaginations of the ectodermal nasal placodes. Lateral palatine processes grow toward the midline to divide the stomodeum into nasal and oral components. The nasal sacs break through to the airway part of the stomodeum, above the lateral palatine processes. The tissue between the nasal sacs and stomodeum is the primary palate, and the lateral palatine processes form the secondary palate. Palate formation is completed when the primary palate, lateral palatine processes of the secondary palate, and the nasal septum all fuse to each other. See Chapter 9 for more details.

Terminology

Alveolus	(L., "hollow") Saclike terminal elements of the distal airway in the lungs, where gas exchange occurs between alveolar air and the bloodstream. They total 300 million.
Bronchopulmonary segments	Subdivisions of lung lobes aerated by tertiary (segmental) bronchi, the third generation of branching of the trachea.
Carina	Cartilaginous ridge at the internal bifurcation point of the trachea into the left and right primary bronchi.
Coelom	(Gr., "hollow") The pericardial, pleural, and peritoneal body cavities.
Epiglottis	Cartilaginous projection of the larynx into the laryngopharynx above the glottis.
Glottis	The aperture between the vocal folds (mucosa over the vocal "cords") in the larynx. It is the entryway into the lower airway.
Lobar bronchus	A bronchus supplying a lung lobe. The second generation of bronchial branching.
Lower airway	Larynx, trachea, and lungs (with the bronchial tree).
Main bronchus (right and left)	Primary (mainstem) bronchus that supplies an entire lung. It is the first order of branching of the trachea.
Mesothelium	The simple squamous epithelium that lines the body cavities. Mesothelia are pleura, peritoneum, and pericardium.
Pseudostratified ciliated columnar epithelium	Respiratory epithelium in the nasal cavities, most of the larynx, trachea, and larger bronchi. The nuclei appear to be stratified in section, but all of the cells touch the basal lamina.
Root of lung	All of the structures that enter and leave each lung—main bronchus, pulmonary artery and veins, bronchial arteries and veins, nerves, and lymphatics.
Segmental bronchus	A bronchus supplying a bronchopulmonary segment. It is the third generation of bronchial branching.
Septum transversum	Thick transverse partition of mesenchyme in the embryo just caudal to the developing heart. It contributes to the diaphragm and stroma of the liver and gallbladder.
Serous fluid	Proteinaceous, watery fluid produced by the mesothelia lining the body cavities. It reduces friction between movements of parietal against visceral layers.
Surfactant	A fluid rich in phospholipids secreted by type II alveolar cells to reduce surface tension in the pulmonary alveoli. This prevents them from collapsing and contributes to the elastic properties of lung tissue.
Types I and II alveolar cells	Type I cells are the simple squamous cells forming most of the gas-exchanging walls of alveoli. Type II cells produce surfactant. They are equal in number to type I cells but occupy much less alveolar area because of their cuboidal shape.
Upper airway	Nasal cavity and pharynx.

6

THE GASTROINTESTINAL SYSTEM AND ABDOMINAL WALL

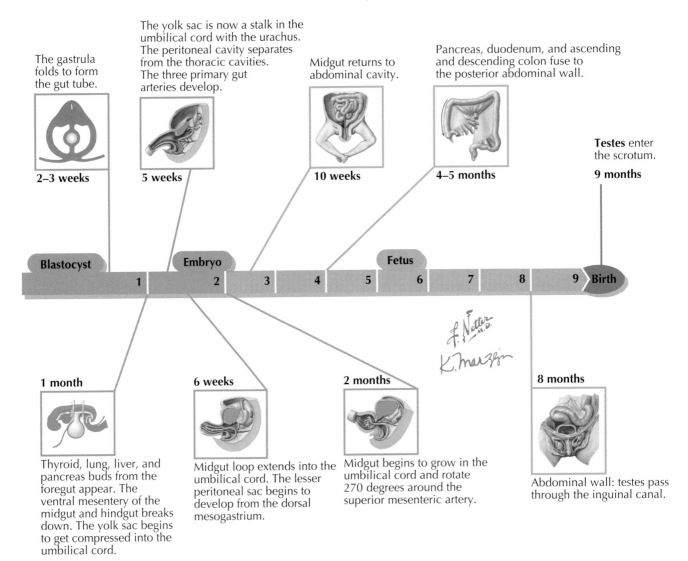

PRENATAL TIME SCALE (MONTHS)

The gastrula folds to form the gut tube.

2–3 weeks

The yolk sac is now a stalk in the umbilical cord with the urachus. The peritoneal cavity separates from the thoracic cavities. The three primary gut arteries develop.

5 weeks

Midgut returns to abdominal cavity.

10 weeks

Pancreas, duodenum, and ascending and descending colon fuse to the posterior abdominal wall.

4–5 months

Testes enter the scrotum.

9 months

Blastocyst   Embryo   Fetus   Birth
1   2   3   4   5   6   7   8   9

1 month

Thyroid, lung, liver, and pancreas buds from the foregut appear. The ventral mesentery of the midgut and hindgut breaks down. The yolk sac begins to get compressed into the umbilical cord.

6 weeks

Midgut loop extends into the umbilical cord. The lesser peritoneal sac begins to develop from the dorsal mesogastrium.

2 months

Midgut begins to grow in the umbilical cord and rotate 270 degrees around the superior mesenteric artery.

8 months

Abdominal wall: testes pass through the inguinal canal.

6.1 TIMELINE

PRIMORDIUM

The foregut, midgut, and hindgut and their associated organs are derived from splanchnopleure (endoderm and splanchnic mesoderm of the lateral plate).

PLAN FOR THE GASTROINTESTINAL SYSTEM

Perhaps nowhere in the body is the organization of an organ system so simple in the embryo and its appearance so complex in the adult than the gastrointestinal (GI) system. The GI system in the abdomen first develops as a tube suspended by dorsal and ventral, sheetlike mesenteries. Blood vessels, autonomic nerves, lymphatic drainage, and mesentery structure are all organized according to abdominal foregut, midgut, and hindgut subdivisions of the GI tract. These basic relationships persist, but the adult anatomy appears complex because of four developments: (1) rotation of the abdominal foregut tube 90 degrees clockwise, (2) development of the greater omentum and lesser peritoneal sac from the dorsal mesentery of the abdominal foregut, (3) rotation of the midgut 270 degrees around the superior mesenteric artery, and (4) tremendous growth of the midgut intestines.

PLAN FOR THE INGUINAL CANAL

The development of the testes plays an important role in the development and organization of the anterior abdominal wall. (This is discussed more extensively in the next chapter.) The testis begins development between parietal peritoneum and the muscles and fascia of the abdominal wall, but must end up in the scrotum, an evagination of the superficial body wall. The testis forms the inguinal canal by pushing its way through the deep body wall. The layers of the wall contribute to the coverings of the spermatic cord of vessels, nerves, and lymphatics supplying the testis.

INCLUSION AND BIAS CONSIDERATION: WEIGHT BIAS AND STIGMA

This chapter focuses extensively on the embryonic and fetal development of the GI system and abdomen, and as such, it does not depict much variation in adiposity or weight. Still, it is important to recognize that weight bias and stigma do exist in clinical practice and can often be heightened in discussion of the GI system. Educators, students, and clinicians need to be mindful and reflective in discussions of weight, as perceived weight stigma and bias prove detrimental to patient engagement in healthcare. There should be focus on person-first language, when agreeable with patients, and attention should be paid to ensuring spaces are inclusionary for patients of all sizes and body habitus.

A. 14 days

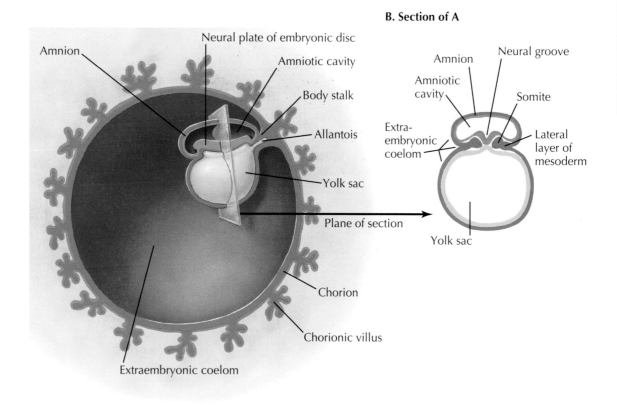

Neural plate of embryonic disc

Amnion

Amniotic cavity

Body stalk

Allantois

Yolk sac

Plane of section

Chorion

Chorionic villus

Extraembryonic coelom

B. Section of A

Amnion

Neural groove

Amniotic cavity

Somite

Extra-embryonic coelom

Lateral layer of mesoderm

Yolk sac

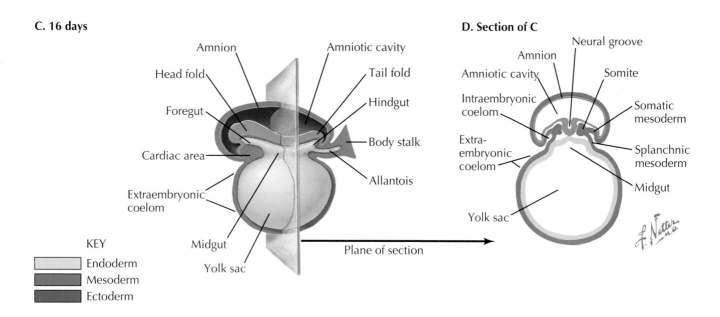

C. 16 days

Amnion

Amniotic cavity

Head fold

Tail fold

Foregut

Hindgut

Cardiac area

Body stalk

Extraembryonic coelom

Allantois

Midgut

Yolk sac

Plane of section

KEY

Endoderm
Mesoderm
Ectoderm

D. Section of C

Neural groove

Amnion

Amniotic cavity

Somite

Intraembryonic coelom

Somatic mesoderm

Extra-embryonic coelom

Splanchnic mesoderm

Midgut

Yolk sac

6.2 EARLY PRIMORDIA

The GI system develops from the endoderm of the gastrula and mesoderm from the lateral plate. The lateral plate becomes hollow to form primitive peritoneal and pleural coelomic cavities. As a result, the lateral plate mesoderm divides into somatic and splanchnic components. The splanchnic component lines the endoderm to form splanchnopleure, the primordium of the GI tract.

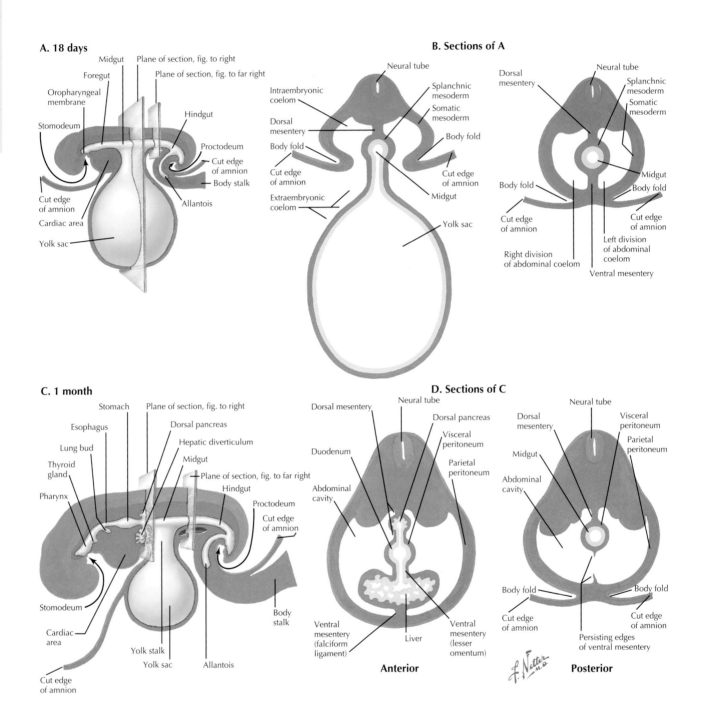

A. 18 days

Midgut
Foregut
Oropharyngeal membrane
Stomodeum
Cut edge of amnion
Cardiac area
Yolk sac
Plane of section, fig. to right
Plane of section, fig. to far right
Hindgut
Proctodeum
Cut edge of amnion
Body stalk
Allantois

B. Sections of A

Neural tube
Intraembryonic coelom
Dorsal mesentery
Body fold
Cut edge of amnion
Extraembryonic coelom
Splanchnic mesoderm
Somatic mesoderm
Body fold
Cut edge of amnion
Midgut
Yolk sac

Dorsal mesentery
Neural tube
Splanchnic mesoderm
Somatic mesoderm
Body fold
Cut edge of amnion
Right division of abdominal coelom
Midgut
Body fold
Cut edge of amnion
Left division of abdominal coelom
Ventral mesentery

C. 1 month

Stomach
Esophagus
Lung bud
Thyroid gland
Pharynx
Stomodeum
Cardiac area
Yolk stalk
Yolk sac
Cut edge of amnion
Plane of section, fig. to right
Dorsal pancreas
Hepatic diverticulum
Midgut
Plane of section, fig. to far right
Hindgut
Proctodeum
Cut edge of amnion
Body stalk
Allantois

D. Sections of C

Dorsal mesentery
Neural tube
Duodenum
Abdominal cavity
Ventral mesentery (falciform ligament)
Dorsal pancreas
Visceral peritoneum
Parietal peritoneum
Liver
Ventral mesentery (lesser omentum)

Anterior

Dorsal mesentery
Neural tube
Midgut
Abdominal cavity
Body fold
Cut edge of amnion
Persisting edges of ventral mesentery
Visceral peritoneum
Parietal peritoneum
Body fold
Cut edge of amnion

Posterior

6.3 FORMATION OF THE GUT TUBE AND MESENTERIES

As the trilaminar disc of the gastrula folds into a cylinder, the splanchnopleure is shaped into a tube with a foregut extending into the head region, a midgut in wide communication with the yolk sac, and a hindgut extending into the tail. It is suspended by dorsal and ventral mesenteries flanked on either side by the coelomic cavities. The lateral plate mesoderm lining these cavities differentiates into the simple squamous epithelium of peritoneum (and pleura). Visceral peritoneum covers the mesenteries and GI organs; parietal peritoneum lines the inner surface of the body wall. By the end of the first month, organ buds grow from the gut tube, and the ventral mesentery of the midgut and hindgut disappears.

5 weeks

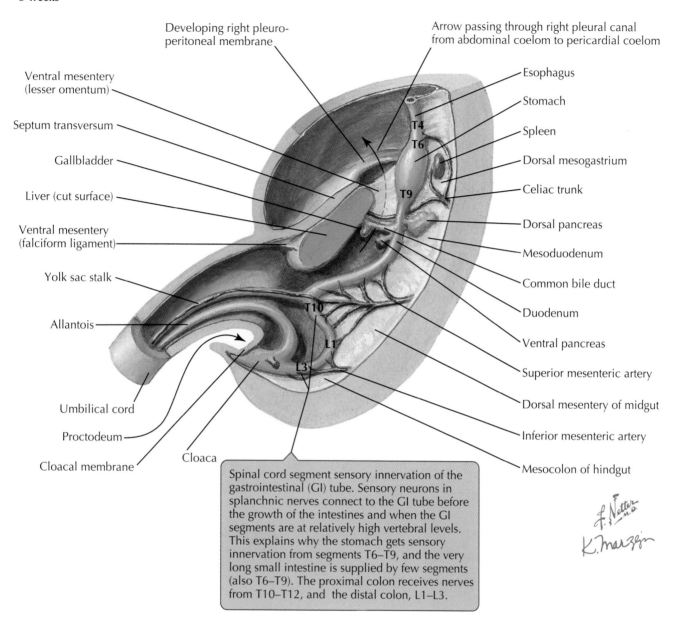

Developing right pleuro-peritoneal membrane

Arrow passing through right pleural canal from abdominal coelom to pericardial coelom

Ventral mesentery (lesser omentum)

Septum transversum

Gallbladder

Liver (cut surface)

Ventral mesentery (falciform ligament)

Yolk sac stalk

Allantois

Umbilical cord

Proctodeum

Cloacal membrane

Cloaca

Esophagus

Stomach

Spleen

Dorsal mesogastrium

Celiac trunk

Dorsal pancreas

Mesoduodenum

Common bile duct

Duodenum

Ventral pancreas

Superior mesenteric artery

Dorsal mesentery of midgut

Inferior mesenteric artery

Mesocolon of hindgut

T4

T6

T9

T10

L1

L3

Spinal cord segment sensory innervation of the gastrointestinal (GI) tube. Sensory neurons in splanchnic nerves connect to the GI tube before the growth of the intestines and when the GI segments are at relatively high vertebral levels. This explains why the stomach gets sensory innervation from segments T6–T9, and the very long small intestine is supplied by few segments (also T6–T9). The proximal colon receives nerves from T10–T12, and the distal colon, L1–L3.

6.4 FOREGUT, MIDGUT, AND HINDGUT

By week 5, the yolk sac is compressed into the umbilical cord as a thin stalk. The ventral mesentery of the midgut and hindgut is gone, and the left and right peritoneal cavities communicate as a single abdominal cavity lined by the **greater peritoneal sac** of parietal peritoneum. The pleuroperitoneal membranes are separating the peritoneal and pleural cavities, and the foregut organ buds are elaborating. The abdominal foregut retains its ventral mesentery (ventral mesogastrium or lesser omentum); its free edge contains the common bile duct component of the portal triad.

The abdominal foregut, midgut, and hindgut each have their own artery off the aorta:

- **Foregut:** celiac trunk
- **Midgut:** superior mesenteric artery
- **Hindgut:** inferior mesenteric artery

CLINICAL POINT

Referred pain. Spinal segment innervation in the developing GI tract (see Fig. 6.4) is the embryonic basis for where pain will be felt from GI organ pathology in spinal nerve dermatomes on the body surface (see Fig. 3.15).

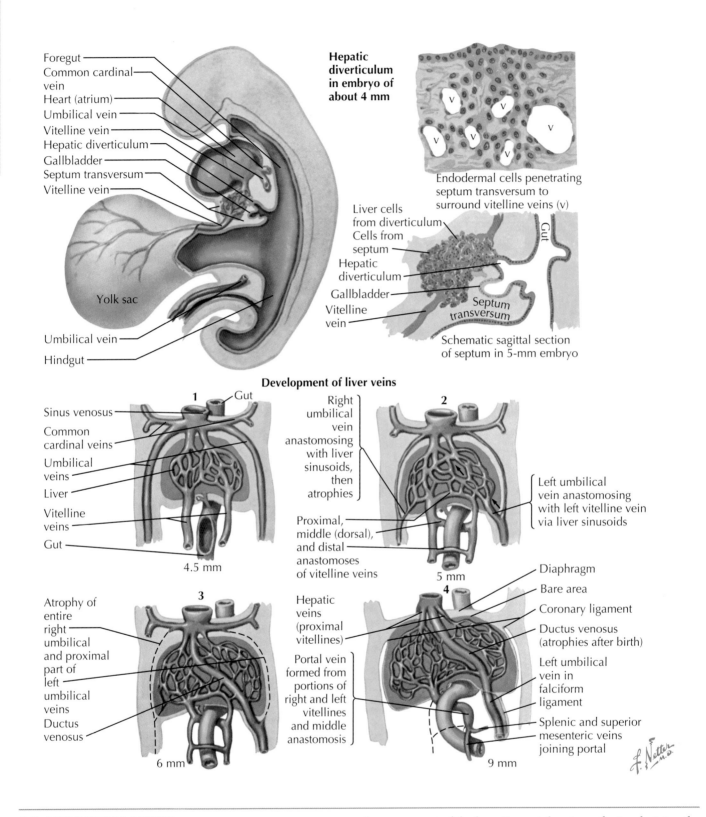

Foregut
Common cardinal vein
Heart (atrium)
Umbilical vein
Vitelline vein
Hepatic diverticulum
Gallbladder
Septum transversum
Vitelline vein

Yolk sac

Umbilical vein

Hindgut

Hepatic diverticulum in embryo of about 4 mm

Endodermal cells penetrating septum transversum to surround vitelline veins (v)

Liver cells from diverticulum
Cells from septum
Hepatic diverticulum
Gallbladder
Vitelline vein

Gut

Septum transversum

Schematic sagittal section of septum in 5-mm embryo

Development of liver veins

1   Gut

Sinus venosus
Common cardinal veins
Umbilical veins
Liver
Vitelline veins
Gut

4.5 mm

2

Right umbilical vein anastomosing with liver sinusoids, then atrophies

Proximal, middle (dorsal), and distal anastomoses of vitelline veins

Left umbilical vein anastomosing with left vitelline vein via liver sinusoids

5 mm

3

Atrophy of entire right umbilical and proximal part of left umbilical veins
Ductus venosus

6 mm

Hepatic veins (proximal vitellines)

Portal vein formed from portions of right and left vitellines and middle anastomosis

4

Diaphragm
Bare area
Coronary ligament
Ductus venosus (atrophies after birth)
Left umbilical vein in falciform ligament
Splenic and superior mesenteric veins joining portal

9 mm

6.5 ABDOMINAL VEINS

Converging on the sinus venosus of the developing heart are the **common cardinal veins** with embryonic blood, the **umbilical veins** carrying oxygenated blood from the placenta, and the **vitelline veins** from the yolk sac. The vitelline veins pass through the developing liver, where they form a network of liver sinusoids. The remainder of the intraembryonic portion of the vitelline veins becomes most of the **hepatic portal system** of veins draining the gut. The right umbilical vein and proximal segment of the left disappear; the remaining part of the left umbilical vein anastomoses with the liver sinusoids to form a liver shunt into the inferior vena cava, the **ductus venosus**. After birth, it becomes the fibrous **ligamentum venosum**.

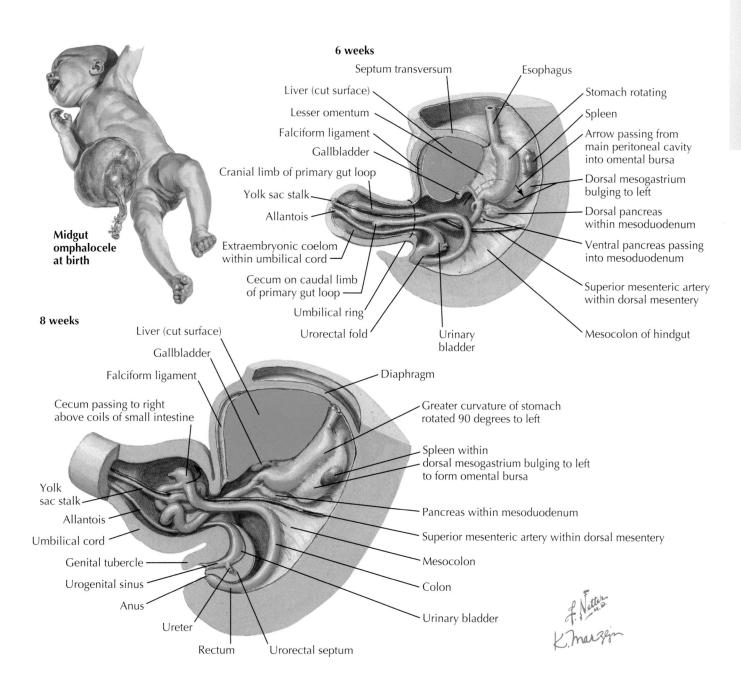

6 weeks

Septum transversum
Liver (cut surface)
Lesser omentum
Falciform ligament
Gallbladder
Cranial limb of primary gut loop
Yolk sac stalk
Allantois
Extraembryonic coelom within umbilical cord
Cecum on caudal limb of primary gut loop
Umbilical ring
Urorectal fold

Esophagus
Stomach rotating
Spleen
Arrow passing from main peritoneal cavity into omental bursa
Dorsal mesogastrium bulging to left
Dorsal pancreas within mesoduodenum
Ventral pancreas passing into mesoduodenum
Superior mesenteric artery within dorsal mesentery
Mesocolon of hindgut
Urinary bladder

Midgut omphalocele at birth

8 weeks

Liver (cut surface)
Gallbladder
Falciform ligament
Cecum passing to right above coils of small intestine
Yolk sac stalk
Allantois
Umbilical cord
Genital tubercle
Urogenital sinus
Anus
Ureter
Rectum
Urorectal septum

Diaphragm
Greater curvature of stomach rotated 90 degrees to left
Spleen within dorsal mesogastrium bulging to left to form omental bursa
Pancreas within mesoduodenum
Superior mesenteric artery within dorsal mesentery
Mesocolon
Colon
Urinary bladder

6.6 FOREGUT AND MIDGUT ROTATIONS

Near the end of week 8, two major events occur. The midgut grows so rapidly that it extends into the umbilical cord and begins to rotate around the superior mesenteric artery. Also, the foregut rotates 90 degrees around its long axis as the enlarging liver in the **ventral mesogastrium** (lesser omentum) moves to the right and the **dorsal mesogastrium** (greater omentum) begins to bulge to the left. This bag of dorsal mesentery will grow extensively to form the **lesser peritoneal sac** (the **omental bursa**). The greater peritoneal sac communicates with the lesser peritoneal sac under the ventral mesogastrium through the **epiploic foramen** of Winslow (dashed arrow in Fig. 6.6).

CLINICAL POINT

Omphalocele. If the midgut intestines do not return to the abdomen after 8 weeks, a newborn will have an omphalocele, a congenital abdominal wall defect with intestines still within a distended umbilical cord. A characteristic feature of the herniated intestines is their covering by the amnion that surrounds the umbilical cord. Omphalocele is associated with a 25% mortality rate, as the condition often occurs with other major malformations.

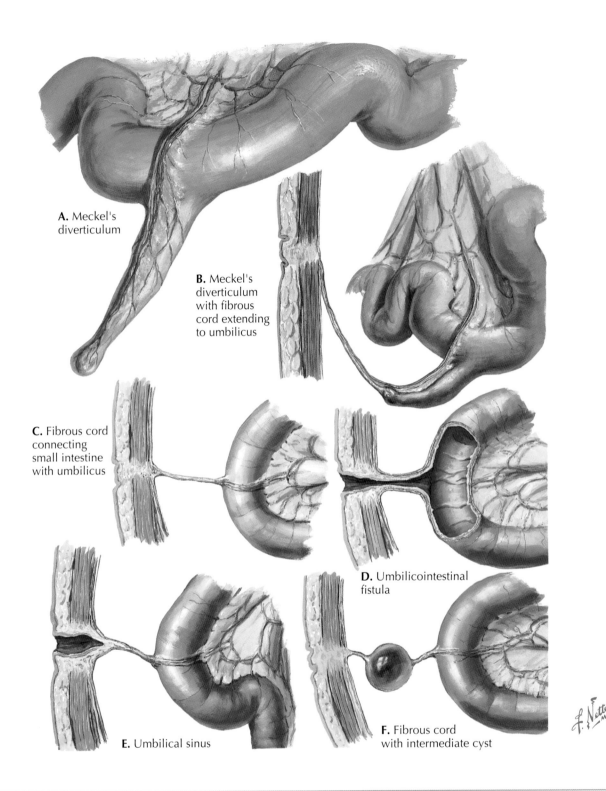

A. Meckel's diverticulum

B. Meckel's diverticulum with fibrous cord extending to umbilicus

C. Fibrous cord connecting small intestine with umbilicus

D. Umbilicointestinal fistula

E. Umbilical sinus

F. Fibrous cord with intermediate cyst

6.7 MECKEL'S DIVERTICULUM

The yolk sac is initially in wide communication with the midgut. It becomes compressed into the umbilical cord when the gastrula folds into the cylindrical embryo. The stalk of the yolk sac may persist as a diverticulum off the ileum (midgut) or a cord from ileum to umbilicus with varying degrees of the persistence of the yolk sac lumen. The cord may be fibrous all the way (no lumen), or it may contain a sinus, cyst, or fistula.

CLINICAL POINT

Umbilicointestinal fistula (Fig. 6.7D). In the case of a fistula, a newborn will have meconium (fetal feces) passing out of the umbilicus (navel). A classic Meckel's diverticulum is asymptomatic unless it becomes infected, in which case it can mimic the pain of appendicitis because it is close to the appendix and innervated by the same visceral spinal segment (T10).

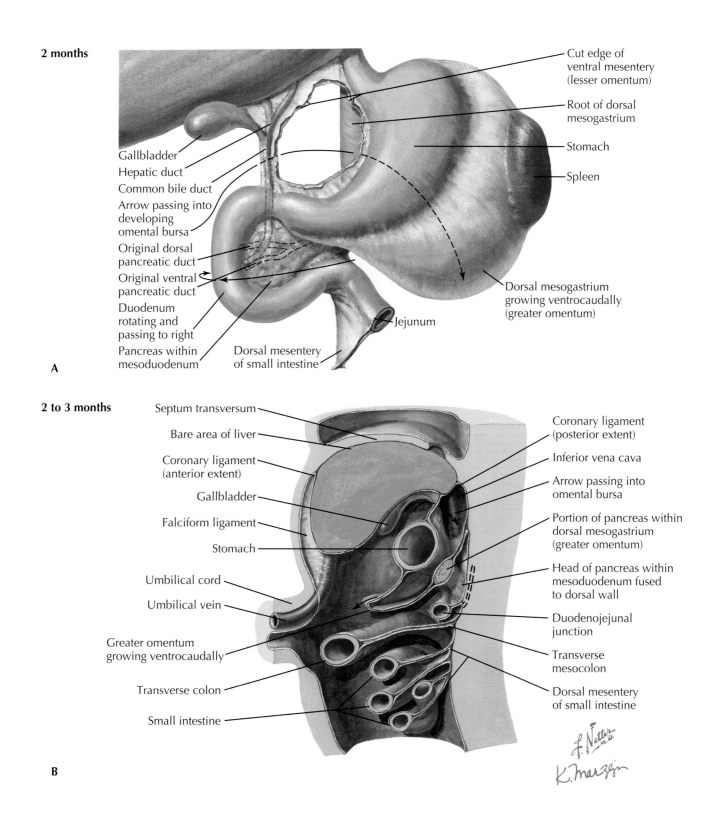

2 months

Cut edge of
ventral mesentery
(lesser omentum)

Root of dorsal
mesogastrium

Stomach

Spleen

Gallbladder

Hepatic duct

Common bile duct

Arrow passing into
developing
omental bursa

Original dorsal
pancreatic duct

Original ventral
pancreatic duct

Duodenum
rotating and
passing to right

Pancreas within
mesoduodenum

Dorsal mesentery
of small intestine

Jejunum

Dorsal mesogastrium
growing ventrocaudally
(greater omentum)

A

2 to 3 months

Septum transversum

Bare area of liver

Coronary ligament
(anterior extent)

Gallbladder

Falciform ligament

Stomach

Umbilical cord

Umbilical vein

Greater omentum
growing ventrocaudally

Transverse colon

Small intestine

Coronary ligament
(posterior extent)

Inferior vena cava

Arrow passing into
omental bursa

Portion of pancreas within
dorsal mesogastrium
(greater omentum)

Head of pancreas within
mesoduodenum fused
to dorsal wall

Duodenojejunal
junction

Transverse
mesocolon

Dorsal mesentery
of small intestine

B

6.8 LESSER PERITONEAL SAC

The Fig. 6.8A shows the lesser peritoneal sac of dorsal mesogastrium growing to the left and the ventral mesogastrium extending to the right. A hole is cut in the lesser omentum to expose the root of the dorsal mesogastrium in the midline. The Fig. 6.8B is a sagittal section that emphasizes the caudal and ventral growth of the lesser sac toward the transverse colon. Both images have arrows passing through the epiploic foramen into the omental bursa of the lesser sac. The surgical epiploic foramen is under the free edge of the lesser omentum; the true epiploic foramen is in the midline.

3 to 4 months

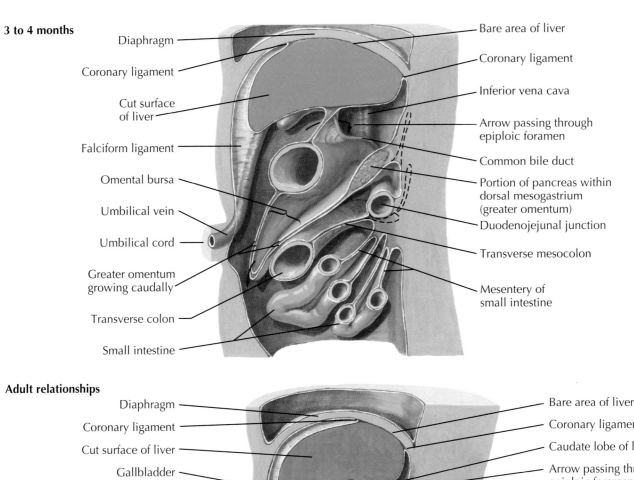

Diaphragm

Coronary ligament

Cut surface of liver

Falciform ligament

Omental bursa

Umbilical vein

Umbilical cord

Greater omentum growing caudally

Transverse colon

Small intestine

Bare area of liver

Coronary ligament

Inferior vena cava

Arrow passing through epiploic foramen

Common bile duct

Portion of pancreas within dorsal mesogastrium (greater omentum)

Duodenojejunal junction

Transverse mesocolon

Mesentery of small intestine

Adult relationships

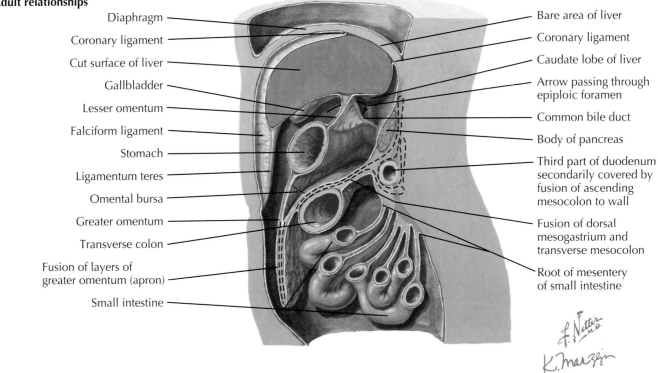

Diaphragm

Coronary ligament

Cut surface of liver

Gallbladder

Lesser omentum

Falciform ligament

Stomach

Ligamentum teres

Omental bursa

Greater omentum

Transverse colon

Fusion of layers of greater omentum (apron)

Small intestine

Bare area of liver

Coronary ligament

Caudate lobe of liver

Arrow passing through epiploic foramen

Common bile duct

Body of pancreas

Third part of duodenum secondarily covered by fusion of ascending mesocolon to wall

Fusion of dorsal mesogastrium and transverse mesocolon

Root of mesentery of small intestine

6.9 INTRODUCTION TO THE RETROPERITONEAL CONCEPT

By 4 months, the lesser sac begins to drape over the transverse colon. With growth of the intestines, the pancreas and duodenum are pressed against the body wall so that it appears they are outside the abdominal cavity in a **retroperitoneal** location (superficial to parietal peritoneum). Because they begin development in a mesentery, they are said to be **secondarily retroperitoneal**.

- **Primarily retroperitoneal organs:** aorta, inferior vena cava, kidneys, suprarenal glands, urinary bladder, prostate, vagina, rectum
- **Secondarily retroperitoneal organs:** pancreas, duodenum, ascending and descending colon

CLINICAL POINT

Somatic pain. Because of their relationship to the body wall, lesions in retroperitoneal organs can elicit intense, local somatic pain from spinal nerves.

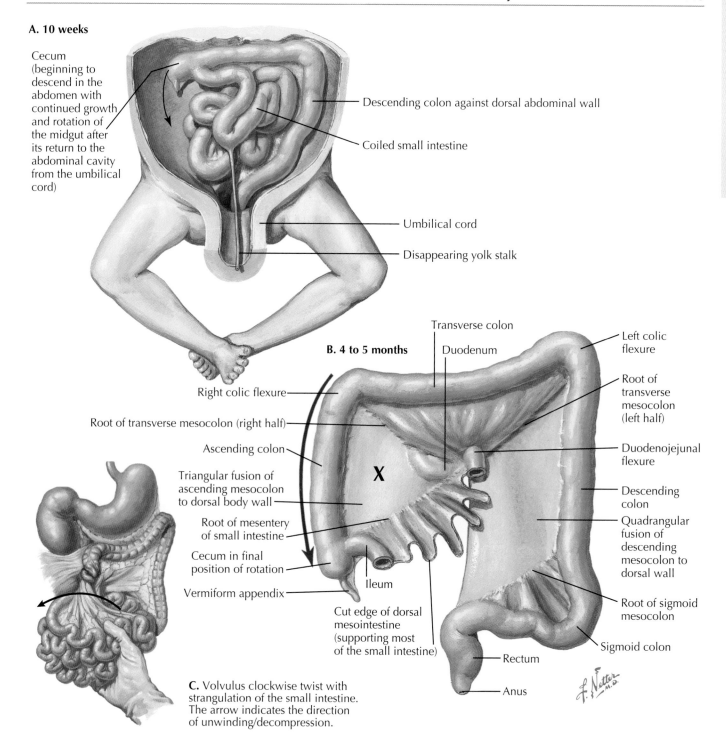

A. 10 weeks

Cecum (beginning to descend in the abdomen with continued growth and rotation of the midgut after its return to the abdominal cavity from the umbilical cord)

Descending colon against dorsal abdominal wall

Coiled small intestine

Umbilical cord

Disappearing yolk stalk

Transverse colon

Duodenum

Left colic flexure

Root of transverse mesocolon (left half)

B. 4 to 5 months

Right colic flexure

Root of transverse mesocolon (right half)

Ascending colon

Triangular fusion of ascending mesocolon to dorsal body wall

Root of mesentery of small intestine

Cecum in final position of rotation

Vermiform appendix

Ileum

Cut edge of dorsal mesointestine (supporting most of the small intestine)

Duodenojejunal flexure

Descending colon

Quadrangular fusion of descending mesocolon to dorsal wall

Root of sigmoid mesocolon

Sigmoid colon

Rectum

Anus

C. Volvulus clockwise twist with strangulation of the small intestine. The arrow indicates the direction of unwinding/decompression.

6.10 MIDGUT LOOP

By week 10, the intestines have returned to the abdominal cavity (Fig. 6.10A), and by week 20 (Fig. 6.10B), the midgut has completed its 270-degree loop. The midgut consists of most of the duodenum, the jejunum, the ileum, the ascending colon, and most of the transverse colon. With growth of the small intestines, the ascending and descending colon are pushed against the body wall in a secondarily retroperitoneal location, such as the pancreas and duodenum. The small intestine, transverse colon, and sigmoid colon are still freely suspended by mesenteries in the abdominal cavity (peritonealized).

CLINICAL POINT

Malrotation of the midgut can be in many forms, from lack of rotation with misplaced organs to extreme rotation resulting in **volvulus**, a twisting of the intestines and their mesenteries that compresses their blood supply (Fig. 6.10C).

CLINICAL POINT

Abdominal fluid flow. A clinical consequence of normal rotation is its effect on the flow of fluids between the abdominal and pelvic cavities. Blood, fluid, and infection to the right of the dorsal mesointestine ("X" in Fig. 6.10B) will be contained by the loop of mesenteries, while fluid, elsewhere has free passage between the abdominal and pelvic cavities.

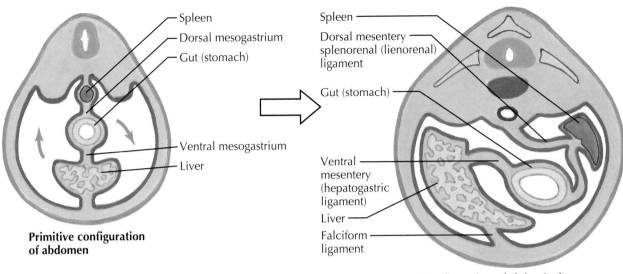

**Primitive configuration
of abdomen**

**Configuration of abdominal organs
and mesenteries after gut rotation**

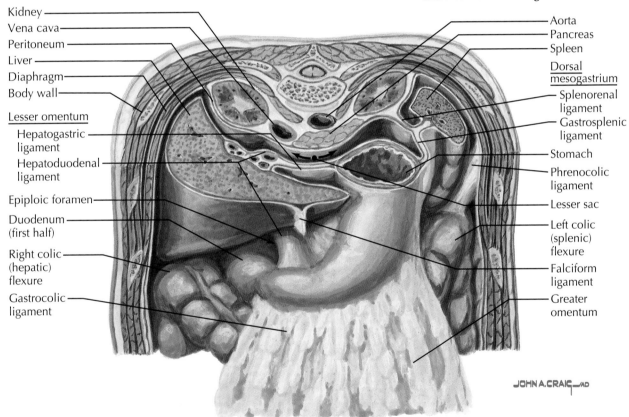

JOHN A. CRAIG—AD

6.11 ABDOMINAL LIGAMENTS

After the rotations of the foregut and midgut and growth of the dorsal mesogastrium (lesser peritoneal sac), the initially straight mesenteries of the abdominal foregut are in a very convoluted S-shaped arrangement from ventral to dorsal body wall. They are referred to as "ligaments," named by their shape or the organs they connect. Other types of ligaments are adhesions of mesenteries involving the transverse colon (phrenicocolic, gastrocolic, and hepatocolic ligaments) or fibrous cords (round ligament of the liver, ovarian ligament, and round ligament of the uterus).

CLINICAL POINT
Adhesion ligaments in surgery. Unlike most mesentery "ligaments," the adhesion ligaments of the transverse colon (e.g., phrenicocolic ligament) do not have neurovascular bundles within them. They can be cut without ligation during surgery to mobilize the transverse colon.

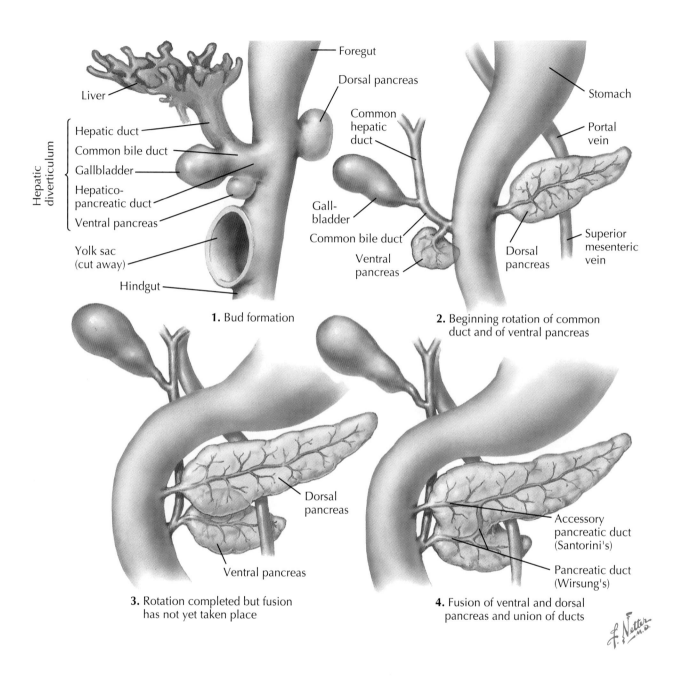

1. Bud formation

2. Beginning rotation of common duct and of ventral pancreas

3. Rotation completed but fusion has not yet taken place

4. Fusion of ventral and dorsal pancreas and union of ducts

6.12 ABDOMINAL FOREGUT ORGAN DEVELOPMENT

Growing off the abdominal foregut are a **dorsal pancreatic bud** and a ventral **liver diverticulum**. Sprouting from the latter are gallbladder and ventral pancreatic buds. The hepatic diverticulum gives rise to hepatocytes, the gallbladder, and the entire biliary apparatus. The ventral **pancreatic bud** and common bile duct migrate clockwise around the duodenum into the dorsal mesentery, where the ventral and dorsal pancreatic buds fuse. Although the ventral bud forms only part of the head of the pancreas, its duct joins that of the dorsal pancreatic bud to become the **major pancreatic duct** (of Wirsung). Vascular endothelial cells play an important role in the induction of endoderm of the liver, pancreas, and other visceral organs.

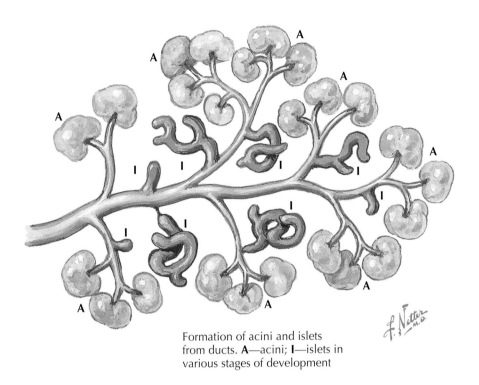

Formation of acini and islets
from ducts. **A**—acini; **I**—islets in
various stages of development

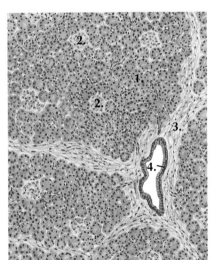

Low-power section of pancreas
1. acini, **2.** islet, **3.** interlobular
septum, **4.** interlobular duct

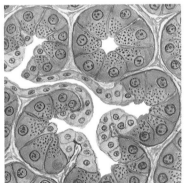

High magnification: relationship of
intercalated duct and centroacinar
cells to acini

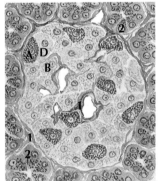

Pancreatic islet
A (= α-), **B** (= β-), and **D**-cells.
1. reticulum, **2.** acini

6.13 DEVELOPMENT OF PANCREATIC ACINI AND ISLETS

The pancreas is an exocrine and endocrine organ with serous **acini** and vascular **islets of Langerhans** that secrete insulin, glucagon, and somatostatin. The duct system begins with **centroacinar cells** within the acini. The pancreatic buds first develop under the inductive influence of endothelial cells, the notochord, and hepatic mesenchyme. Subsequent branching and elaboration of the ducts and acini involve numerous reciprocal interactions between endoderm and mesoderm typical of the development of gut-related glands. The inductive role of the mesenchyme is nonspecific and more important for the formation of acini than ducts. The endocrine islet cells are derived from early duct epithelium.

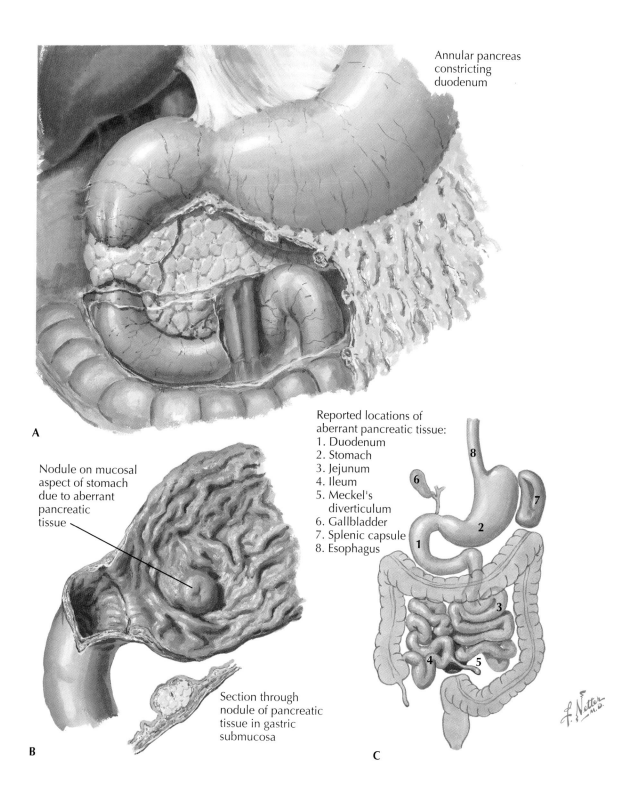

Annular pancreas constricting duodenum

A

Nodule on mucosal aspect of stomach due to aberrant pancreatic tissue

Section through nodule of pancreatic tissue in gastric submucosa

B

Reported locations of aberrant pancreatic tissue:
1. Duodenum
2. Stomach
3. Jejunum
4. Ileum
5. Meckel's diverticulum
6. Gallbladder
7. Splenic capsule
8. Esophagus

C

6.14 CONGENITAL PANCREATIC ANOMALIES

The pancreas may encircle and constrict the duodenum (Fig. 6.14A) if the ventral pancreatic bud is bifid and passes around both sides of the duodenum. Peristalsis through the duodenum will be impaired. Pancreatic tissue may develop abnormally in many locations in the GI tract, the spleen, and even the lungs. The sites are ranked in approximate order of frequency. The most common pancreatic anomaly is failure of fusion of the two pancreatic buds. Although typically asymptomatic, there is a higher risk of infection.

Segmental distribution of myotomes in fetus of 6 weeks

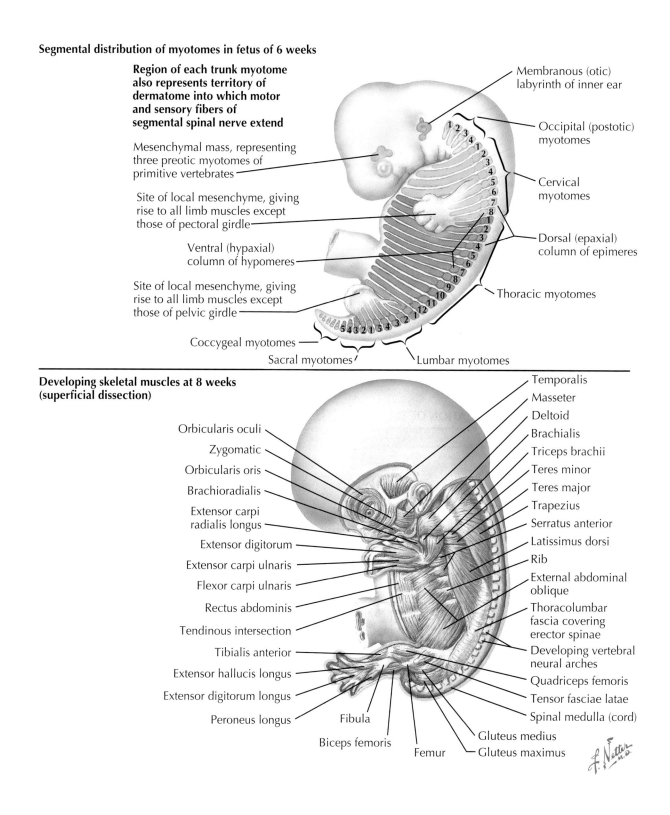

Region of each trunk myotome also represents territory of dermatome into which motor and sensory fibers of segmental spinal nerve extend

Mesenchymal mass, representing three preotic myotomes of primitive vertebrates

Site of local mesenchyme, giving rise to all limb muscles except those of pectoral girdle

Ventral (hypaxial) column of hypomeres

Site of local mesenchyme, giving rise to all limb muscles except those of pelvic girdle

Coccygeal myotomes

Sacral myotomes

Lumbar myotomes

Membranous (otic) labyrinth of inner ear

Occipital (postotic) myotomes

Cervical myotomes

Dorsal (epaxial) column of epimeres

Thoracic myotomes

Developing skeletal muscles at 8 weeks (superficial dissection)

Orbicularis oculi
Zygomatic
Orbicularis oris
Brachioradialis
Extensor carpi radialis longus
Extensor digitorum
Extensor carpi ulnaris
Flexor carpi ulnaris
Rectus abdominis
Tendinous intersection
Tibialis anterior
Extensor hallucis longus
Extensor digitorum longus
Peroneus longus

Temporalis
Masseter
Deltoid
Brachialis
Triceps brachii
Teres minor
Teres major
Trapezius
Serratus anterior
Latissimus dorsi
Rib
External abdominal oblique
Thoracolumbar fascia covering erector spinae
Developing vertebral neural arches
Quadriceps femoris
Tensor fasciae latae
Spinal medulla (cord)

Fibula
Biceps femoris
Femur
Gluteus medius
Gluteus maximus

6.19 DEVELOPMENT OF THE ABDOMINAL WALL

Muscles of the abdominal wall develop from the hypomeres of somites from spinal segments T7 to L1, with dermatome T10 at the level of umbilicus. As with the thoracic musculature, the abdominal muscles develop in three layers. There is a single vertical muscle anteriorly—the rectus abdominis.

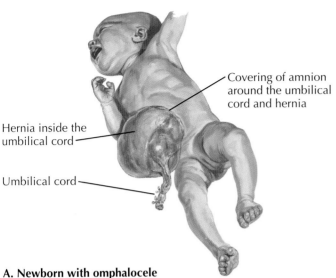

A. Newborn with omphalocele

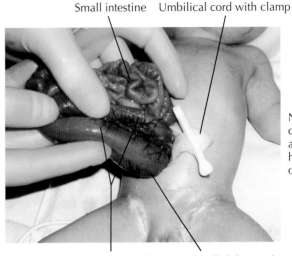

B. Newborn with gastroschisis
(Reused with permission from Polites S, Nathan JD. Newborn Abdominal Wall Defects. In Pediatric Gastrointestinal and Liver Disease, 6th edition. Edited by Wyllie R, Hyams JS, Kay M. Elsevier, Philadelphia 2020.)

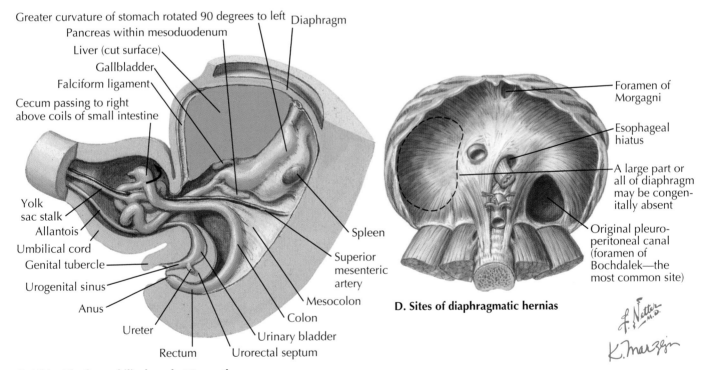

C. Midgut in the umbilical cord at 2 months

D. Sites of diaphragmatic hernias

6.20 ABDOMINAL HERNIAS

A **hernia** is typically the protrusion of an internal organ in a **sac of parietal peritoneum** through a weak spot in the abdominal wall (or other site). Potential sites include umbilicus (Figs. 6.20A and 6.20C), the ventral midline where the left and right sides must fuse (Fig. 6.20B), weak areas between muscles, the inguinal and femoral canals, and sites related to the diaphragm (Fig. 6.20D). Fig. 6.20 is a comparison of omphalocele (Figs. 6.20A with gastroschisis (Fig. 6.20B). The former is a herniation of the midgut into the umbilical cord (see Fig. 6.6); the organs are covered by the amnion that surrounds the umbilical cord. The latter is a defect in the abdominal wall where the left and right sides fail to fuse, usually to the right of the umbilical cord as seen in the figure. The herniated organs are not enclosed by a membrane; they are directly bathed in amniotic fluid.

11 weeks (43-mm crown–rump)

4 months (107-mm crown–rump)

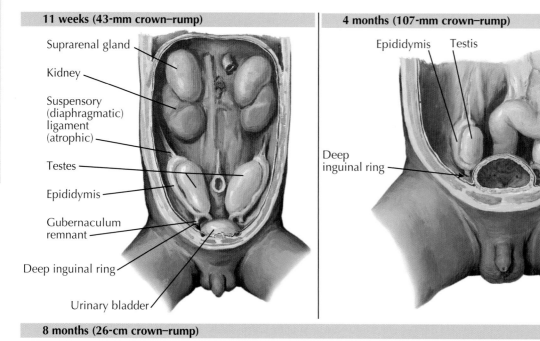

Suprarenal gland
Kidney
Suspensory (diaphragmatic) ligament (atrophic)
Testes
Epididymis
Gubernaculum remnant
Deep inguinal ring
Urinary bladder

Epididymis Testis
Deep inguinal ring
Gubernaculum

8 months (26-cm crown–rump)

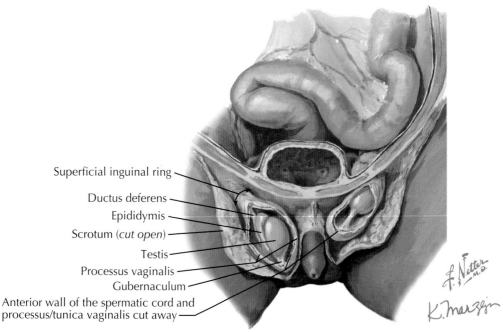

Superficial inguinal ring
Ductus deferens
Epididymis
Scrotum (cut open)
Testis
Processus vaginalis
Gubernaculum
Anterior wall of the spermatic cord and processus/tunica vaginalis cut away

6.21 TESTES' DESCENT THROUGH THE DEEP BODY WALL

The testes develop from the intermediate mesoderm that develops against the parietal peritoneum deep to the abdominal wall. They must pass through the deep muscle and fascial layers via the **inguinal canal** to end up in the scrotum for the proper temperature regulation required for sperm development. The openings at each end of the inguinal canal are the **deep and superficial inguinal rings**. The testes are "guided" into the scrotum by the fibrous **gubernaculum**, and they pull their **spermatic cord** of vessels and nerves along their path of descent. They pass through the inguinal canal behind an extension of parietal peritoneum, the **processus vaginalis**. It pinches off around each testis in the scrotum as its coelomic **tunica vaginalis testis**.

CLINICAL POINT

Cryptorchidism ("hidden testis"). Undescended testes are the most common congenital defects of the male genital system. In the fetus, the testes descend along the posterior abdominal wall, enter the inguinal canal after 28 weeks, and pass into the scrotum by 36 weeks, although it may take up to a year postnatally for the testes to reach the scrotum. One or both testes remain in the inguinal canal (or other less likely locations) at birth in 30% of premature male infants, 3% of full-term male infants, and 1% of male infants by the end of the first year. Undescended testes are associated with infertility and increased risk of testicular germ-cell tumors, inguinal hernia, testicular torsion with subsequent infarction, and psychological problems later in life.

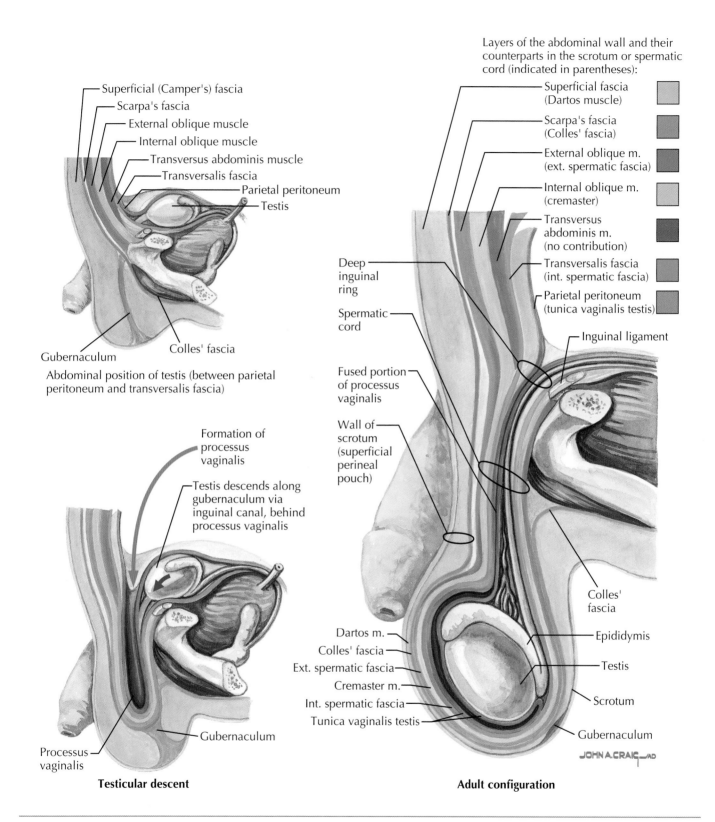

Layers of the abdominal wall and their counterparts in the scrotum or spermatic cord (indicated in parentheses):

- Superficial fascia (Dartos muscle)
- Scarpa's fascia (Colles' fascia)
- External oblique m. (ext. spermatic fascia)
- Internal oblique m. (cremaster)
- Transversus abdominis m. (no contribution)
- Transversalis fascia (int. spermatic fascia)
- Parietal peritoneum (tunica vaginalis testis)

Superficial (Camper's) fascia
Scarpa's fascia
External oblique muscle
Internal oblique muscle
Transversus abdominis muscle
Transversalis fascia
Parietal peritoneum
Testis
Colles' fascia
Gubernaculum

Abdominal position of testis (between parietal peritoneum and transversalis fascia)

Deep inguinal ring
Spermatic cord
Fused portion of processus vaginalis
Wall of scrotum (superficial perineal pouch)

Inguinal ligament
Colles' fascia
Epididymis
Testis
Scrotum
Gubernaculum

Dartos m.
Colles' fascia
Ext. spermatic fascia
Cremaster m.
Int. spermatic fascia
Tunica vaginalis testis

Formation of processus vaginalis
Testis descends along gubernaculum via inguinal canal, behind processus vaginalis
Gubernaculum
Processus vaginalis

Testicular descent

Adult configuration

JOHN A.CRAIG—AD

6.22 COVERINGS OF THE SPERMATIC CORD

As the testis passes through the inguinal canal, the layers of the deep body wall contribute to coverings of the spermatic cord (**external and internal spermatic fascia** with the **cremaster muscle** in between). The scrotum is an evagination of the superficial body wall. The superficial fascia and **Scarpa's fascia** of the latter extend into the scrotum as the **Dartos muscle** and **Colles'** fascia, respectively. Females have an inguinal canal that contains the remnant of the gubernaculum. Descent of the ovaries stops in the pelvis, and the gubernaculum attaches to the uterus. From the ovary to the uterus, it is the **ovarian ligament**, and from the uterus through the inguinal canal, it becomes the **round ligament of the uterus**.

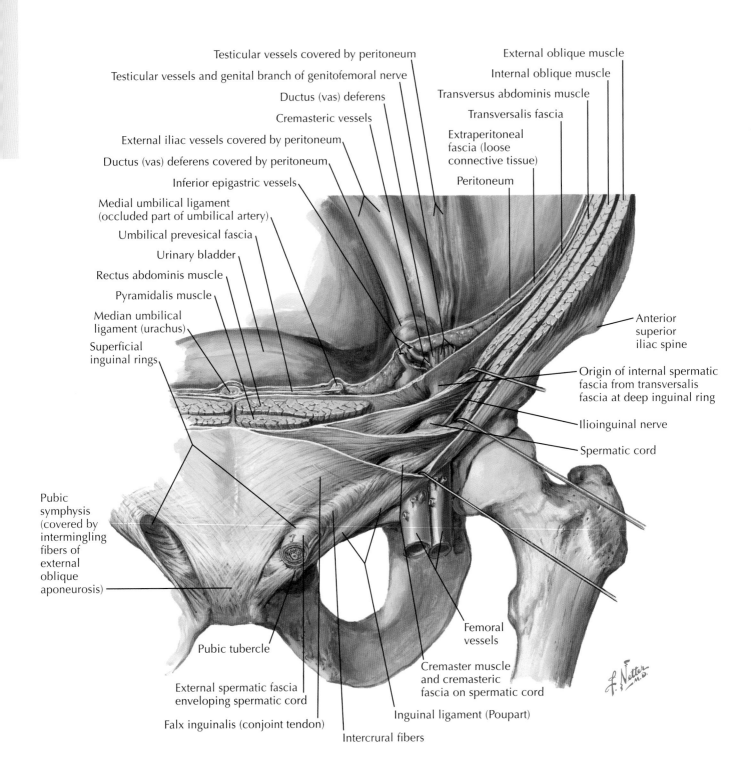

Testicular vessels covered by peritoneum

Testicular vessels and genital branch of genitofemoral nerve

Ductus (vas) deferens

Cremasteric vessels

External iliac vessels covered by peritoneum

Ductus (vas) deferens covered by peritoneum

Inferior epigastric vessels

Medial umbilical ligament (occluded part of umbilical artery)

Umbilical prevesical fascia

Urinary bladder

Rectus abdominis muscle

Pyramidalis muscle

Median umbilical ligament (urachus)

Superficial inguinal rings

Pubic symphysis (covered by intermingling fibers of external oblique aponeurosis)

External oblique muscle

Internal oblique muscle

Transversus abdominis muscle

Transversalis fascia

Extraperitoneal fascia (loose connective tissue)

Peritoneum

Anterior superior iliac spine

Origin of internal spermatic fascia from transversalis fascia at deep inguinal ring

Ilioinguinal nerve

Spermatic cord

Pubic tubercle

External spermatic fascia enveloping spermatic cord

Falx inguinalis (conjoint tendon)

Intercrural fibers

Inguinal ligament (Poupart)

Cremaster muscle and cremasteric fascia on spermatic cord

Femoral vessels

6.23 THE ADULT INGUINAL REGION

Fig. 6.23 is an anterior view of the left inguinal canal showing how the layers of the abdominal wall become the coverings of the spermatic cord. The testis begins its descent from the deepest location in the body wall just superficial to the parietal peritoneum. The first layer it encounters is the transversalis fascia that evaginates

to form the internal spermatic fascia. The rim of evagination is the deep inguinal ring. The transversus abdominis muscle has no contribution to the cord. The internal oblique gives rise to the cremaster muscle, and the external oblique aponeurosis continues as the external spermatic fascia just deep to an opening in the aponeurosis, the superficial inguinal ring.

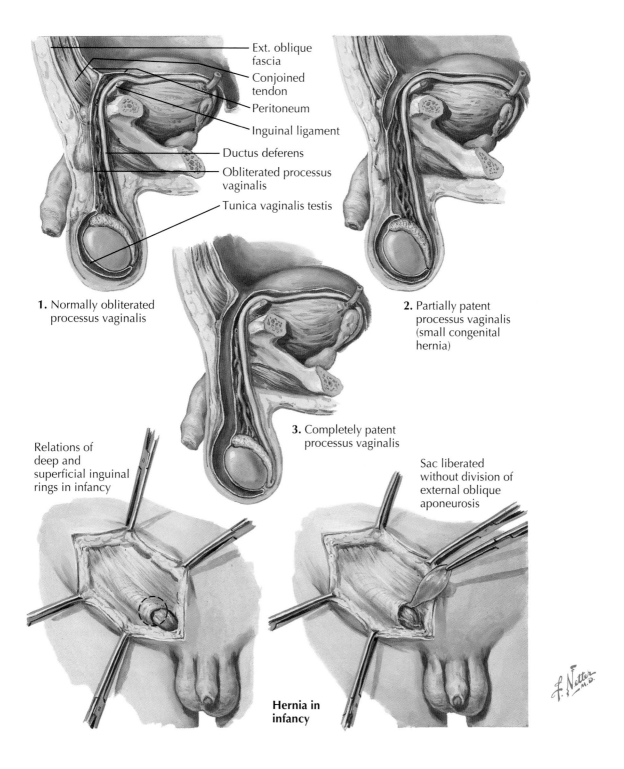

1. Normally obliterated processus vaginalis

2. Partially patent processus vaginalis (small congenital hernia)

3. Completely patent processus vaginalis

Ext. oblique fascia
Conjoined tendon
Peritoneum
Inguinal ligament
Ductus deferens
Obliterated processus vaginalis
Tunica vaginalis testis

Relations of deep and superficial inguinal rings in infancy

Sac liberated without division of external oblique aponeurosis

Hernia in infancy

6.24 ANOMALIES OF THE PROCESSUS VAGINALIS

The **processus vaginalis**, a finger-like extension of parietal peritoneum into the scrotum, usually becomes obliterated as it pinches off to become the tunica vaginalis testis. It may persist either completely or in part as a ready-made hernial sac passing through the inguinal canal. This is a congenital **indirect inguinal hernia**.

A section of the processus vaginalis may also persist as a cyst or hydrocele (not shown in Fig. 6.24). A **direct inguinal hernia** passes medial to the spermatic cord and inferior epigastric vessels. It does not go through the inguinal canal, but rather forces its way through the body wall under the conjoined tendon.

Terminology

Acinus	(L., "grape") A saclike dilation or cluster of cells found in many exocrine glands.
Alveolus	(L., "hollow") Sometimes used interchangeably with *acinus*.
Biliary apparatus	The bile system. Bile is a fat emulsifier produced in the liver by hepatocytes. It is secreted into bile canaliculi that converge on larger ducts until a single common bile duct joins the pancreatic duct to empty into the duodenum. The gallbladder stores and concentrates bile.
Cloaca	(L., "sewer") Chamber at the caudal end of the hindgut and allantois that divides in most mammals into the urinary bladder and rectum and related organs and structures. Other animals retain this common urinary, GI, and genital receptacle with one external opening.
Colles' fascia	Membranous inner lining of the scrotum and perineum. It is continuous with Scarpa's fascia, the deepest layer of the superficial body wall.
Deep inguinal ring	The margin of evagination of the transversalis fascia where it becomes the internal spermatic fascia. All of the constituents of the spermatic cord (and an indirect inguinal hernia) pass through the deep ring.
Exocrine	(G., "outside," "to separate") Usually refers to glands that secrete "outwardly" into a duct. Endocrine glands secrete their product "inwardly" into the bloodstream. Paracrine glands or cells secrete their product into the tissue around them to affect adjacent cells. Holocrine glands slough off cellular contents into ducts.
Greater omentum	In the embryo, it is the dorsal mesogastrium. Common use in the adult is restricted to the fused layers of the dorsal mesogastrium that cover the intestines below the transverse colon (the "apron" of the dorsal mesogastrium).
Greater peritoneal sac	Parietal peritoneum enclosing the abdominal cavity. It is the inner lining of the muscular abdominal wall.
Gubernaculum	(L., "helm or rudder") The fibrous cord that guides the descent of the testis from the abdominal cavity to the scrotum.
Hemorrhoids	Varicose dilations of veins in the anal canal. Internal hemorrhoids are above the pectinate line and related to the gut. External hemorrhoids are below the pectinate line and associated with the body wall.
Hepatocytes	Liver cells arranged in epithelial sheets. One cell type is responsible for all of the liver's metabolic functions.
Intercalate	(L., "to insert between") Intercalated ducts drain secretory acini in glands. In the pancreas, the duct system begins with centroacinar cells within acini then continues with intercalated, intralobular, and interlobular ducts that unite to form the main and accessory pancreatic ducts. In salivary glands (but not the pancreas), there are also striated (secretory) ducts.
Lesser omentum	In the embryo, it is the ventral mesogastrium. In the adult, it refers to the hepatogastric and hepatoduodenal ligaments.
Lesser peritoneal sac	A sac of dorsal mesogastrium that initially grows to the left and eventually drapes down over the transverse colon to form the greater omentum. Its cavity is the omental bursa.
Mesentery	Two opposing layers of visceral peritoneum anchoring the organs of the GI tract to the body wall. They contain fat and serve as a route for vessels, nerves, and lymphatics supplying the organs.
Mesothelium	A developmental term for the mesoderm-derived, simple squamous epithelium that lines the body cavities.
Omental bursa	The cavity of the lesser peritoneal sac.
Omental (epiploic) foramen	(G., epiploon = "omentum") Foramen of Winslow. Entry into the lesser peritoneal sac under the free edge of the lesser omentum (hepatoduodenal ligament).
Omentum (lesser and greater omentum)	(L., "fat skin") The fat-filled dorsal and ventral mesenteries of the stomach. The term is not used for other mesenteries. The ventral mesogastriuim is the lesser omentum, and the dorsal mesogastrium is the greater omentum.

Terminology—cont'd

Omphalocele	Hernia of the midgut in the umbilical cord. The midgut intestines naturally enter the umbilical cord as they begin their tremendous growth in length. Omphalocele results if they fail to return to the abdominal cavity.
Peristalsis	(G., "around" + "constriction") Wavelike contractions of the smooth muscle wall of the intestines or other tubular structures to propel its contents. It involves the coordinated contraction of circular muscle fibers to constrict the lumen and longitudinal fibers to shorten and dilate the organ tube.
Peritoneum	Layer of simple squamous epithelium (mesothelium) with underlying connective tissue. It lines the abdominopelvic cavity. Parietal peritoneum is against the body wall; visceral peritoneum covers the mesenteries and organs.
Portal triad	Common bile duct, common hepatic artery, and hepatic portal vein located in the free edge of the lesser omentum.
Processus vaginalis	(L., "sheathlike process") A fingerlike projection of parietal peritoneum extending through the inguinal canal that pinches off to form the tunica vaginalis testis, a coelomic sac covering the testis. The proximal part usually disappears but may persist as a congenital, indirect, inguinal hernial sac.
Root of a mesentery	Where an intestinal mesentery attaches to the body wall—the site where visceral peritoneum becomes parietal peritoneum.
Scarpa's fascia	The deepest layer of the superficial body wall. Thickest in the lower abdomen, it is a membrane continuous with Colles' fascia in the scrotum.
Serous	(Pertaining to serum—L., "whey"—the clear part of any body fluid) Membranes and glands in the body are serous or mucous. Serosa (versus mucosa) are the peritoneal, pleural, and pericardial linings of the body cavities that produce a proteinaceous, watery, lubricating fluid.
Situs inversus	(L., "site" + "reversed") A left-right reversal in symmetry where the organs are in mirror-image opposite locations of their normal position. Can involve only the thorax or abdomen, or the entire body.
Superficial inguinal ring	Opening in the external oblique muscle aponeurosis through which the spermatic cord passes. Just deep to the right, the aponeurosis gives rise to the external spermatic fascia.
Zymogen	(Gr., "leaven" + "born") Zymogen granules (vesicles) in the pancreas and other glands contain the inactive precursors of their secretory enzymes.

7

THE UROGENITAL SYSTEM

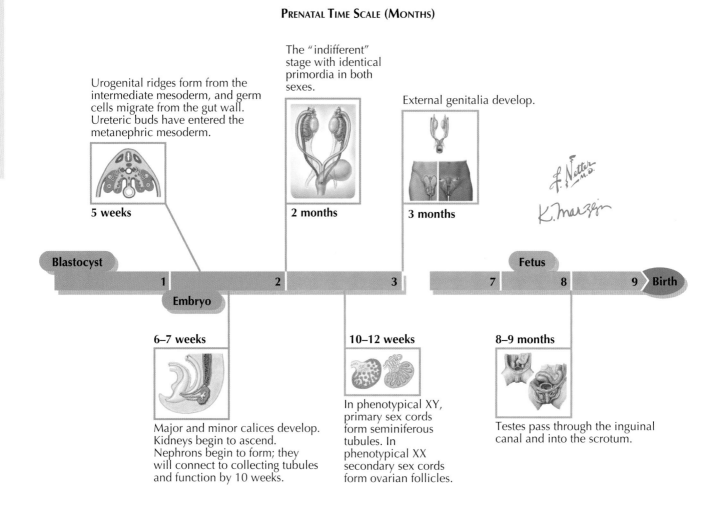

PRENATAL TIME SCALE (MONTHS)

Urogenital ridges form from the intermediate mesoderm, and germ cells migrate from the gut wall. Ureteric buds have entered the metanephric mesoderm.

5 weeks

The "indifferent" stage with identical primordia in both sexes.

2 months

External genitalia develop.

3 months

Blastocyst

Embryo

Fetus

1 2 3 7 8 9 **Birth**

6–7 weeks

Major and minor calices develop. Kidneys begin to ascend. Nephrons begin to form; they will connect to collecting tubules and function by 10 weeks.

10–12 weeks

In phenotypical XY, primary sex cords form seminiferous tubules. In phenotypical XX secondary sex cords form ovarian follicles.

8–9 months

Testes pass through the inguinal canal and into the scrotum.

7.1 TIMELINE

PRIMORDIA

Hindgut splanchnopleure and intermediate mesoderm of the gastrula (with somatopleure contributing to the external genitalia).

PLAN

At 8 weeks, all embryos have identical primordia in the indifferent stage of urogenital development, with gonads capable of developing into testes or ovaries. The process of sexual differentiation (influenced by genetic and hormonal factors) results in either phenotypical XY (male) or phenotypical XX (female) internal and external genital structures to develop. The kidneys develop from the intermediate mesoderm in three successive waves, from cranial to caudal, with the third, most inferior pair of kidneys (metanephros) becoming the permanent kidneys. Complicating factors are the relatively huge size of the middle, mesonephric kidney (the first functioning kidney) and the change in function of the mesonephric duct in phenotypical XY (male) development from urinary (a temporary ureter) to genital (the ductus deferens and related structures).

INCLUSION AND BIAS CONSIDERATION: SEXUAL DIFFERENTIATION AND VARIATION

There have been calls for the scientific and anatomical community to move beyond the binary categorizations of "anatomical sex" (or just female and male, representing the most frequent anatomical genital organ variants of the XX and XY genotypes). Presentation of sex as this binary does not allow for representation of sex as a continuum, which scientific advances suggest is a more accurate understanding. Examples of this include individuals with the XX or XY genotype who have undifferentiated gonads and/or external genital organs typically similar phenotypically to the opposite genetic sex. This is particularly important for embryology education—as noted, all early developing embryos have an "indifferent" stage. It is only the complex interaction of chromosomal, genetic, hormonal, and structural development that result in "typical" sexual differentiation. Throughout this chapter, this spectrum of sex is acknowledged frequently with the terms phenotypical XY (male) and phenotypical XX (female). An individual's sex is determined, in part, by the internal and external genitalia that develop. These terms aim to recognize that phenotypic sex is just a common variation of sexual differentiation but allow for understanding that it does not always align with genotypic sex or with gender.

Finally, it is critical to always be clear about the differences between sex (often sex assigned at birth) and gender. Gender is a social, psychological, and cultural construct that includes self-identification elements. This is independent of physical structures that can inform sex assigned at birth or chromosomal/genetic sex. There are entire articles, chapters and books dedicated to addressing these concepts with more depth, and we encourage readers to explore them. But, in the context of this chapter, we hope to recognize how even seemingly small changes in terminology can be steps in the right direction for inclusive practice and representation.

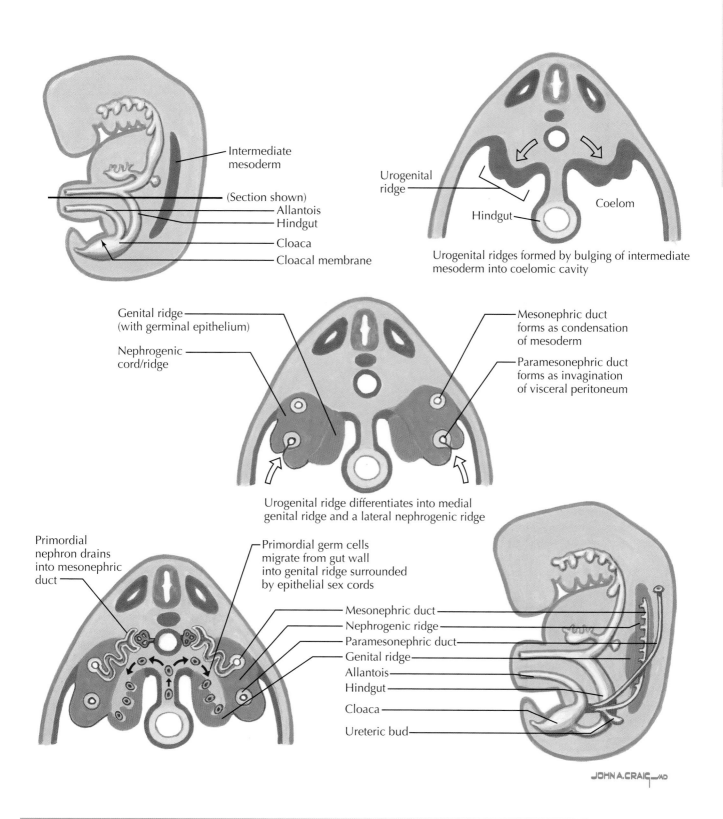

Urogenital ridges formed by bulging of intermediate mesoderm into coelomic cavity

Urogenital ridge differentiates into medial genital ridge and a lateral nephrogenic ridge

JOHN A.CRAIG—AD

7.2 EARLY PRIMORDIA

The caudal end of the **hindgut** has a dilated chamber, the **cloaca**. Its endoderm is in tight contact with the surface ectoderm, and together they form the **cloacal membrane**. Extending from the cloaca into the umbilical cord is the **allantois**. The intermediate mesoderm of the gastrula bulges into the dorsal aspect of the intraembryonic coelom as a **urogenital ridge** on each side. It develops into two ridges: a medial **genital (gonadal) ridge** and a lateral **nephrogenic ridge** or **cord**. Primordial germ cells begin to migrate from the endoderm of the hindgut toward the genital ridge through the dorsal mesentery. A **mesonephric (wolffian) duct** and **paramesonephric (Müllerian) duct** form in the nephrogenic ridge (cord).

Abdominal foregut, midgut, and hindgut at 5 weeks

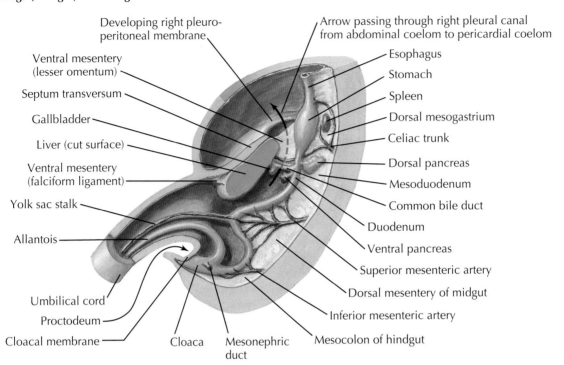

Developing right pleuro-peritoneal membrane

Ventral mesentery (lesser omentum)

Septum transversum

Gallbladder

Liver (cut surface)

Ventral mesentery (falciform ligament)

Yolk sac stalk

Allantois

Umbilical cord

Proctodeum

Cloacal membrane

Cloaca

Mesonephric duct

Arrow passing through right pleural canal from abdominal coelom to pericardial coelom

Esophagus

Stomach

Spleen

Dorsal mesogastrium

Celiac trunk

Dorsal pancreas

Mesoduodenum

Common bile duct

Duodenum

Ventral pancreas

Superior mesenteric artery

Dorsal mesentery of midgut

Inferior mesenteric artery

Mesocolon of hindgut

Division of the cloaca by the urorectal septum

Urogenital sinus and rectum

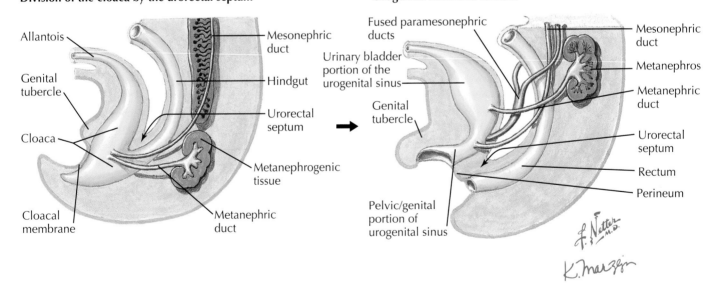

Allantois

Genital tubercle

Cloaca

Cloacal membrane

Mesonephric duct

Hindgut

Urorectal septum

Metanephrogenic tissue

Metanephric duct

Fused paramesonephric ducts

Urinary bladder portion of the urogenital sinus

Genital tubercle

Pelvic/genital portion of urogenital sinus

Mesonephric duct

Metanephros

Metanephric duct

Urorectal septum

Rectum

Perineum

7.3 DIVISION OF THE CLOACA

The **urorectal septum** between the allantois and hindgut divides the cloaca in the frontal plane into an anterior **urogenital sinus** and posterior **rectum** (Fig. 7.3B). The septum divides the cloacal membrane into a urogenital membrane and anal membrane. The upper part of the urogenital (UG) sinus is the fusiform urinary bladder. The lower pelvic and phallic parts of the UG sinus

(UG sinus proper) form the urethra and related glands and structures in each sex. The genital portion of the urogenital sinus is closely related to the **genital tubercle**, a swelling of somatopleure (Fig. 7.3C). The metanephric duct (future ureter) opens into the developing urinary bladder; the male (mesonephric) and female (paramesonephric) genital ducts shift to a more caudal position on the UG sinus.

A. Phenotypical XY exstrophy of the bladder

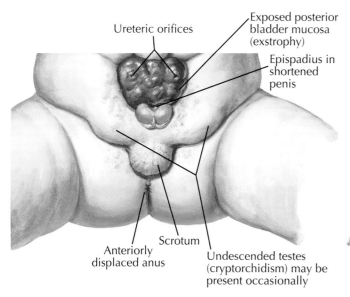

Ureteric orifices

Exposed posterior bladder mucosa (exstrophy)

Epispadius in shortened penis

Anteriorly displaced anus

Scrotum

Undescended testes (cryptorchidism) may be present occasionally

B. Phenotypical XX exstrophy of the bladder

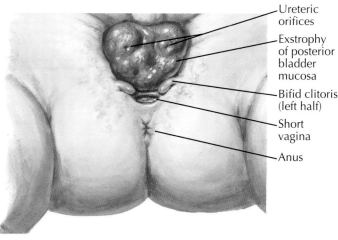

Ureteric orifices

Exstrophy of posterior bladder mucosa

Bifid clitoris (left half)

Short vagina

Anus

C. Basis for exstrophy of the bladder (5 weeks)

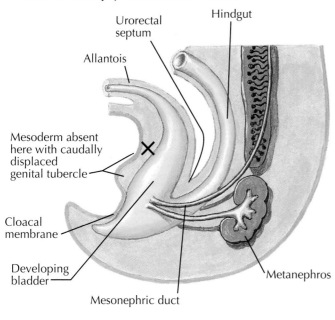

Urorectal septum

Hindgut

Allantois

Mesoderm absent here with caudally displaced genital tubercle

Cloacal membrane

Developing bladder

Mesonephric duct

Metanephros

D. Basis for exstrophy of the cloaca (4 weeks; newborn not shown). Cloacal membrane and adjacent mesoderm breaks down for exstrophy of combined bladder and hindgut mucosa. Separated pubic bones, omphalocele, hypoplastic genital organs, and spina bifida often result as well.

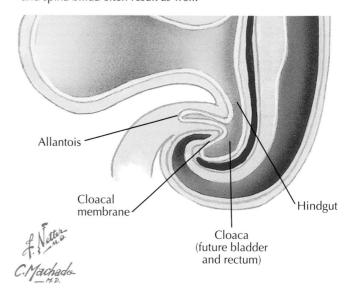

Allantois

Cloacal membrane

Hindgut

Cloaca (future bladder and rectum)

7.4 EXSTROPHY OF THE BLADDER AND CLOACA

Exstrophy of the bladder and cloaca are lower abdominal wall defects that have parallels with ectopia cordis in the thorax and gastroschisis in the midabdomen. The lower abdominal wall is open, the anterior wall of the bladder or cloaca is absent, and the posterior mucosal wall of the bladder or cloaca protrudes through the defect. Exstrophy of the bladder occurs in 1/10,000 to 1/40,000 births (twice as common in males), and exstrophy of the cloaca occurs in 1/250,000 births. Exstrophy of the cloaca can appear similar to exstrophy of the bladder, but the defect occurs earlier (see Fig. 7.4D), resulting in more severe multisystem consequences.

FISTULAS RESULTING FROM THE INCOMPLETE DIVISION OF THE CLOACA

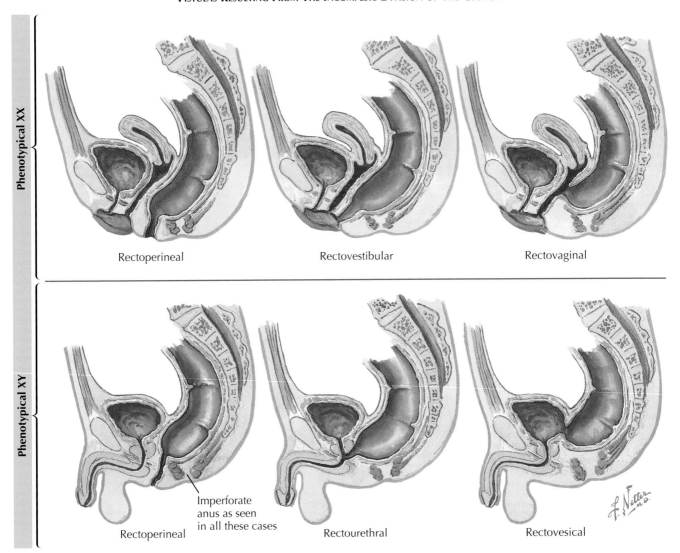

Phenotypical XX

Rectoperineal · Rectovestibular · Rectovaginal

Phenotypical XY

Rectoperineal · Imperforate anus as seen in all these cases · Rectourethral · Rectovesical

7.5 CONGENITAL CLOACAL ANOMALIES

If the urorectal septum does not completely divide the cloaca, the rectum will connect anteriorly with urinary or genital structures derived from the urogenital sinus. The resulting fistulas are all associated with an imperforate anus. A rectoperineal fistula opens to the surface. It is an abnormal connection anterior to the external anal sphincter (and anus) through the central tendon of the perineum (perineal body).

Section through pronephros

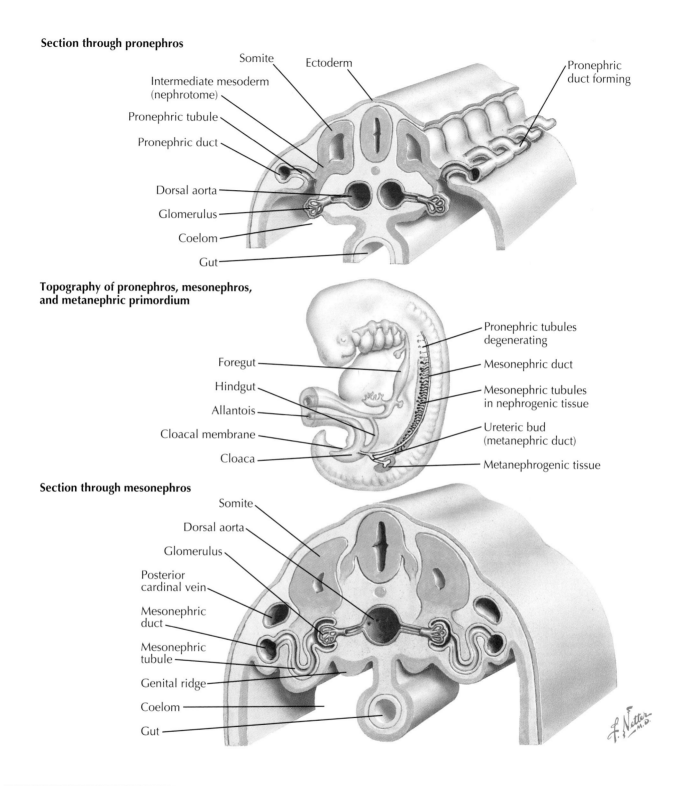

Somite
Ectoderm
Pronephric duct forming
Intermediate mesoderm (nephrotome)
Pronephric tubule
Pronephric duct
Dorsal aorta
Glomerulus
Coelom
Gut

Topography of pronephros, mesonephros, and metanephric primordium

Foregut
Hindgut
Allantois
Cloacal membrane
Cloaca
Pronephric tubules degenerating
Mesonephric duct
Mesonephric tubules in nephrogenic tissue
Ureteric bud (metanephric duct)
Metanephrogenic tissue

Section through mesonephros

Somite
Dorsal aorta
Glomerulus
Posterior cardinal vein
Mesonephric duct
Mesonephric tubule
Genital ridge
Coelom
Gut

7.6 PRONEPHROS, MESONEPHROS, AND METANEPHROS

The intermediate mesoderm differentiates into nephrogenic tissue in the nephrogenic ridge lateral to the genital ridge. From cranial to caudal it forms three successive kidneys.

- The **pronephros** never fully develops and quickly diminishes.
- The **mesonephros** is the first functioning kidney, with glomeruli, **mesonephric tubules**, and a **mesonephric duct** that drains embryonic urine into the dividing cloaca.

- The **metanephros** becomes the permanent kidney.

The **metanephric duct** (future ureter) develops from a **ureteric bud** that grows from the caudal end of the mesonephric duct into the metanephric mesoderm. It quickly shifts inferiorly to make its own connection with the cloaca.

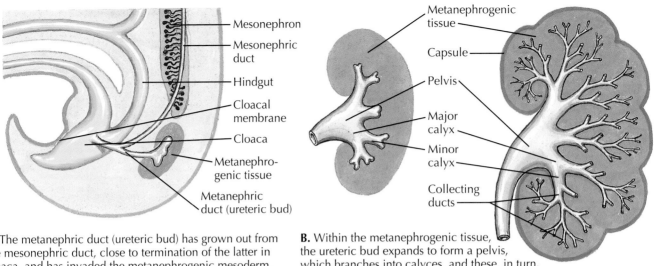

A. The metanephric duct (ureteric bud) has grown out from the mesonephric duct, close to termination of the latter in cloaca, and has invaded the metanephrogenic mesoderm.

B. Within the metanephrogenic tissue, the ureteric bud expands to form a pelvis, which branches into calyces, and these, in turn, bud into successive generations of collecting ducts.

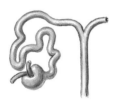

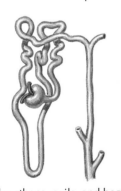

C. The distal ends of the collecting ducts connect with the tubule system of the nephron developing from the metanephric mesoderm. The nephron extends from the collecting duct to the renal corpuscle.

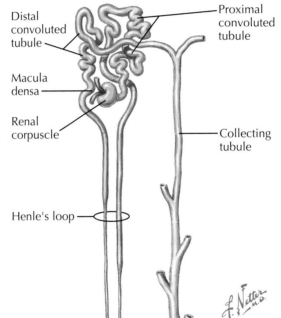

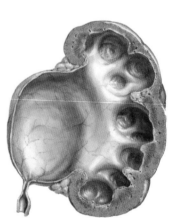

D. The tubule lengthens, coils, and begins to dip down toward the renal pelvis, as Henle's loop; one area of the tubule remains close to the glomerular mouth, as the future macula densa.

E. The loop elongates; renal corpuscle, proximal tubule, Henle's loop, distal tubule, and macula densa of mature nephron are thus derived from metanephrogenic mesoderm and collecting tubules from the metanephric duct.

F. Polycystic kidney sectioned: only a shell of renal parenchyma remains

7.7 DEVELOPMENT OF THE METANEPHROS

The metanephric kidneys become the permanent kidneys. Each kidney develops from two primordia: a **ureteric bud** from a mesonephric duct that grows into the **metanephric mesoderm** at the caudal end of the intermediate mesoderm of the gastrula. The ureteric bud (metanephric duct) soon makes its own connection to the urinary bladder. The ureter, renal pelvis, calyces, and collecting ducts of each kidney develop from the ureteric bud. The tubule system of the nephron (proximal and distal convoluted tubules, Henle's loop, and Bowman's capsule of the renal corpuscle) develops from the metanephric mesoderm.

CLINICAL POINT

Polycystic kidney (Fig. 7.7F) is a condition where multiple urinary cysts form and renal parenchyma diminishes. Included are autosomal dominant and recessive forms that can develop any time between the fetal period and adulthood. Pathogenesis in both is based on ciliary dysfunction, not obstruction from the lack of connection between the two primordia that must fuse.

Ascent and rotation of the kidneys in embryological development

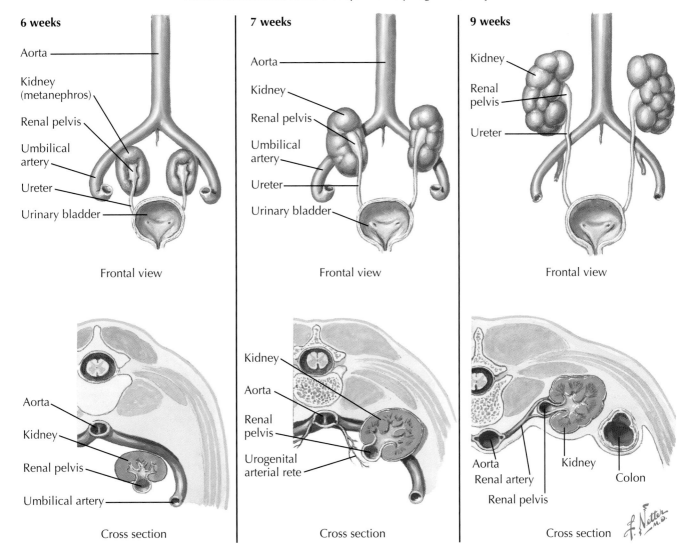

6 weeks

Aorta

Kidney
(metanephros)

Renal pelvis

Umbilical
artery

Ureter

Urinary bladder

Frontal view

Aorta

Kidney

Renal pelvis

Umbilical artery

Cross section

7 weeks

Aorta

Kidney

Renal pelvis

Umbilical
artery

Ureter

Urinary bladder

Frontal view

Kidney

Aorta

Renal
pelvis

Urogenital
arterial rete

Cross section

9 weeks

Kidney

Renal
pelvis

Ureter

Frontal view

Aorta
Renal artery

Renal pelvis

Kidney

Colon

Cross section

7.8 ASCENT AND ROTATION OF THE METANEPHRIC KIDNEYS

After week 8, the mesonephric mesoderm begins to disappear. In phenotypical XX (females), the mesonephric (Wolffian) duct disappears; in phenotypical XY (males), it connects to the developing testis as the ductus (vas) deferens. The metanephric, permanent kidney is in the pelvis at the caudal end of the intermediate mesoderm. It ascends to the posterior wall of the abdomen. The renal hilum of the metanephric kidneys faces anteriorly in the pelvis; the smooth, convex surface is posterior. As the kidneys ascend to the posterior abdominal wall, each rotates 90 degrees so that the renal pelvis and blood vessels in the hilum are medial as in adults. The kidneys are in a retroperitoneal location during the entire process.

Anomalies of renal rotation

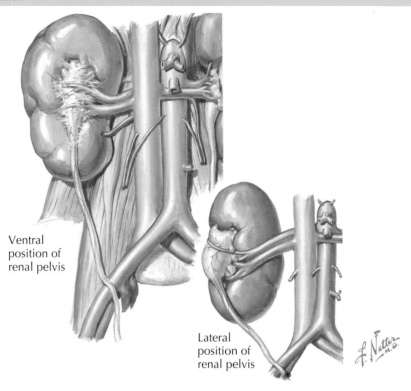

Ventral position of renal pelvis

Lateral position of renal pelvis

Renal fusion

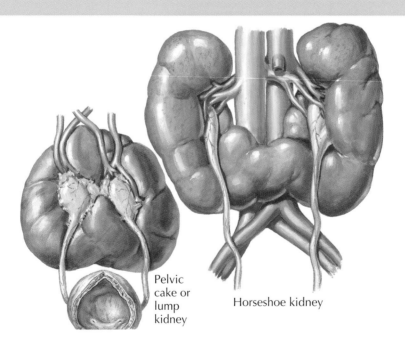

Pelvic cake or lump kidney

Horseshoe kidney

7.9 KIDNEY ROTATION ANOMALIES AND RENAL FUSION

Anomalies include failure of the metanephric kidneys to ascend, failure to rotate, excessive rotation, and rotation in the opposite direction. The ureteric buds may also fuse in the pelvis. If a fused kidney ascends, it encounters the inferior mesenteric artery (not shown in Fig. 7.9) and assumes the shape of a horseshoe as it extends around it.

Ectopia of the kidney

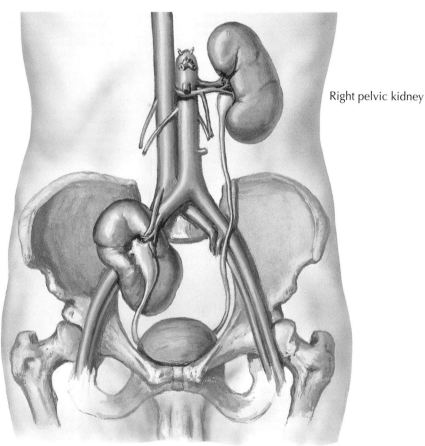

Right pelvic kidney

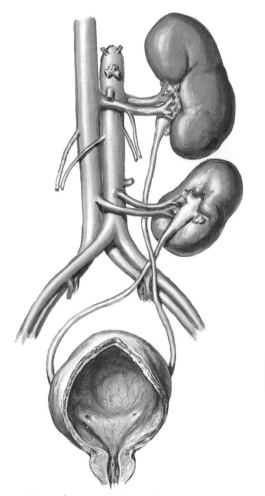

Crossed ectopia of the right kidney

7.10 KIDNEY MIGRATION ANOMALIES AND BLOOD VESSEL FORMATION

A kidney can fail to ascend on one side only, or a kidney can migrate to the opposite side of the body. The development of renal blood vessels is unique. Most organs "trail" their blood supply as they migrate. As the kidneys ascend, new blood vessels form at higher levels of the aorta and inferior vena cava and connect to the kidneys as lower vessels disappear. Renal arteries of pelvic kidneys originate near the bifurcation of the aorta. For normal adult kidneys, they are at the level of the superior mesenteric arteries of the midgut. Sometimes, more inferior renal vessels fail to disappear. This is the embryonic basis of multiple renal arteries and veins in adults.

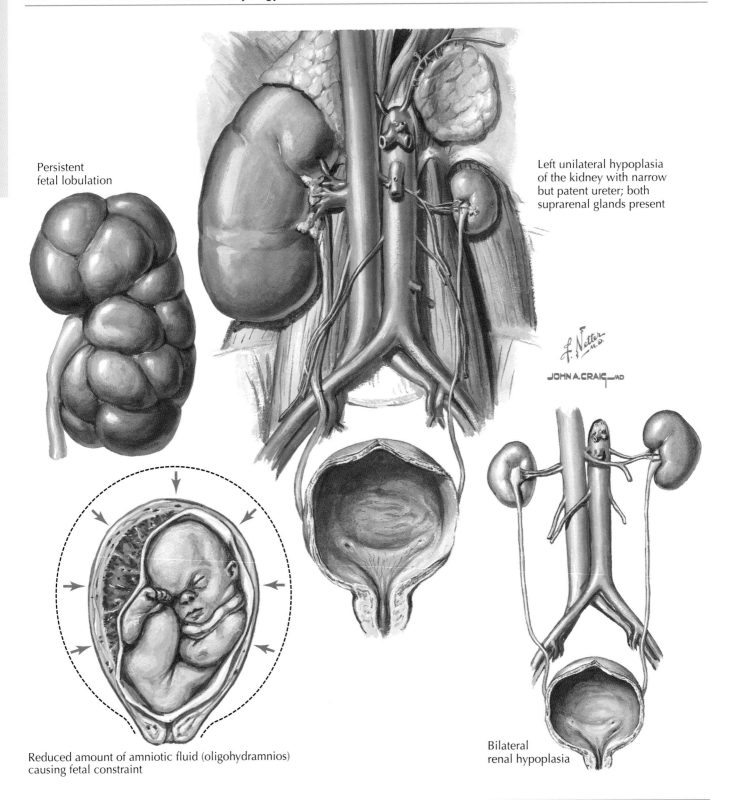

Persistent
fetal lobulation

Left unilateral hypoplasia
of the kidney with narrow
but patent ureter; both
suprarenal glands present

Reduced amount of amniotic fluid (oligohydramnios)
causing fetal constraint

Bilateral
renal hypoplasia

7.11 HYPOPLASIA

A kidney may be underdeveloped (hypoplasia) or completely absent (agenesis), and either condition may be unilateral or bilateral. Development of the suprarenal (adrenal) glands is unrelated to the development of the kidneys. The suprarenal glands are usually normal in size and location if the kidneys are ectopic or hypoplastic. Another kidney abnormality is persistent fetal lobulation. Fetal kidneys do not have the smooth surface of adult kidneys.

CLINICAL POINT

Oligohydramnios. This is a deficiency of amniotic fluid, which is fetal urine. Although there can be maternal causes related to placental insufficiency, an important fetal cause is renal agenesis. Amniotic fluid is important for cushioning the fetus, allowing for normal movement, and for proper development of the lungs, upper airway, and facial swallowing muscles. An outcome of severe oligohydramnios is the **Potter deformation sequence** (see Fig. 1.21), where fetal constraint leads to many secondary anomalies, such as facial variations and club feet.

Incomplete duplication of ureter

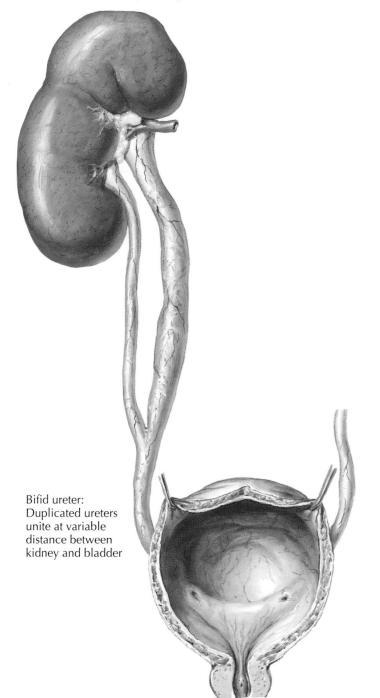

Bifid ureter:
Duplicated ureters
unite at variable
distance between
kidney and bladder

Anomalies of renal pelvis and calyces

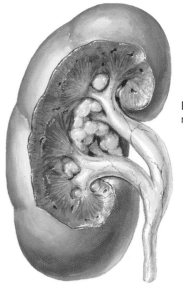

Duplicated
renal pelvis

Anomalies in number of kidneys

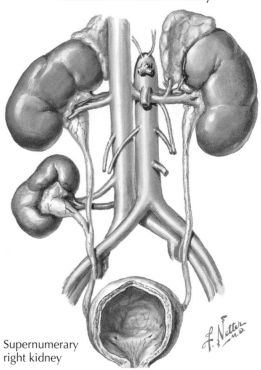

Supernumerary
right kidney

7.12 URETERIC BUD DUPLICATION

The effects of division of the ureteric bud range from bifurcation of the renal pelvis or ureter to complete duplication of the ureter and kidney. The greater the extent of division of the ureteric bud, the more likely the metanephric mesoderm will also divide and form two kidneys. Like most of the other anomalies, duplication can be unilateral or bilateral.

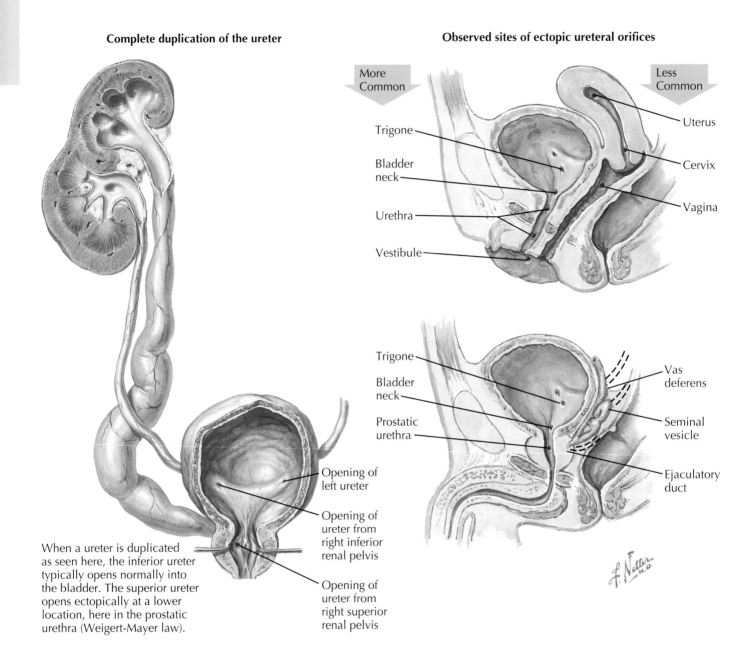

Complete duplication of the ureter

Observed sites of ectopic ureteral orifices

More Common

Less Common

Trigone

Bladder neck

Urethra

Vestibule

Uterus

Cervix

Vagina

When a ureter is duplicated as seen here, the inferior ureter typically opens normally into the bladder. The superior ureter opens ectopically at a lower location, here in the prostatic urethra (Weigert-Mayer law).

Opening of left ureter

Opening of ureter from right inferior renal pelvis

Opening of ureter from right superior renal pelvis

Trigone

Bladder neck

Prostatic urethra

Vas deferens

Seminal vesicle

Ejaculatory duct

7.13 ECTOPIC URETERS

The ureteric buds originate from the mesonephric duct instead of the cloaca, and this is often the embryonic basis for the ectopic location of the distal ureter in pelvic organs. The mesonephric duct migrates to a lower position on the UG sinus in both sexes before it disappears in the phenotypical XX (female) and becomes the vas deferens in the phenotypical XY development (male). The ureters can be carried with it to open on the urethra, prostate, vestibule, or other structures inferior to the bladder.

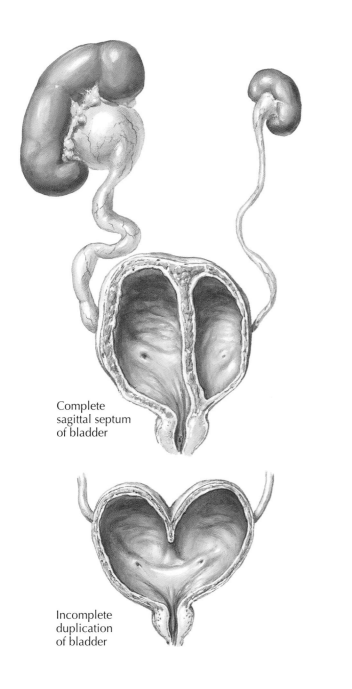

Complete
sagittal septum
of bladder

Incomplete
duplication
of bladder

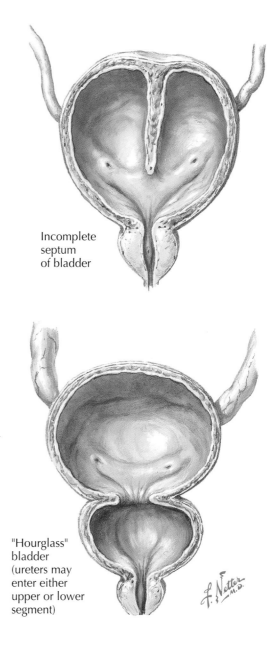

Incomplete
septum
of bladder

"Hourglass"
bladder
(ureters may
enter either
upper or lower
segment)

7.14 BLADDER ANOMALIES

The urinary bladder separates from the rectum when the urorectal septum divides the cloaca in a coronal plane between the allantois and hindgut. Partial or complete septa in a sagittal plane within the urinary bladder are unrelated to this process. They usually result from duplication of the cloaca, and the rectum and part of the colon are often affected as well. The mechanisms for other types of division or constriction of the bladder are not as well understood.

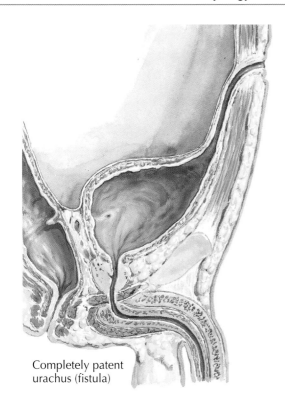

Completely patent
urachus (fistula)

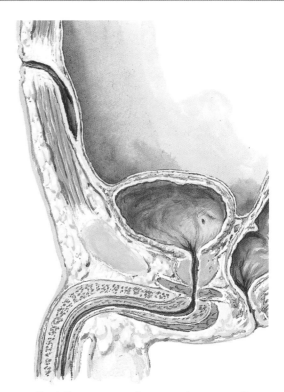

Partially patent urachus; opening externally
(external sinus), blind internally

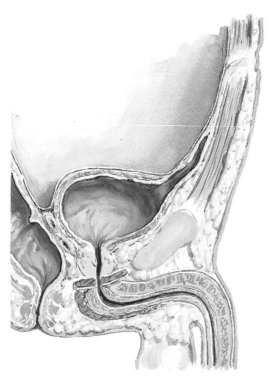

Partially patent urachus; opening internally
(internal sinus), blind externally

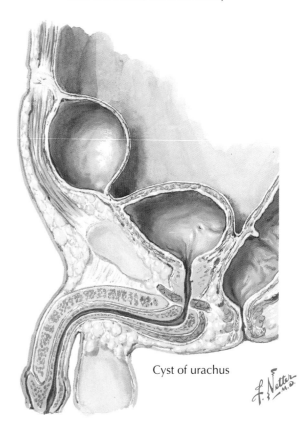

Cyst of urachus

7.15 ALLANTOIS/URACHUS ANOMALIES

The **urachus** is the fibrous remnant of the **allantois**, an extension of the cloaca/UG sinus into the umbilical cord. The lumen of the allantois may persist as a **fistula** (completely patent lumen), **sinus** (blind pit at either end), or **cyst** (enclosed swelling). These types of congenital defects may occur in any tubular primordium in the embryo that is supposed to form a fibrous cord or disappear. See Fig. 6.6 for an example of the yolk sac stalk.

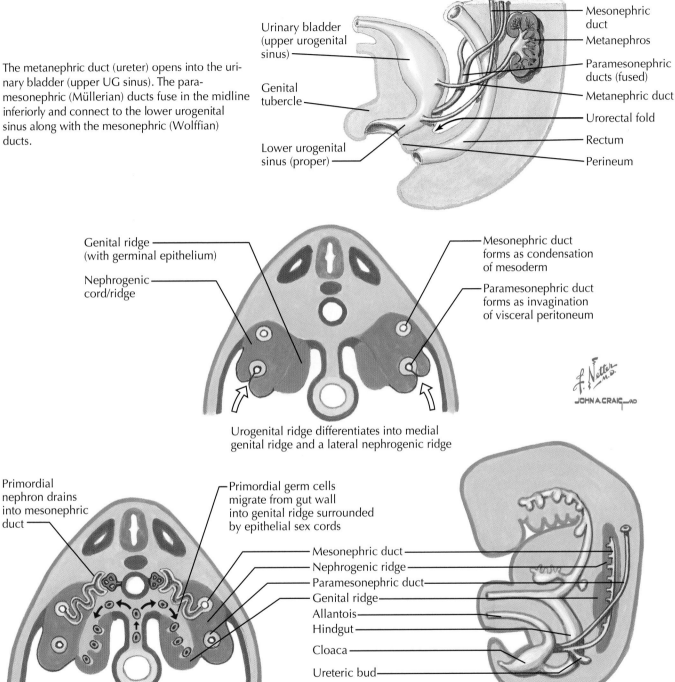

The metanephric duct (ureter) opens into the urinary bladder (upper UG sinus). The paramesonephric (Müllerian) ducts fuse in the midline inferiorly and connect to the lower urogenital sinus along with the mesonephric (Wolffian) ducts.

Urinary bladder (upper urogenital sinus)

Genital tubercle

Lower urogenital sinus (proper)

Mesonephric duct

Metanephros

Paramesonephric ducts (fused)

Metanephric duct

Urorectal fold

Rectum

Perineum

Genital ridge (with germinal epithelium)

Nephrogenic cord/ridge

Mesonephric duct forms as condensation of mesoderm

Paramesonephric duct forms as invagination of visceral peritoneum

Urogenital ridge differentiates into medial genital ridge and a lateral nephrogenic ridge

Primordial nephron drains into mesonephric duct

Primordial germ cells migrate from gut wall into genital ridge surrounded by epithelial sex cords

Mesonephric duct

Nephrogenic ridge

Paramesonephric duct

Genital ridge

Allantois

Hindgut

Cloaca

Ureteric bud

7.16 PRIMORDIA OF THE GENITAL SYSTEM

The genital primordia include the **genital tubercle** of somatopleure associated with the lower portion of the **urogenital sinus** and the **gonad** developing from the **genital ridge** of intermediate mesoderm. The **paramesonephric duct** develops beside the **mesonephric duct** by an invagination of the peritoneum. The gonads are closely applied to the mesonephric kidneys, a relationship that is very important in the development of testicular-associated structures. When the mesonephric kidneys disappear, the mesonephric duct and tubules connect with the developing testis and change their function from urinary (mesonephric ureter) to genital (ductus deferens, seminal vesicle, ejaculatory duct, and related structures).

Anterior view of 8-week indifferent stage. The mesonephric kidney will disappear in both sexes.

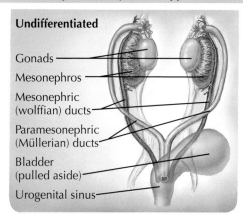

Undifferentiated

- Gonads
- Mesonephros
- Mesonephric (wolffian) ducts
- Paramesonephric (Müllerian) ducts
- Bladder (pulled aside)
- Urogenital sinus

Lateral view of differentiation in both sexes from the identical primordia in the indifferent stage.

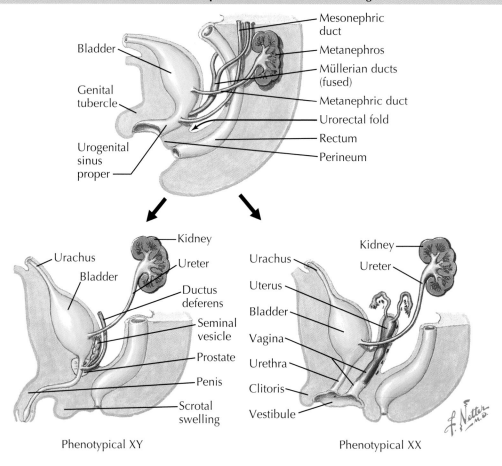

Bladder
Genital tubercle
Urogenital sinus proper

Mesonephric duct
Metanephros
Müllerian ducts (fused)
Metanephric duct
Urorectal fold
Rectum
Perineum

Urachus
Bladder
Kidney
Ureter
Ductus deferens
Seminal vesicle
Prostate
Penis
Scrotal swelling

Phenotypical XY

Urachus
Uterus
Bladder
Vagina
Urethra
Clitoris
Vestibule
Kidney
Ureter

Phenotypical XX

7.17 8-WEEK UNDIFFERENTIATED (INDIFFERENT) STAGE

All embryos have the same primordia in the undifferentiated stage at the end of the embryonic period (8 weeks). In phenotypical XY (males), the paramesonephric ducts degenerate. The mesonephric ducts become the ductus deferens, ejaculatory ducts, and seminal vesicles. The urogenital sinus develops into the urinary bladder, prostate gland, bulbourethral (Cowper's) and paraurethral glands,

and prostatic, membranous, and penile (spongy) urethra. In phenotypical XX (females), the mesonephric ducts degenerate, and the paramesonephric ducts develop into the uterine tubes, uterus, and upper part of the vagina. The UG sinus forms the bladder, urethra, greater vestibular and paraurethral glands, vestibule, and lower part of the vagina. The allantois becomes the fibrous urachus in both sexes.

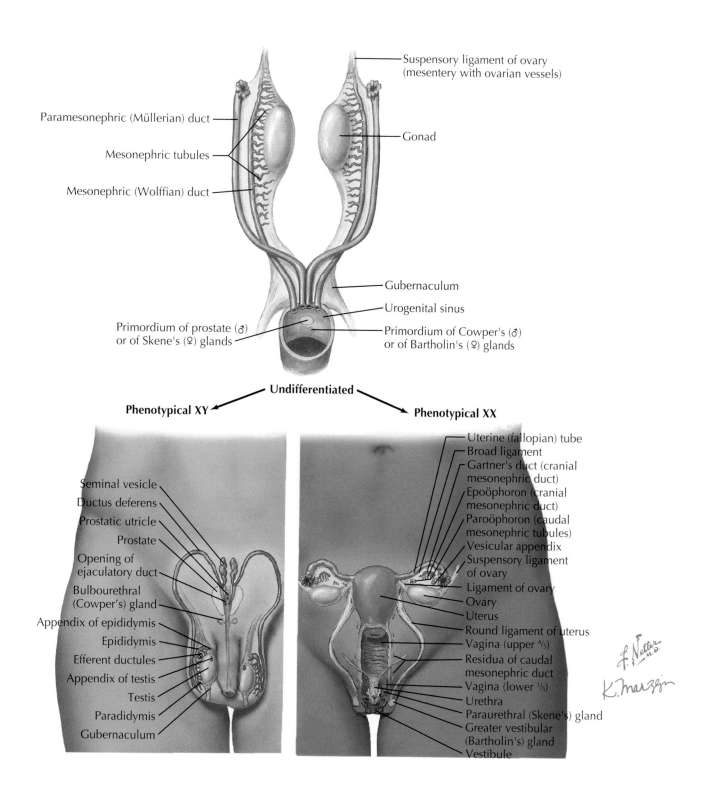

- Suspensory ligament of ovary (mesentery with ovarian vessels)
- Paramesonephric (Müllerian) duct
- Mesonephric tubules
- Mesonephric (Wolffian) duct
- Gonad
- Gubernaculum
- Urogenital sinus
- Primordium of prostate (♂) or of Skene's (♀) glands
- Primordium of Cowper's (♂) or of Bartholin's (♀) glands

Undifferentiated

Phenotypical XY

Phenotypical XX

- Seminal vesicle
- Ductus deferens
- Prostatic utricle
- Prostate
- Opening of ejaculatory duct
- Bulbourethral (Cowper's) gland
- Appendix of epididymis
- Epididymis
- Efferent ductules
- Appendix of testis
- Testis
- Paradidymis
- Gubernaculum

- Uterine (fallopian) tube
- Broad ligament
- Gartner's duct (cranial mesonephric duct)
- Epoöphoron (cranial mesonephric duct)
- Paroöphoron (caudal mesonephric tubules)
- Vesicular appendix
- Suspensory ligament of ovary
- Ligament of ovary
- Ovary
- Uterus
- Round ligament of uterus
- Vagina (upper ⁴/₅)
- Residua of caudal mesonephric duct
- Vagina (lower ¹/₅)
- Urethra
- Paraurethral (Skene's) gland
- Greater vestibular (Bartholin's) gland
- Vestibule

7.18 ANTERIOR VIEW OF THE DERIVATIVES

The genetic sex of the embryo determines the sexual path of differentiation. The **sex regulatory (SRY) gene** on the Y chromosome codes for a **testis-determining factor (TDF)** that causes the gonad to become a testis. Testosterone secreted by Leydig cells in the testis during week 9 causes external genital development and the mesonephric ducts to develop into the phenotypical XY (male) genital duct system. The glycoprotein **anti-Müllerian hormone (AMH)** causes the degeneration of the paramesonephric ducts and promotes growth of the mesonephric ducts. Phenotypical XX (female) development is the "default" system. The absence of testosterone and AMH in an embryo causes the mesonephric ducts to regress and the paramesonephric ducts to develop into the phenotypical XX (female) genital structures.

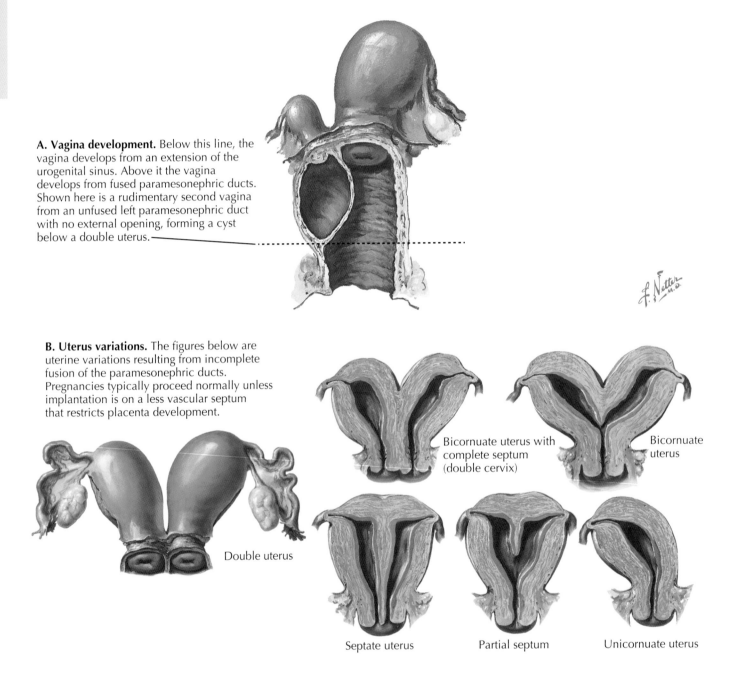

A. Vagina development. Below this line, the vagina develops from an extension of the urogenital sinus. Above it the vagina develops from fused paramesonephric ducts. Shown here is a rudimentary second vagina from an unfused left paramesonephric duct with no external opening, forming a cyst below a double uterus.

B. Uterus variations. The figures below are uterine variations resulting from incomplete fusion of the paramesonephric ducts. Pregnancies typically proceed normally unless implantation is on a less vascular septum that restricts placenta development.

Double uterus

Bicornuate uterus with complete septum (double cervix)

Bicornuate uterus

Septate uterus

Partial septum

Unicornuate uterus

7.19 PARAMESONEPHRIC DUCT ANOMALIES

The left and right paramesonephric (Müllerian) ducts fuse in the midline as they connect with the UG sinus. Anomalies of the uterus, uterine tubes (Fig. 7.19B), and upper vagina (Fig. 7.19A) result from the absence of one duct, complete absence of fusion, or varying degrees of fusion of the left and right ducts. The lower vagina develops from **sinovaginal bulbs** that are endodermal extensions of the UG sinus (Fig. 7.19A). An epithelial **vaginal plate** occludes the lumen of the vaginal primordium. It becomes hollow, except for a membranous **hymen** that separates the vaginal lumen from the vestibule.

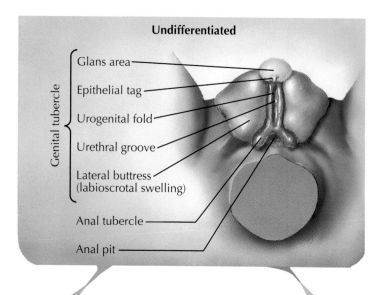

Undifferentiated

Genital tubercle
- Glans area
- Epithelial tag
- Urogenital fold
- Urethral groove
- Lateral buttress (labioscrotal swelling)

Anal tubercle

Anal pit

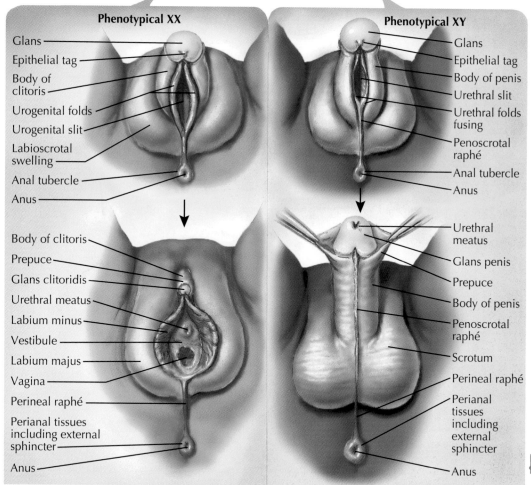

Phenotypical XX

- Glans
- Epithelial tag
- Body of clitoris
- Urogenital folds
- Urogenital slit
- Labioscrotal swelling
- Anal tubercle
- Anus

- Body of clitoris
- Prepuce
- Glans clitoridis
- Urethral meatus
- Labium minus
- Vestibule
- Labium majus
- Vagina
- Perineal raphé
- Perianal tissues including external sphincter
- Anus

Phenotypical XY

- Glans
- Epithelial tag
- Body of penis
- Urethral slit
- Urethral folds fusing
- Penoscrotal raphé
- Anal tubercle
- Anus

- Urethral meatus
- Glans penis
- Prepuce
- Body of penis
- Penoscrotal raphé
- Scrotum
- Perineal raphé
- Perianal tissues including external sphincter
- Anus

7.20 HOMOLOGUES OF THE EXTERNAL GENITAL ORGANS

The earliest primordium for the external genital organs is the **genital tubercle**, a swelling of somatopleure dorsal to the caudal end of the UG sinus. **UG folds** flank the external genital part of the UG sinus, and **labioscrotal folds** of somatopleure appear lateral to the UG folds. The genital tubercle forms the penis and clitoris.

The UG folds become the labia minora, and the labioscrotal folds become the labia majora and scrotum. The UG sinus develops into the vestibule and urethra, and related glands, in phenotypical XX (female). In phenotypical XY (male), the UG sinus folds within the genital tubercle to become most of the penile urethra (except the navicular fossa in the glans). The UG folds in the male may contribute a bit to the ventral surface of the penis.

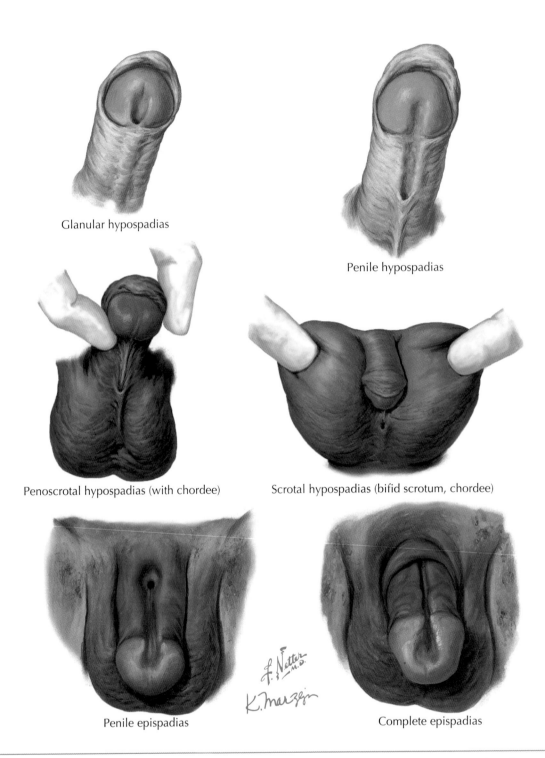

Glanular hypospadias

Penile hypospadias

Penoscrotal hypospadias (with chordee)

Scrotal hypospadias (bifid scrotum, chordee)

Penile epispadias

Complete epispadias

7.21 **HYPOSPADIAS AND EPISPADIAS**

The penile urethra is formed by two mechanisms. Most of the penile urethra develops as the UG folds fuse on the ventral surface of the penis to enclose the distal UG sinus as the penile (spongy) urethra. The ectoderm at the tip of the glans penis invaginates as a cord that connects to the end of the spongy urethra, then becomes hollow to form the navicular fossa. Hypospadias results from failure of fusion of the UG folds to varying degrees caused by insufficient production of androgens from the fetal testes or lack of hormone receptors. Epispadias results from the improper location of the genital tubercle relative to the UG sinus, and the

UG membrane breaks open on its dorsal surface instead of on the ventral.

CLINICAL POINT

Hypospadias is the second most common anomaly of the phenotypical XY (male) reproductive system (1/250 male births) and most often occurs in isolation. It sometimes has a controversial designation as an intersex condition. Epispadias can occur in both sexes and almost always is associated with exstrophy of the bladder or cloaca (see Fig. 7.4). It is often associated with an opening on a bifid penis or clitoris or cranial to it. Surgery typically has a good outcome, although sexual dysfunction, depression, and psychosocial challenges are often experienced in adults.

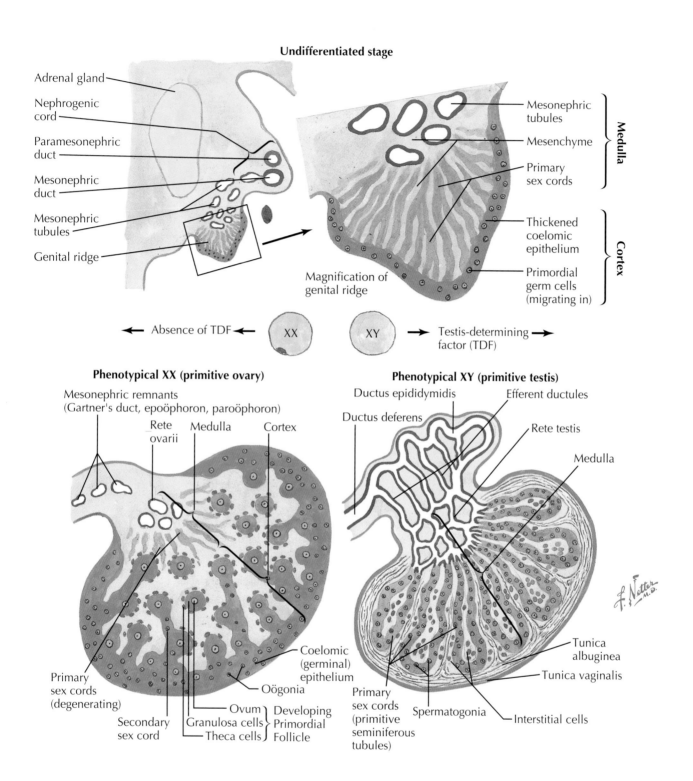

Undifferentiated stage

Adrenal gland

Nephrogenic cord

Paramesonephric duct

Mesonephric duct

Mesonephric tubules

Genital ridge

Mesonephric tubules

Mesenchyme

Primary sex cords

Thickened coelomic epithelium

Primordial germ cells (migrating in)

Medulla

Cortex

Magnification of genital ridge

←── Absence of TDF ←── XX   XY ──→ Testis-determining factor (TDF) ──→

Phenotypical XX (primitive ovary)

Mesonephric remnants (Gartner's duct, epoöphoron, paroöphoron)

Rete ovarii   Medulla   Cortex

Primary sex cords (degenerating)

Secondary sex cord

Ovum
Granulosa cells
Theca cells

Developing Primordial Follicle

Oögonia

Coelomic (germinal) epithelium

Phenotypical XY (primitive testis)

Ductus epididymidis   Efferent ductules

Ductus deferens

Rete testis

Medulla

Primary sex cords (primitive seminiferous tubules)

Spermatogonia

Tunica albuginea

Tunica vaginalis

Interstitial cells

7.22 GONADAL DIFFERENTIATION

The gonads develop from the **gonadal ridge** mesoderm derived from the intermediate mesoderm of the gastrula. The epithelium on the ridge is continuous with the parietal peritoneum (mesothelium). It thickens and projects into the developing gonad in two waves of epithelial sex cords. The **primary sex cords** extend into the medulla and become the **seminiferous tubules** of the testis. They diminish in phenotypical XX (female) and may persist as a vestigial **rete ovarii**. **Secondary sex cords** (cortical cords) extend into the ovarian cortex to become **primordial follicles** surrounding the oogonia. Primordial germ cells migrate into the gonads from the gut tube.

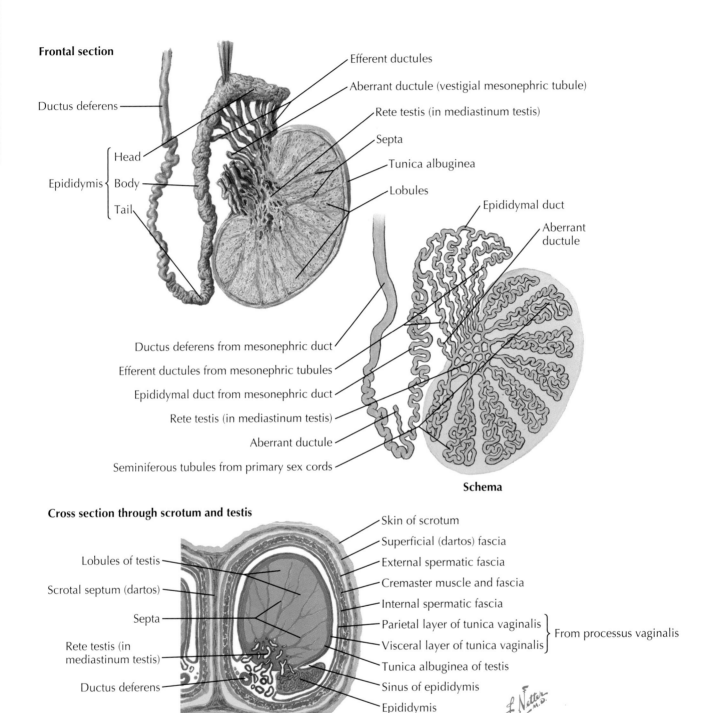

Frontal section

Ductus deferens

Epididymis
- Head
- Body
- Tail

Efferent ductules

Aberrant ductule (vestigial mesonephric tubule)

Rete testis (in mediastinum testis)

Septa

Tunica albuginea

Lobules

Epididymal duct

Aberrant ductule

Ductus deferens from mesonephric duct

Efferent ductules from mesonephric tubules

Epididymal duct from mesonephric duct

Rete testis (in mediastinum testis)

Aberrant ductule

Seminiferous tubules from primary sex cords

Schema

Cross section through scrotum and testis

Lobules of testis

Scrotal septum (dartos)

Septa

Rete testis (in mediastinum testis)

Ductus deferens

Skin of scrotum

Superficial (dartos) fascia

External spermatic fascia

Cremaster muscle and fascia

Internal spermatic fascia

Parietal layer of tunica vaginalis

Visceral layer of tunica vaginalis

} From processus vaginalis

Tunica albuginea of testis

Sinus of epididymis

Epididymis

7.23 TESTIS, EPIDIDYMIS, AND DUCTUS DEFERENS

Spermatogonia (primitive male germ cells) are dormant in the seminiferous tubules until puberty, when they increase in number by mitosis and enlarge to become **primary spermatocytes**. Two rounds of meiotic divisions produce two haploid **secondary spermatocytes** and four haploid **spermatids**. The latter are gradually transformed into four mature sperm cells in the process of **spermiogenesis**. The whole process takes approximately 2 months and continues throughout adult life. The gubernaculum guides the descent of the testes through the inguinal canal into the scrotum. They pass behind the peritoneal extension of the **processus vaginalis** that forms the parietal and visceral layers of the tunica vaginalis testis. The visceral layer is closely applied to the tunica albuginea.

A. Undifferentiated gonads

Paramesonephric
(mullerian) duct

Future ovary

Mesonephric
(wolffian) duct

Gubernaculum

Urogenital sinus

B. Ovaries and gubernaculum in the pelvis

Attachment of gubernaculum to the uterus

**Gubernaculum
derivatives:**

Ovarian ligament

Uterine
tube

Uterus

Ovary

Round ligament
of the uterus

Suspensory
ligament of
the ovary

Remnants of the
mesonephric duct

Termination in
the labia majora

Vagina

C. Superior view of adult female pelvic organs

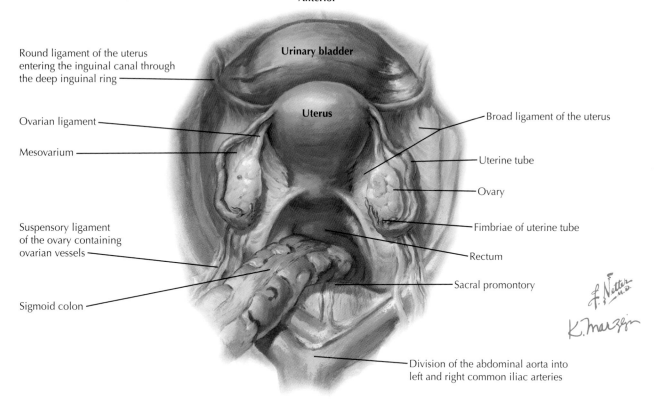

Anterior

Urinary bladder

Round ligament of the uterus
entering the inguinal canal through
the deep inguinal ring

Uterus

Broad ligament of the uterus

Ovarian ligament

Uterine tube

Mesovarium

Ovary

Fimbriae of uterine tube

Suspensory ligament
of the ovary containing
ovarian vessels

Rectum

Sacral promontory

Sigmoid colon

Division of the abdominal aorta into
left and right common iliac arteries

7.24 DESCENT OF OVARIES

The gonads descend in both sexes and are guided by the fibrous **gubernaculum** (Fig. 7.24A). The testis passes through the deep body wall into the scrotum via the **inguinal canal** that extends between the deep and superficial inguinal rings (see Chapter 6 and Fig. 7.17 for details). It descends behind a fingerlike extension of parietal peritoneum, the **processus vaginalis**, which pinches off around the testis as a coelomic sac in the scrotum called the **tunica vaginalis testis**. Descent of the ovary stops in the pelvis where it ends up in the mesovarium, a posterior extension of the broad ligament of the uterus in the pelvis (Fig. 7.24C). The gubernaculum attaches to the uterus to become two ligaments (Fig. 7.24B). The part of it extending from the ovary to the uterus is the **ovarian ligament**, and from the uterus through the inguinal canal it is called the **round ligament of the uterus**. As in males, the latter passes through the inguinal canal; in phenotypical XX (females), it terminates in the superficial fascia of the labia majora.

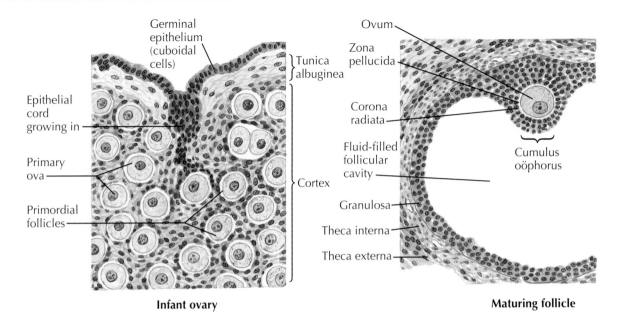

Infant ovary

Maturing follicle

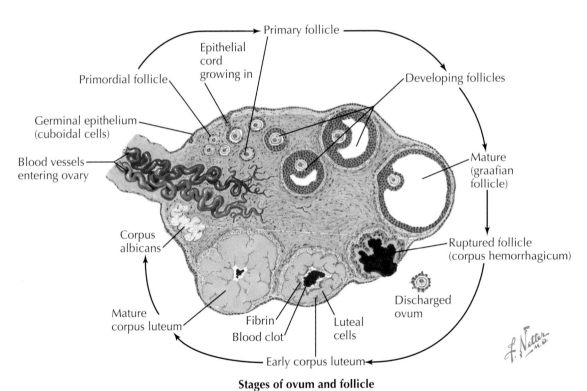

Stages of ovum and follicle

7.25 OVA AND FOLLICLES

Oogonia (primitive oocytes) divide by mitosis in the fetal ovary. Many degenerate, but approximately 700,000 are present at birth and 400,000 at puberty. No new oocytes are produced postnatally. Oogonia become primary oocytes as they complete prophase of the first meiotic division before birth; they remain in that state until after puberty. The first meiotic division is completed just before ovulation and results in a secondary oocyte and a small, nonfunctional, polar body. The second meiotic division is arrested in metaphase and is not completed until after fertilization by a sperm.

Oocytes develop in follicles that originate from secondary sex cords of epithelium extending from the surface of the ovary.

Primordial follicles have a simple squamous epithelium. Mature follicles have a stratified epithelium and may be a centimeter in diameter. The germinal epithelium is continuous with and functionally equivalent to visceral peritoneum.

CLINICAL POINT

Trisomy 21 (Down syndrome) is the most common result of maternal meiosis **nondisjunction** (0.3% of newborns and much higher in spontaneous abortions) and is correlated with advanced maternal age. The arrest of meiosis for many decades increases the chance that chromatids will not properly separate.

Undifferentiated

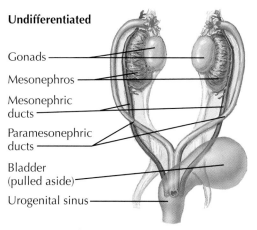

Gonads

Mesonephros

Mesonephric ducts

Paramesonephric ducts

Bladder (pulled aside)

Urogenital sinus

8-week indifferent stage, anterior view

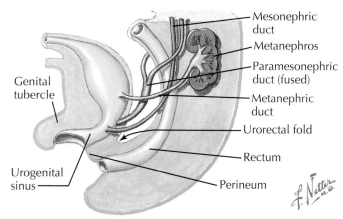

Genital tubercle

Urogenital sinus

Mesonephric duct

Metanephros

Paramesonephric duct (fused)

Metanephric duct

Urorectal fold

Rectum

Perineum

8-week indifferent stage, lateral view (gonad not shown)

Urogenital primordia and derivatives

Phenotypical XX	Phenotypical XY
From the Urogenital Sinus	
Urinary bladder Urethra Lower vagina (and vaginal epithelium) Vestibule Greater vestibular/urethral glands	Urinary bladder Urethra (except navicular fossa) Prostate gland Bulbourethral glands
	Vestigial: prostatic utricle
From the Mesonephric Duct and Tubules	

Ureteric bud from mesonephric duct forms:
  Ureter
  Renal pelvis
  Major and minor calices
  Collecting tubules
	Efferent ductules
	Duct of epididymis
	Ductus deferens
	Ejaculatory duct
	Seminal vesicles
	Ureter, renal pelvis, calices, and collecting tubules

Vestigial: epoophoron, paoophoron, appendix vesiculosa, Gartner's duct	Vestigial: appendix of epididymis
From the Paramesonephric Duct	
Uterine tubes, uterus, upper vagina	Vestigial: appendix of testis
Vestigial: hydatid	

Summary of Sexual Differentiation

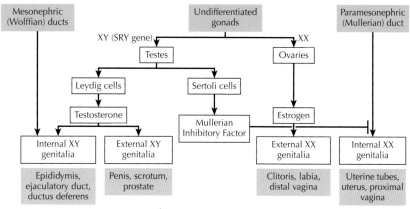

7.26 SUMMARY OF UROGENITAL PRIMORDIA AND DERIVATIVES

A summary of the major concepts of UG system development:

1. Gonads and kidneys develop from intermediate mesoderm of the gastrula (genital and nephrogenic ridges).
2. Kidneys form in three successive waves from cranial to caudal. The huge mesonephros is the first functioning kidney. The caudal metanephros is the permanent kidney.
3. Urinary structures develop from the cloaca, a dilation of hindgut splanchnopleure.
4. All sexes have identical primordia in the 8-week embryo.
5. The mesonephric ducts develop into the epididymis, ductus deferens, and ejaculatory duct; the paramesonephric ducts develop into the uterine tubes, uterus, and proximal vagina.
6. The mesonephric duct changes its function in the phenotypical XY (male) from urinary (mesonephric kidney ureter) to genital (ductus deferens). The flow chart in Fig. 7.26 provides an overview of sexual differentiation, including key genetic factors and hormones that influence the embryonic development of structures.

10-week external genitalia primordia

Glans

Urogenital fold

Urogenital groove

Corpus or
shaft of phallus

Labioscrotal swelling

Anus

Indifferent gonad developing from genital ridge

Mesonephric
tubules

Mesenchyme

Primary
sex cords

Medulla

Thickened
coelomic
epithelium

Primordial
germ cells
(migrating in)

Cortex

Genital primordia and derivatives

Phenotypical XX	Phenotypical XY
From the Genital Tubercle/Phallus	

Clitoris:
  Glans clitoridis
  Corpora cavernosa clitoridis
Bulb of the vestibule
	Penis:
	  Glans penis (and navicular fossa)
	  Corpora cavernosum penis
	  Corpus spongiosum penis

From the Urogenital Folds	
Labia minora Perineal raphé Perianal tissue (and external anal sphincter)	Ventral aspect of penis Most of the penile urethra Perineal raphé Perianal tissue (and external sphincter)
From the Labioscrotal Folds	
Labia majora	Scrotum
From the Indifferent Gonad	

Ovary: follicles from secondary sex
  cords in cortex
	Testis: seminiferous tubules from
	  primary sex cords

Vestigial: rete ovarii in medulla	Rete testis in medulla
From the Gubernaculum	
Ovarian ligament Round ligament of the uterus	Gubernaculum testis

7.27 SUMMARY OF GENITAL PRIMORDIA AND DERIVATIVES

A summary of major concepts of genital development:

1. The external genital organs develop from three swellings of somatopleure: a genital tubercle, UG folds, and labioscrotal folds.
2. The urethra in the phenotypical XY (male) comes from two primordia: the UG sinus that closes on the ventral surface of the penis and an invagination of ectoderm at the end of the glans.
3. The urethra, vestibule, and lower vagina come from the UG sinus in phenotypical XX (females).
4. There are two waves of epithelial sex cords in the primitive gonad. The primary wave forms the seminiferous tubules of the testis. A secondary wave forms follicles surrounding oocytes in the ovary. The epithelium of the original genital ridge persists as the "germinal" epithelium of the ovary.

Terminology

Allantois	(G., "sausage-like") A vestigial, endodermal extension of the cloaca into the umbilical cord in mammals. In egg-laying animals, it lines the inner surface of the egg for gas exchange.
Appendix of the testis	A remnant of the paramesonephric duct in the male. It is attached to the superior pole of the testis.
Appendix vesiculosa	Persistence of the cranial end of the mesonephric (Wolffian) duct in females lateral to the ovary/epoöphoron.
Bicornuate	(L, "two horns") Double uterus characteristic of most mammals, but an anomaly in primates whose single uterus comes from fused paramesonephric (Müllerian) ducts.
Bowman's capsule	The epithelial covering of the glomerular capillaries. It has a visceral layer of podocytes and simple squamous parietal layer. The urinary space between the two continues into the proximal convoluted tubule of the nephron.
Cloaca	(L., "sewer") A dilation at the caudal end of the hindgut that divides to form the rectum, urinary bladder, urethra, vestibule, prostate, and related structures.
Cryptorchidism	(G., "hidden testis") An undescended testis not in the scrotum.
Epoöphoron	Remnants of mesonephric tubules and a segment of mesonephric duct between the ovary and uterine tube. These correspond to efferent ductules and duct of the epididymis in males.
Gartner's duct	Remnants of the mesonephric duct in the broad ligament of the uterus. They may form cysts.
Germinal epithelium	A term for the epithelium on the surface of the ovary. It was thought that this epithelium gave rise to primordial germ cells (oogonia). Follicular cells come from ovarian epithelium, but the germ cells migrate from the wall of the gut tube into the ovary.
Glomerulus	Tuft of capillaries in the in the renal corpuscle of a nephron where urine is filtered from the blood.
Hydatid (of Morgagni)	A persistent part of the cranial end of the paramesonephric (Müllerian) duct that does not contribute to the uterine tube.
Hymen	A membrane that is a remnant from a secondary cavitation of the vagina after endodermal cells from the urogenital sinus fill the lumen of lower part of the uterovaginal primordium (from the fused paramesonephric ducts). It is not a vestige of the cloacal membrane.
Hypospadias	Failure of the urogenital folds to fuse completely on the ventral surface of the penis in the formation of the penile urethra. Urine escapes from a ventral opening in the newborn penis.
Indifferent stage	The 8-week embryo that has identical primordial in both sexes. As embryos of each sex develop, they lose the primordial of the opposite sex.
Intermediate mesoderm	Mesoderm in the gastrula between the paraxial column and lateral plate that gives rise to the kidneys and gonads.
Klinefelter's syndrome	A chromosomal condition where individuals have karyotype 47 XXY; they are phenotypically male, but with an extra X chromosome that can come from the mother or father for a total of 47 chromosomes instead of 46. The main indications are infertility and small, poorly functioning testes. Other signs and symptoms are subtle, but may include breast development, less body hair, and diminished muscle strength and coordination. Individuals often have less interest in sex. Cognitive development is usually unaffected, though some individuals may have symptoms associated with special senses and reading comprehension.
Mesonephros	(G., "middle kidney") The first functioning kidney in the embryo, it develops from the intermediate mesoderm of the gastrula and is closely applied to the primitive gonad. It disappears as the permanent metanephric kidney forms. In the male, the mesonephric duct and tubules become connected to the testis to form the male genital duct system (e.g., ductus deferens, ejaculatory duct).
Nephron	The structural and functional unit of the kidney where urine is filtered from the blood, concentrated, processed, and transported. In sequence, it consists of a glomerulus, proximal convoluted tubule, Henle's loop, and a distal convoluted tubule that connects with a collecting tubule.
Paramesonephric (Müllerian) duct	Primordium of the uterine tubes, uterus, and upper vagina.

Terminology—cont'd

Paroöphoron	Remnants of mesonephric tubules medial to the ovary and the location of the vestigial epoöphoron.
Pronephros	(G., "first kidney") The first kidney to develop at the cranial end of the intermediate mesoderm. It has a brief existence and never functions.
Prostatic utricle	A midline, blind pouch off the prostatic urethra that is the remnant of the caudal end of the paramesonephric duct. The male equivalent of the vagina.
Renal corpuscle	Glomerular capillaries surrounded by Bowman's capsule, the site of filtration of urine from the bloodstream in the cortex of the kidney.
Sinovaginal bulbs	Paired outgrowths of the sinus tubercle of the urogenital sinus at the base of the uterovaginal primordium that are induced by contact of the fused paramesonephric ducts with the urogenital sinus. They form a solid endodermal vaginal plate at the bottom of the vagina that cavitates and gives rise to all of the vaginal epithelium.
Sinus tubercle	Swelling of the urogenital sinus in which the left and right paramesonephric ducts contact the sinus.
Turner's syndrome	A chromosomal condition where individuals have karyotype 45,XO (or 45,X); they have only one X sex chromosome for a total of 45 chromosomes rather than the typical 46. They have XX (female) genitalia, but are infertile and do not have breast development or menstrual periods without hormonal therapy. Presentation may include short stature, short neck with webbed skin, visual and hearing issues, heart problems, and other minor morphological variations. Cognitive development is usually unaffected.
Urachus	Fibrous remnant of the allantois extending from the top of the bladder to the umbilicus.
Urogenital sinus	The anterior product of the division of the cloaca that consists of the primitive urinary bladder, a pelvic portion, and a lower genital portion (urogenital sinus proper) that gives rise to the urethra and all related glands in both sexes and the vestibule and lower vagina in the phenotypical XX (female).
Urogenital folds	Primordia that give rise to the labia minora surrounding the vestibule in the phenotypical XX (female) and the penile urethra and ventral penis in the phenotypical XY (male).
Urorectal septum	The tissue in the natural cleft between the allantois and hindgut tube. It extends inferiorly to divide the cloaca into the rectum and a urogenital sinus that becomes urinary bladder, urethra, vestibule, prostate, and related structures.

8

THE MUSCULOSKELETAL SYSTEM

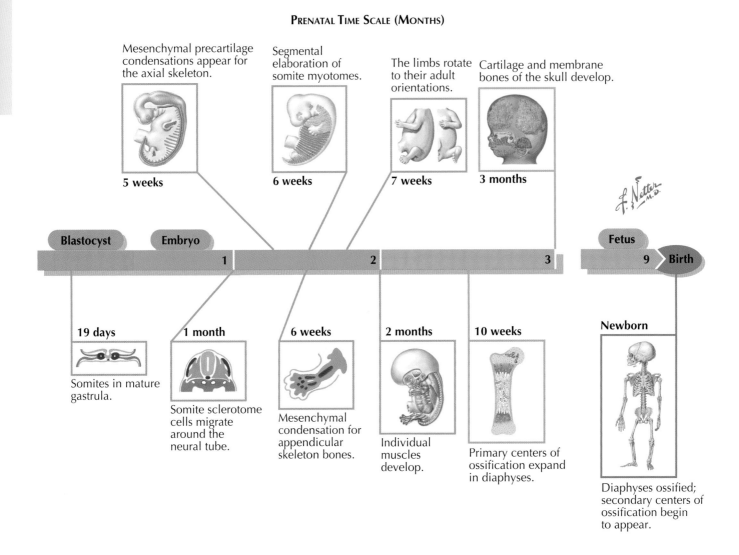

PRENATAL TIME SCALE (MONTHS)

Mesenchymal precartilage condensations appear for the axial skeleton.

Segmental elaboration of somite myotomes.

The limbs rotate to their adult orientations.

Cartilage and membrane bones of the skull develop.

5 weeks

6 weeks

7 weeks

3 months

Blastocyst   Embryo   1   2   3   Fetus   9   Birth

19 days

Somites in mature gastrula.

1 month

Somite sclerotome cells migrate around the neural tube.

6 weeks

Mesenchymal condensation for appendicular skeleton bones.

2 months

Individual muscles develop.

10 weeks

Primary centers of ossification expand in diaphyses.

Newborn

Diaphyses ossified; secondary centers of ossification begin to appear.

8.1 TIMELINE

PRIMORDIA FOR THE SKELETAL SYSTEM

(1) Sclerotome of somites, (2) somatopleure mesoderm, and (3) neural crest cells in the head (forming pharyngeal arch mesenchyme and general head mesenchyme).

PRIMORDIA FOR SKELETAL MUSCLES

(1) Myotome of somites and somitomeres; (2) somatopleure mesoderm and (3) neural crest–derived head and pharyngeal arch mesenchyme.

PRIMORDIA FOR HEART AND SMOOTH MUSCLE

(1) Cardiogenic mesoderm from the primitive streak for the heart and (2) most all sources of mesoderm for smooth muscle.

PLAN

Most bones of the postcranial skeleton form as cartilaginous models that are replaced by bone tissue. Most bones of the skull form in mesenchyme membranes because cartilage is not suitable to accommodate the dynamic forces of the growing brain and face.

The pattern of the developing muscular system is intimately involved with the plan of the peripheral nerves. The two primary themes are the segmental nature of muscle formation from somite myotomes and the division of myotomes to form muscle groups, each with its own branch of a spinal nerve. Each myotome divides to form an epimere (with its dorsal nerve ramus) and a hypomere (with its ventral ramus). The epimere forms the intrinsic back muscles, whereas the hypomere forms the lateral and ventral trunk muscles, including all limb muscles. The hypomere in the limbs further divides to form the flexor and extensor compartment muscles of the limbs (with their anterior and posterior division nerves, respectively).

DIFFERENTIATION OF SOMITES INTO MYOTOMES, DERMATOMES, AND SCLEROTOMES: CROSS SECTION OF HUMAN EMBRYOS

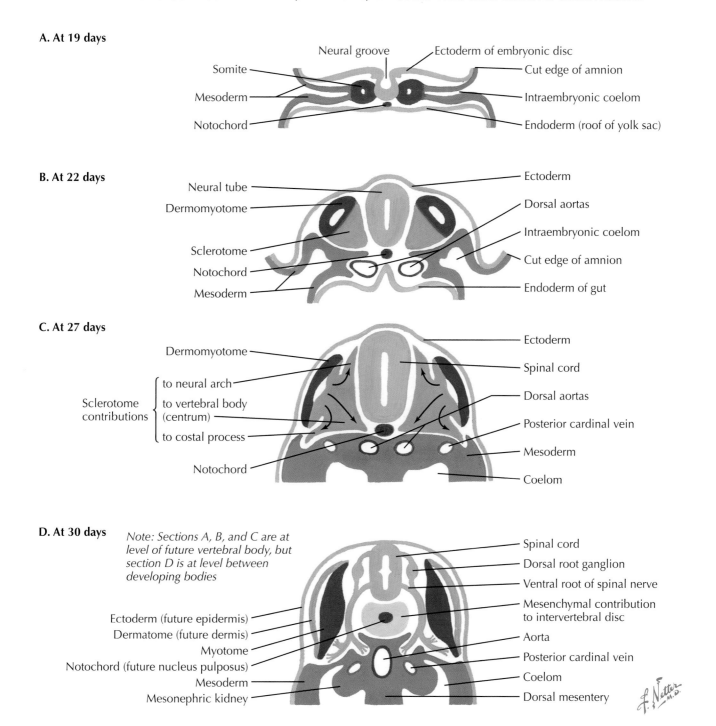

A. At 19 days

Somite
Mesoderm
Notochord
Neural groove
Ectoderm of embryonic disc
Cut edge of amnion
Intraembryonic coelom
Endoderm (roof of yolk sac)

B. At 22 days

Neural tube
Dermomyotome
Sclerotome
Notochord
Mesoderm
Ectoderm
Dorsal aortas
Intraembryonic coelom
Cut edge of amnion
Endoderm of gut

C. At 27 days

Dermomyotome
Sclerotome contributions
{ to neural arch
to vertebral body (centrum)
to costal process
Notochord
Ectoderm
Spinal cord
Dorsal aortas
Posterior cardinal vein
Mesoderm
Coelom

D. At 30 days

Note: Sections A, B, and C are at level of future vertebral body, but section D is at level between developing bodies

Ectoderm (future epidermis)
Dermatome (future dermis)
Myotome
Notochord (future nucleus pulposus)
Mesoderm
Mesonephric kidney
Spinal cord
Dorsal root ganglion
Ventral root of spinal nerve
Mesenchymal contribution to intervertebral disc
Aorta
Posterior cardinal vein
Coelom
Dorsal mesentery

8.2 MYOTOMES, DERMATOMES, AND SCLEROTOMES

Bone, muscle, and connective tissue primarily come from primitive streak mesoderm, including somites, lateral plate mesoderm, and diffuse mesenchyme produced during gastrulation. Cells on the deep aspect of the somites begin to dissociate and migrate around the neural tube and notochord and into the somatopleure. These sclerotome cells differentiate into chondroblasts that form the cartilaginous precursors of the axial skeleton and bones of the cranial base. The remnant of each somite is a dermomyotome that separates into a dermatome and a muscle-forming myotome. The dermatome becomes the connective tissue dermis of the skin.

PROGRESSIVE STAGES IN FORMATION OF VERTEBRAL COLUMN, DERMATOMES, AND MYOTOMES

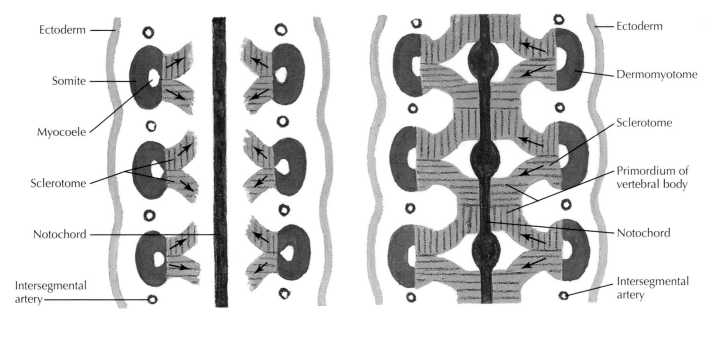

Ectoderm — Somite — Myocoele — Sclerotome — Notochord — Intersegmental artery

Ectoderm — Dermomyotome — Sclerotome — Primordium of vertebral body — Notochord — Intersegmental artery

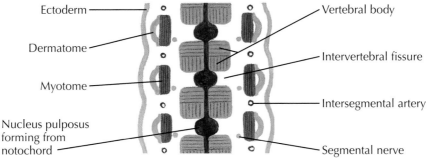

Ectoderm — Dermatome — Myotome — Nucleus pulposus forming from notochord

Vertebral body — Intervertebral fissure — Intersegmental artery — Segmental nerve

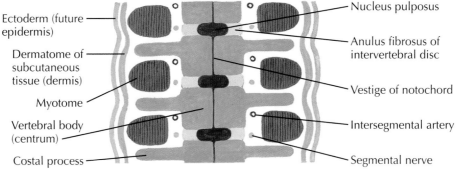

Ectoderm (future epidermis) — Dermatome of subcutaneous tissue (dermis) — Myotome — Vertebral body (centrum) — Costal process

Nucleus pulposus — Anulus fibrosus of intervertebral disc — Vestige of notochord — Intersegmental artery — Segmental nerve

8.3 MUSCLE AND VERTEBRAL COLUMN SEGMENTATION

The dermatomes form connective tissue beneath the surface ectoderm, the primordium of the epidermis of the skin. The myotomes differentiate into segmental muscle masses, and the sclerotome and notochord form the vertebral column. The body (centrum) of a vertebra comes not from a single sclerotome, but from the fusion of two halves of adjacent sclerotomes. This is the most notable morphological example of segmental gene products expressed as **parasegments** that overlap adjacent early segments. The result is that the intervals between the vertebral bodies are at the level of the myotomes, and the spinal nerves that exit the vertebral column have a direct path to their muscle targets.

Mesenchymal precartilage primordia of axial and appendicular skeletons at 5 weeks

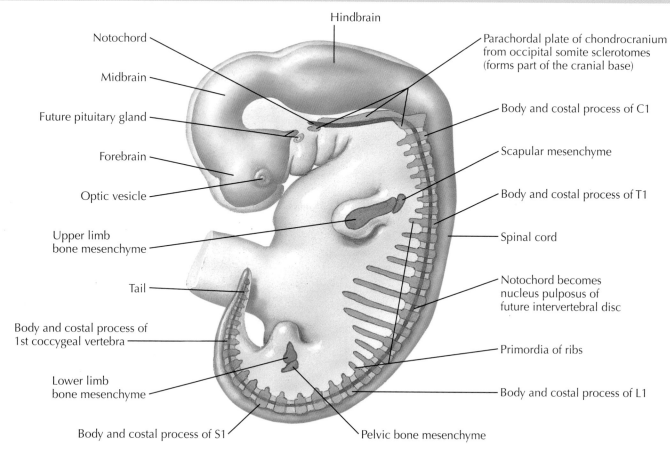

Hindbrain

Notochord

Midbrain

Future pituitary gland

Forebrain

Optic vesicle

Upper limb bone mesenchyme

Tail

Body and costal process of 1st coccygeal vertebra

Lower limb bone mesenchyme

Body and costal process of S1

Parachordal plate of chondrocranium from occipital somite sclerotomes (forms part of the cranial base)

Body and costal process of C1

Scapular mesenchyme

Body and costal process of T1

Spinal cord

Notochord becomes nucleus pulposus of future intervertebral disc

Primordia of ribs

Body and costal process of L1

Pelvic bone mesenchyme

Precartilage mesenchymal cell condensations of appendicular skeleton at 6 weeks

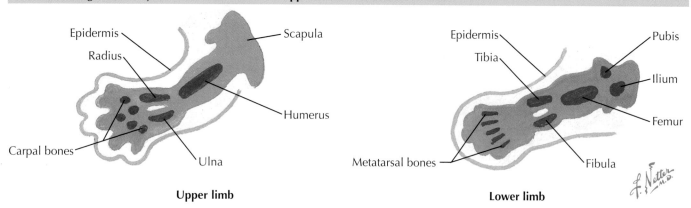

Epidermis

Radius

Scapula

Carpal bones

Humerus

Ulna

Upper limb

Epidermis

Tibia

Pubis

Ilium

Femur

Metatarsal bones

Fibula

Lower limb

8.4 MESENCHYMAL PRIMORDIA AT 5 AND 6 WEEKS

Bone development begins with condensations of mesenchyme from sclerotomes (for the axial skeleton) and somatopleure (for the appendicular skeleton). Cells from these condensations differentiate into chondroblasts that convert the mesenchymal primordia into cartilaginous precursors of the bones. The cartilage eventually is replaced by bone through **endochondral ossification**. The sclerotomes extend into the embryonic head to form endochondral bone at the base of the neurocranium. Most other bones of the skull form by **intramembranous (mesenchymal) ossification**, the direct deposition of bone in mesenchyme derived from the neural crest.

FATE OF BODY, COSTAL PROCESS, AND NEURAL ARCH COMPONENTS OF VERTEBRAL COLUMN, WITH SITES AND TIME OF APPEARANCE OF OSSIFICATION CENTERS

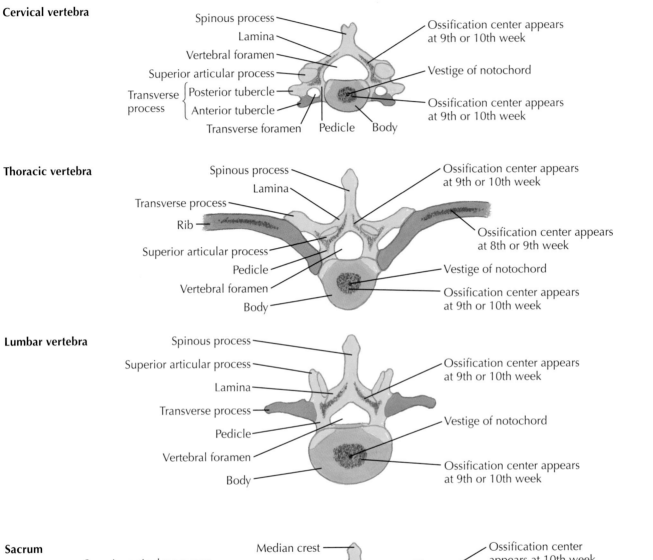

Cervical vertebra

Spinous process
Lamina
Vertebral foramen
Superior articular process
Transverse process { Posterior tubercle
Anterior tubercle }
Transverse foramen   Pedicle   Body

Ossification center appears at 9th or 10th week
Vestige of notochord
Ossification center appears at 9th or 10th week

Thoracic vertebra

Spinous process
Lamina
Transverse process
Rib
Superior articular process
Pedicle
Vertebral foramen
Body

Ossification center appears at 9th or 10th week
Ossification center appears at 8th or 9th week
Vestige of notochord
Ossification center appears at 9th or 10th week

Lumbar vertebra

Spinous process
Superior articular process
Lamina
Transverse process
Pedicle
Vertebral foramen
Body

Ossification center appears at 9th or 10th week
Vestige of notochord
Ossification center appears at 9th or 10th week

Sacrum

Median crest
Superior articular process
Sacral canal
Lateral part (Ala)

Promontory   Body

Ossification center appears at 10th week
Ossification center appears at 6th month (prenatal)
Vestige of notochord
Ossification center appears at 10th week

KEY
- ▨ Body
- ▨ Costal process
- ▨ Neural arch

f. Netter M.D.

8.5 OSSIFICATION OF THE VERTEBRAL COLUMN

Bone first appears in the hyaline cartilage models in local **ossification centers**, where the cartilage is broken down and removed and osteoblasts begin to deposit bone tissue. Most bones develop from a number of ossification centers. The vertebral column develops from ossification centers in the body, the neural arch, and the costal process of cartilage of each vertebra and pair of ribs. In vertebrae without rib articulations, the costal processes contribute to the transverse processes of the vertebrae or the lateral alae (wings) of the sacrum. The notochord mostly disappears; it persists only as the nucleus pulposus, the gelatinous center of an intervertebral disc.

A. Embryonic basis of spina bifida

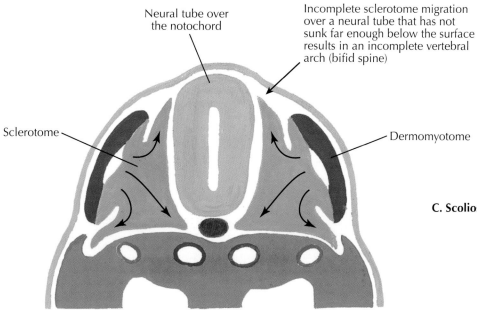

Neural tube over the notochord

Incomplete sclerotome migration over a neural tube that has not sunk far enough below the surface results in an incomplete vertebral arch (bifid spine)

Sclerotome

Dermomyotome

B. Spina bifida with meningomyelocele

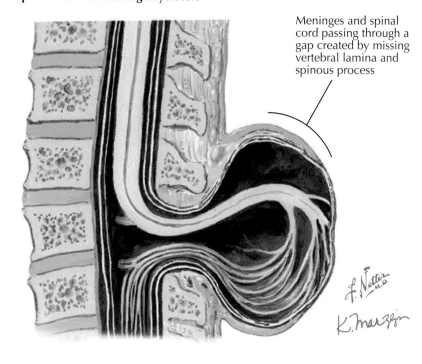

Meninges and spinal cord passing through a gap created by missing vertebral lamina and spinous process

C. Scoliosis

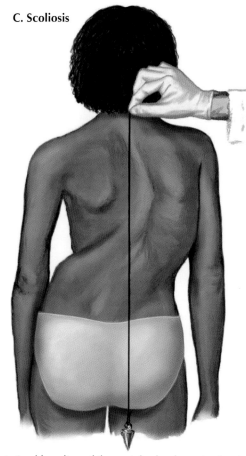

Lateral bending of the vertebral column to the right from increased tone in the left intrinsic back muscles. Affected vertebra are also rotated via the transversospinalis group of intrinsic muscles.

8.6 VERTEBRAL COLUMN ANOMALIES

Spina bifida is a relatively common vertebral column defect related to anomalies of meninges and the spinal cord (see Fig. 3.5). The primary cause is failure of the neural tube primordium of the spinal cord to sink completely beneath the surface ectoderm during neurulation. The somite sclerotomes cannot fully migrate over a more superficial neural tube, resulting in an incomplete vertebral arch (Fig. 8.6A). The spinal cord and/or meninges are exposed on the surface of the back to varying degrees, but, in all cases, spina bifida is present (Fig. 8.6B). **Scoliosis** is lateral curvature of the vertebral column in the coronal plane (Fig. 8.6C). A congenital cause is a hemivertebra, the absence of half a vertebra from a defect in sclerotome migration around the neural tube on one side. More typically it is an imbalance of muscle tone in the intrinsic back muscles, where vertebral column rotation (via the transversospinalis muscle group) accompanies the lateral bending. Scoliosis is often present in some types of dwarfism, particularly variations of achondroplasia.

First and second cervical vertebrae at birth

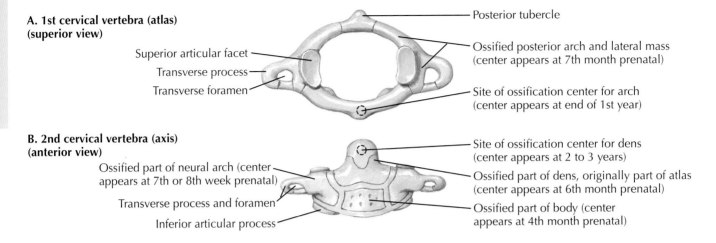

**A. 1st cervical vertebra (atlas)
(superior view)**

Superior articular facet

Transverse process

Transverse foramen

Posterior tubercle

Ossified posterior arch and lateral mass
(center appears at 7th month prenatal)

Site of ossification center for arch
(center appears at end of 1st year)

**B. 2nd cervical vertebra (axis)
(anterior view)**

Ossified part of neural arch (center
appears at 7th or 8th week prenatal)

Transverse process and foramen

Inferior articular process

Site of ossification center for dens
(center appears at 2 to 3 years)

Ossified part of dens, originally part of atlas
(center appears at 6th month prenatal)

Ossified part of body (center
appears at 4th month prenatal)

Development of sternum

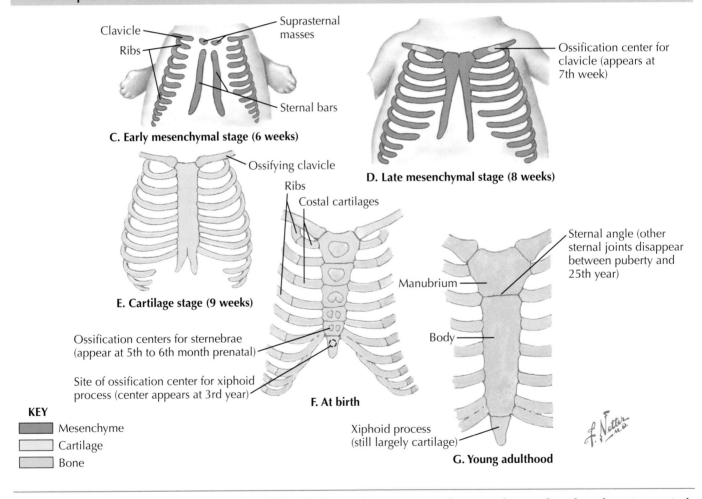

Clavicle

Ribs

Suprasternal
masses

Sternal bars

C. Early mesenchymal stage (6 weeks)

Ossification center for
clavicle (appears at
7th week)

D. Late mesenchymal stage (8 weeks)

Ossifying clavicle

E. Cartilage stage (9 weeks)

Ribs

Costal cartilages

Ossification centers for sternebrae
(appear at 5th to 6th month prenatal)

Site of ossification center for xiphoid
process (center appears at 3rd year)

F. At birth

Manubrium

Body

Sternal angle (other
sternal joints disappear
between puberty and
25th year)

Xiphoid process
(still largely cartilage)

G. Young adulthood

KEY

Mesenchyme
Cartilage
Bone

8.7 DEVELOPMENT OF THE ATLAS, AXIS, RIBS, AND STERNUM

The atlas (C1) and axis (C2) differ from typical vertebrae in that the body (centrum) of the atlas fuses to the body of the axis as the odontoid process (dens), the "axis" around which the atlas and skull rotate. The clavicle is the only postcranial bone that develops in mesenchyme instead of cartilage. Sternum development is unusual in that it progresses from paired mesenchymal condensations, a single piece of cartilage, and a vertical series of ossification centers that are also paired. Rib ossification is also unique. Hyaline cartilage remains between the rib bodies and sternum as the **costal cartilages**. The joint between a costal cartilage and a bony rib is a solid cartilaginous joint; between the cartilages and sternum it is synovial to permit the elevation and depression of the ribs during respiration.

Composition of bone

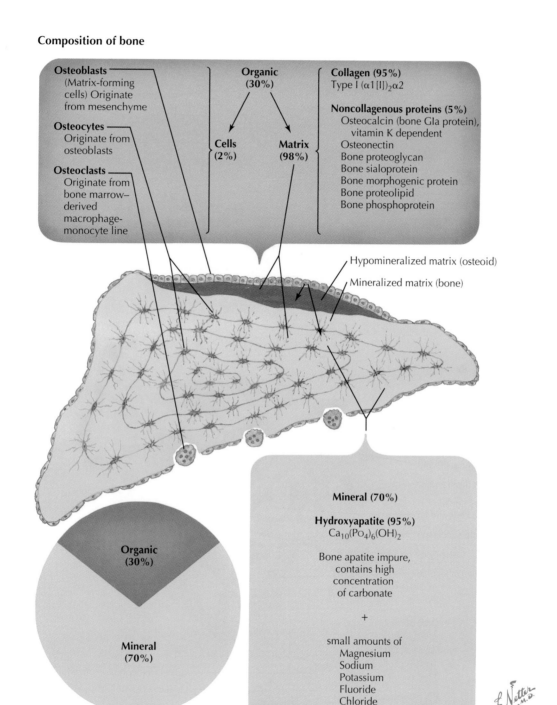

Osteoblasts (Matrix-forming cells) Originate from mesenchyme

Osteocytes Originate from osteoblasts

Osteoclasts Originate from bone marrow–derived macrophage-monocyte line

Organic (30%)

Cells (2%)   **Matrix (98%)**

Collagen (95%) Type I $(\alpha 1\,[I])_2\alpha 2$

Noncollagenous proteins (5%)
Osteocalcin (bone Gla protein), vitamin K dependent
Osteonectin
Bone proteoglycan
Bone sialoprotein
Bone morphogenic protein
Bone proteolipid
Bone phosphoprotein

Hypomineralized matrix (osteoid)

Mineralized matrix (bone)

Mineral (70%)

Hydroxyapatite (95%) $Ca_{10}(PO_4)_6(OH)_2$

Bone apatite impure, contains high concentration of carbonate

+

small amounts of
Magnesium
Sodium
Potassium
Fluoride
Chloride

Organic (30%)

Mineral (70%)

8.8 BONE CELLS AND BONE DEPOSITION

The development of bone and the remodeling of adult bone involve the cellular processes of bone deposition and resorption. **Osteoblasts** deposit bone on surfaces, **osteocytes** maintain bone in spaces called lacunae within the bone matrix, and multinucleated **osteoclasts** resorb bone on surfaces. The organic component of bone, called **osteoid**, is deposited first and later mineralized by membrane-bound packets of **hydroxyapatite crystals** left in the osteoid by the osteoblasts.

Cortical (compact) bone

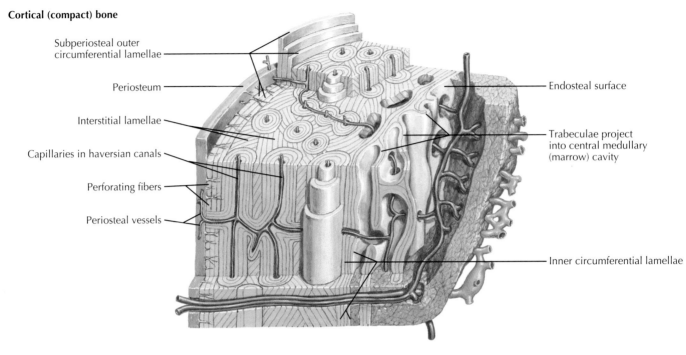

Subperiosteal outer circumferential lamellae

Periosteum

Interstitial lamellae

Capillaries in haversian canals

Perforating fibers

Periosteal vessels

Endosteal surface

Trabeculae project into central medullary (marrow) cavity

Inner circumferential lamellae

Trabecular bone (schematic)

On cut surfaces (as in sections), trabeculae may appear as discontinuous spicules

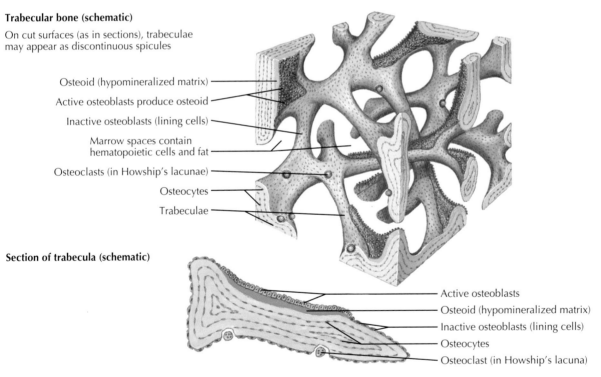

Osteoid (hypomineralized matrix)

Active osteoblasts produce osteoid

Inactive osteoblasts (lining cells)

Marrow spaces contain hematopoietic cells and fat

Osteoclasts (in Howship's lacunae)

Osteocytes

Trabeculae

Section of trabecula (schematic)

Active osteoblasts

Osteoid (hypomineralized matrix)

Inactive osteoblasts (lining cells)

Osteocytes

Osteoclast (in Howship's lacuna)

8.9 HISTOLOGY OF BONE

Endochondral and intramembranous ossification produce the same bone tissues. Most adult bones have **compact bone** on the outside and **spongy** (**trabecular** or **cancellous**) **bone** on the inside. Adult compact bone consists of layers of bone called **lamellae** that are separated from each other by thin layers of aligned collagen fibers. **Circumferential lamellae** envelop the compact layer and long, cylindrical, concentric lamellae form **osteons** (**Haversian systems**), the structural units of compact bone. Between osteons are **interstitial lamellae** that are the remaining segments of older osteons. Surrounding the bone is **periosteum** consisting of an outer fibrous layer and inner osteogenic layer with osteoblasts. **Endosteum** lines the inner, more irregular surface of compact bone.

EARLY DEVELOPMENT OF SKULL

Chondrocranium at 9 weeks

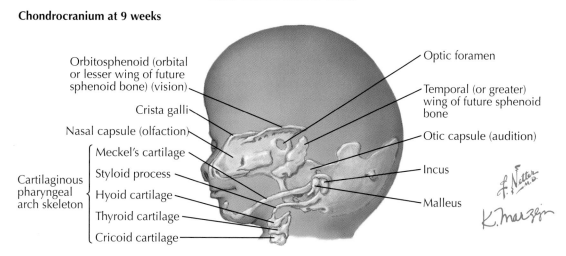

Orbitosphenoid (orbital or lesser wing of future sphenoid bone) (vision)

Crista galli

Nasal capsule (olfaction)

Cartilaginous pharyngeal arch skeleton
- Meckel's cartilage
- Styloid process
- Hyoid cartilage
- Thyroid cartilage
- Cricoid cartilage

Optic foramen

Temporal (or greater) wing of future sphenoid bone

Otic capsule (audition)

Incus

Malleus

Membrane bones at 9 weeks

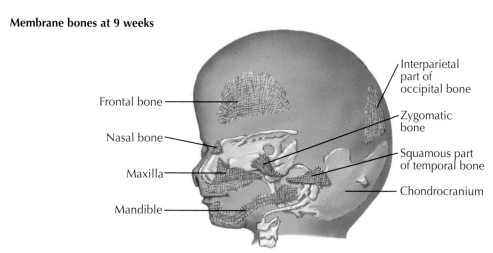

Frontal bone

Nasal bone

Maxilla

Mandible

Interparietal part of occipital bone

Zygomatic bone

Squamous part of temporal bone

Chondrocranium

Membrane bones at 12 weeks

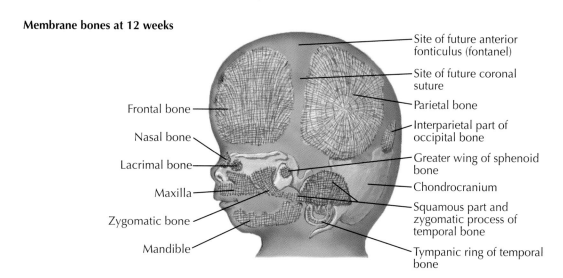

Frontal bone

Nasal bone

Lacrimal bone

Maxilla

Zygomatic bone

Mandible

Site of future anterior fonticulus (fontanel)

Site of future coronal suture

Parietal bone

Interparietal part of occipital bone

Greater wing of sphenoid bone

Chondrocranium

Squamous part and zygomatic process of temporal bone

Tympanic ring of temporal bone

8.10 MEMBRANE BONE AND SKULL DEVELOPMENT

Most postcranial bones and the bones of the cranial base develop via endochondral ossification, whereas most bones of the neurocranium and viscerocranium develop directly from mesenchyme. **Mesenchymal bone formation** is often called **intramembranous ossification**, a misleading term derived from the connective tissue membrane surrounding the developing brain in which ossification centers develop for the flat neurocranial bones. The bones of the facial skeleton and part of the clavicles develop in mesenchyme that does not have a membranous appearance, and the term "membrane" does not characterize the microscopic environment of mesenchymal bone development.

Initial bone formation in mesenchyme

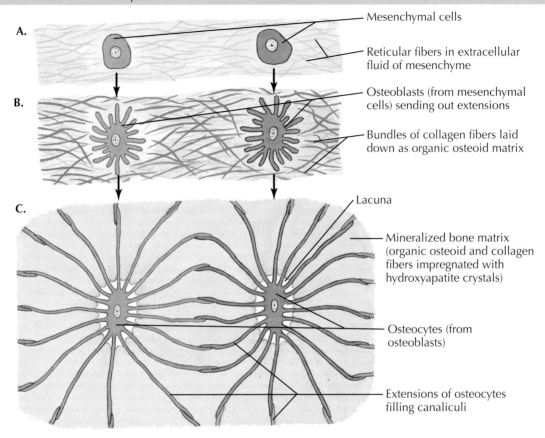

A.
— Mesenchymal cells
— Reticular fibers in extracellular fluid of mesenchyme

B.
— Osteoblasts (from mesenchymal cells) sending out extensions
— Bundles of collagen fibers laid down as organic osteoid matrix

C.
— Lacuna
— Mineralized bone matrix (organic osteoid and collagen fibers impregnated with hydroxyapatite crystals)
— Osteocytes (from osteoblasts)
— Extensions of osteocytes filling canaliculi

Early stages of flat (membrane or dermal) bone formation

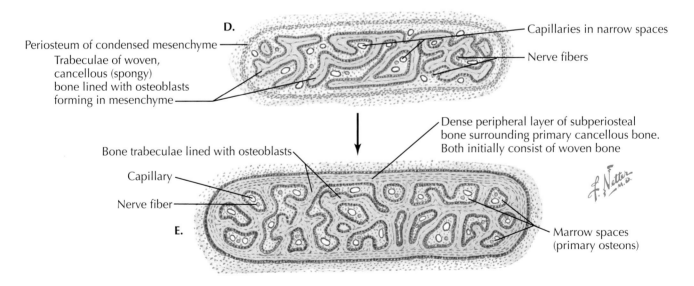

D.
Periosteum of condensed mesenchyme
Trabeculae of woven, cancellous (spongy) bone lined with osteoblasts forming in mesenchyme
— Capillaries in narrow spaces
— Nerve fibers

Bone trabeculae lined with osteoblasts
Capillary
Nerve fiber
E.
— Dense peripheral layer of subperiosteal bone surrounding primary cancellous bone. Both initially consist of woven bone
— Marrow spaces (primary osteons)

8.11 BONE DEVELOPMENT IN MESENCHYME

Mesenchymal cells in the embryonic head differentiate into osteoblasts that develop processes and deposit **osteoid**, the organic matrix of bone. Inorganic hydroxyapatite crystals are incorporated into the osteoid to form mineralized, true bone tissue. The osteoblasts become osteocytes in spaces called **lacunae**, and their processes are metabolically coupled with those of other cells in **canaliculi**. Trabecular bone with thin spicules surrounded by vascular marrow is the first bone to form. This bone is also called **woven bone** because it lacks lamellae—the collagen fibers have a random, "woven" arrangement. All bone is woven bone when first deposited.

PRIMARY OSTEON FORMATION IN MESENCHYMAL BONE DEVELOPMENT

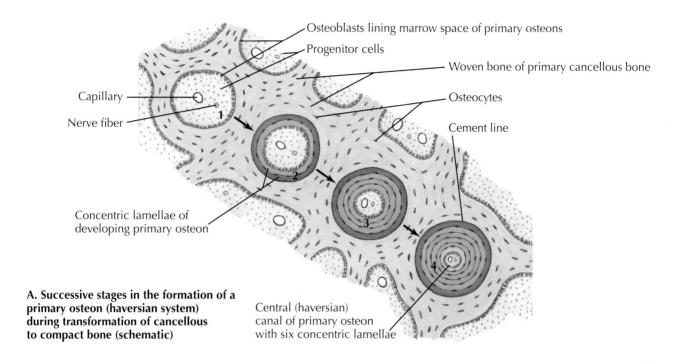

Osteoblasts lining marrow space of primary osteons

Progenitor cells

Woven bone of primary cancellous bone

Capillary

Nerve fiber

Osteocytes

Cement line

Concentric lamellae of developing primary osteon

A. Successive stages in the formation of a primary osteon (haversian system) during transformation of cancellous to compact bone (schematic)

Central (haversian) canal of primary osteon with six concentric lamellae

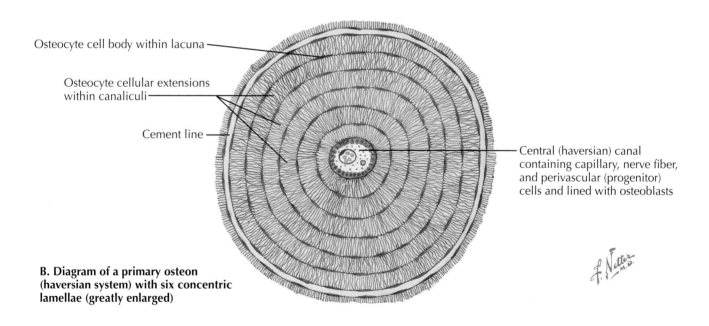

Osteocyte cell body within lacuna

Osteocyte cellular extensions within canaliculi

Cement line

Central (haversian) canal containing capillary, nerve fiber, and perivascular (progenitor) cells and lined with osteoblasts

B. Diagram of a primary osteon (haversian system) with six concentric lamellae (greatly enlarged)

8.12 OSTEON FORMATION

Osteons form in developing compact bone as a way to bring a blood supply into thicker compact bone regions via their central **haversian canals** and interconnecting **Volkmann's canals**. Primary osteons are the first osteons to form in tunnel-shaped marrow spaces within the original trabecular bone; these marrow spaces will be filled in with concentric layers of lamellae. Subsequently, secondary osteons are formed by a remodeling process (see Fig. 8.13). In both primary and secondary osteon formation, the outermost lamellae are deposited first, followed by successive layers toward the central canal.

GROWTH IN WIDTH OF A BONE AND OSTEON REMODELING

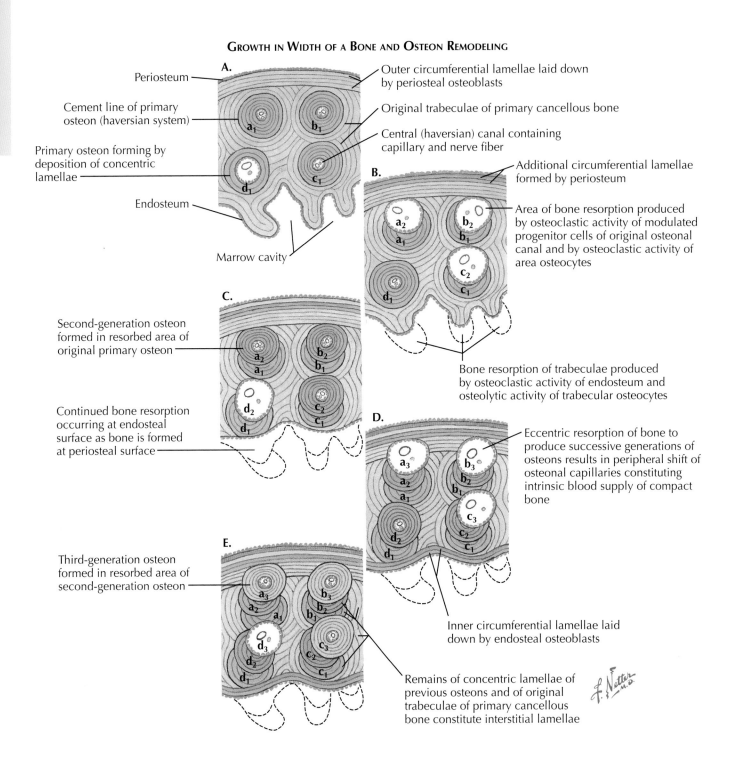

A.

Periosteum

Cement line of primary osteon (haversian system)

Primary osteon forming by deposition of concentric lamellae

Endosteum

Marrow cavity

Outer circumferential lamellae laid down by periosteal osteoblasts

Original trabeculae of primary cancellous bone

Central (haversian) canal containing capillary and nerve fiber

B.

Additional circumferential lamellae formed by periosteum

Area of bone resorption produced by osteoclastic activity of modulated progenitor cells of original osteonal canal and by osteoclastic activity of area osteocytes

C.

Second-generation osteon formed in resorbed area of original primary osteon

Continued bone resorption occurring at endosteal surface as bone is formed at periosteal surface

Bone resorption of trabeculae produced by osteoclastic activity of endosteum and osteolytic activity of trabecular osteocytes

D.

Eccentric resorption of bone to produce successive generations of osteons results in peripheral shift of osteonal capillaries constituting intrinsic blood supply of compact bone

E.

Third-generation osteon formed in resorbed area of second-generation osteon

Inner circumferential lamellae laid down by endosteal osteoblasts

Remains of concentric lamellae of previous osteons and of original trabeculae of primary cancellous bone constitute interstitial lamellae

8.13 COMPACT BONE DEVELOPMENT AND REMODELING

Cartilage can expand by **interstitial growth** (i.e., the addition of a new matrix from within). Bone can grow only by deposition of bone on surfaces (**appositional growth**). When a bone grows in width, new circumferential lamellae are deposited on the outer surface of compact bone by the osteogenic layer of periosteum; the trabeculae and the inner surface are resorbed by osteoclasts. New **secondary osteons** form near the surface by a remodeling process similar to the natural turnover in osteons that occurs throughout life. New generations of osteons form when osteoclasts excavate a tunnel the diameter of the new haversian system, and lamellae are deposited from the outside to the inside in a manner similar to the formation of primary osteons.

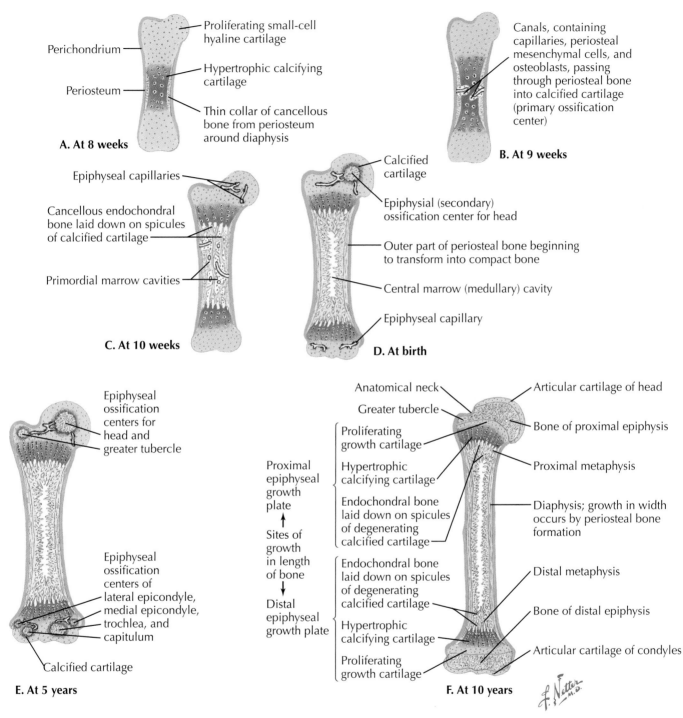

GROWTH AND OSSIFICATION OF LONG BONES (HUMERUS, MIDFRONTAL SECTIONS)

Perichondrium

Periosteum

Proliferating small-cell hyaline cartilage

Hypertrophic calcifying cartilage

Thin collar of cancellous bone from periosteum around diaphysis

A. At 8 weeks

Canals, containing capillaries, periosteal mesenchymal cells, and osteoblasts, passing through periosteal bone into calcified cartilage (primary ossification center)

B. At 9 weeks

Epiphyseal capillaries

Cancellous endochondral bone laid down on spicules of calcified cartilage

Primordial marrow cavities

C. At 10 weeks

Calcified cartilage

Epiphysial (secondary) ossification center for head

Outer part of periosteal bone beginning to transform into compact bone

Central marrow (medullary) cavity

Epiphyseal capillary

D. At birth

Epiphyseal ossification centers for head and greater tubercle

Epiphyseal ossification centers of lateral epicondyle, medial epicondyle, trochlea, and capitulum

Calcified cartilage

E. At 5 years

Proximal epiphyseal growth plate

↑

Sites of growth in length of bone

↓

Distal epiphyseal growth plate

Anatomical neck

Greater tubercle

Proliferating growth cartilage

Hypertrophic calcifying cartilage

Endochondral bone laid down on spicules of degenerating calcified cartilage

Endochondral bone laid down on spicules of degenerating calcified cartilage

Hypertrophic calcifying cartilage

Proliferating growth cartilage

Articular cartilage of head

Bone of proximal epiphysis

Proximal metaphysis

Diaphysis; growth in width occurs by periosteal bone formation

Distal metaphysis

Bone of distal epiphysis

Articular cartilage of condyles

F. At 10 years

8.14 ENDOCHONDRAL OSSIFICATION IN A LONG BONE

Perichondrium differentiates into periosteum, and a **periosteal collar** of bone forms around the diaphysis (shaft). The cartilage becomes calcified in the center of the diaphysis; the cartilage cells hypertrophy and die, and the cartilage breaks up. Blood vessels invade the area, and osteoblasts begin to deposit bone on the remaining cartilage spicules as a **primary center of ossification**. Bone replaces cartilage, and the ossification extends toward each end of the diaphysis. The process is repeated in the epiphyses as **secondary centers of ossification** appear. Bone fills the epiphyses except for cartilage on articular surfaces and the growth plate between the epiphysis and the diaphysis. The metaphysis is the flaring part of the bone near the growth plate.

CLOSE-UP VIEW OF DEVELOPING EPIPHYSIS AND EPIPHYSEAL GROWTH PLATE

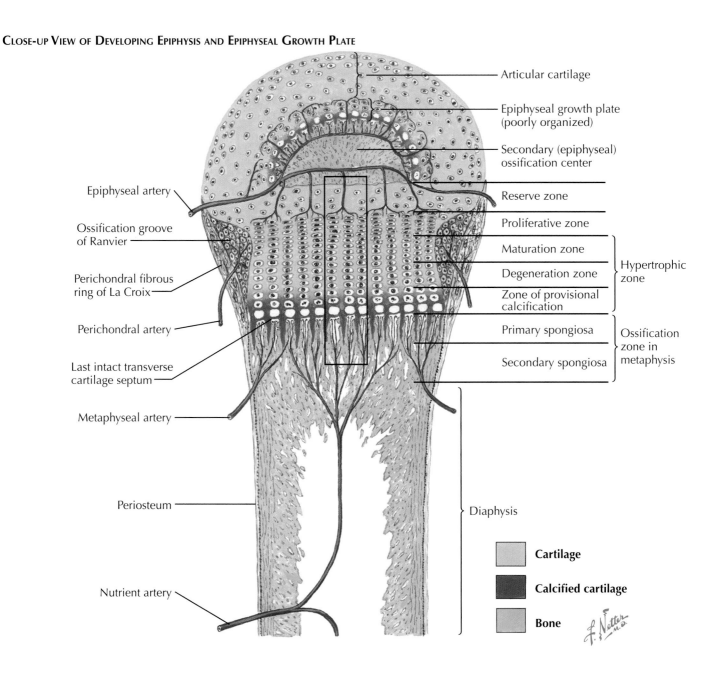

Articular cartilage

Epiphyseal growth plate (poorly organized)

Secondary (epiphyseal) ossification center

Epiphyseal artery

Reserve zone

Proliferative zone

Ossification groove of Ranvier

Maturation zone

Degeneration zone — Hypertrophic zone

Perichondral fibrous ring of La Croix

Zone of provisional calcification

Perichondral artery

Primary spongiosa — Ossification zone in metaphysis

Last intact transverse cartilage septum

Secondary spongiosa

Metaphyseal artery

Periosteum

Diaphysis

Cartilage

Calcified cartilage

Bone

Nutrient artery

8.15 EPIPHYSEAL GROWTH PLATE

The **metaphysis** and bony portion of the growth plate are well supplied with blood, but only the uppermost portion of the cartilage cell columns (proliferative zone) is vascularized. The hypertrophic zone is avascular; cells are poorly oxygenated and nourished, and the lowermost cells degenerate and die. These vascular phenomena have profound physiological significance. Blood is present where new cartilage is added for growth in bone length at the epiphyseal end of the plate and where bone forms at the diaphyseal end. It is absent where cartilage needs to be eliminated.

Zones / Structures	Histology	Functions	Blood supply	Po₂	Cell (chondrocyte) health	Cell respiration	Cell glycogen
Secondary bony epiphysis — Epiphyseal artery							
Reserve zone		Matrix production / Storage	Vessels pass through, do not supply this zone	Poor (low)	Good, active. Much endoplasmic reticulum, vacuoles, mitochondria	Anaerobic	High concentration
Proliferative zone		Matrix production / Cellular proliferation (longitudinal growth)	Excellent	Excellent / Fair	Excellent. Much endoplasmic reticulum, ribosomes, mitochondria. Intact cell membrane	Aerobic / Progressive change to anaerobic	High concentration (less than in above) / Glycogen consumed until depleted
Hypertrophic zone — Maturation zone		Preparation of matrix for calcification	Progressive decrease	Poor (low) / Progressive decrease	Still good / Progressive deterioration	Anaerobic glycolysis	
Hypertrophic zone — Degenerative zone						Anaerobic glycolysis	
Hypertrophic zone — Zone of provisional calcification		Calcification of matrix	Nil	Poor (very low)	Cell death		Nil
Ossification zone — Last intact transverse septum / Primary spongiosa		Vascular invasion and resorption of transverse septa / Bone formation	Closed capillary loops / Good	Poor / Good		Progressive reversion to aerobic	?
Ossification zone — Secondary spongiosa / Branches of metaphyseal and nutrient arteries		Remodeling — Internal: removal of cartilage bars, replacement of fiber bone with lamellar bone. External: funnelization	Excellent	Excellent		Aerobic	?

8.16 STRUCTURE AND FUNCTION OF THE GROWTH PLATE

The endochondral ossification process in the zones of the epiphyseal growth plate involves the same general steps that occur within the primary and secondary ossification centers. These include the calcification of cartilage matrix, the death of cartilage cells, the removal of cartilage, and bone deposition on remaining cartilage spicules. The primary difference is the production of new cartilage cells in the zone of proliferation. This is the ultimate source of new tissue for the growth in length of long bones and the resultant increase in stature of the body.

Zones / Structures	Proteoglycans in matrix	Mitochondrial activity	Matrix calcification	Matrix vesicles	Exemplary diseases	Defect (if known)
Secondary bony epiphysis						
Reserve zone		High Ca²⁺ content	Mito-chondria / Cell membrane / Ca²⁺ intracellular	Few vesicles, contain little Ca²⁺	Diastrophic dwarfism (also, defects in other zones)	Defective type II collagen synthesis
					Pseudoachondroplasia (also, defects in other zones)	Defective processing and transport of proteoglycans
					Kniest's syndrome (also, defects in other zones)	Defective processing of proteoglycans
Proliferative zone	Aggregated proteoglycans (neutral mucopolysaccharides) inhibit calcification	ATP made	Ca²⁺ intracellular	Few vesicles, contain little Ca²⁺	Gigantism	Increased cell proliferation (growth hormone increased)
					Achondroplasia	Deficiency of cell proliferation
					Hypochondroplasia	Less severe deficiency of cell proliferation
					Malnutrition, irradiation injury, glucocorticoid excess	Decreased cell proliferation and/or matrix synthesis
Hypertrophic zone — Maturation zone	Progressively disaggregated	Ca²⁺ uptake, no ATP made	Ca²⁺ intracellular	Contain little Ca²⁺	Mucopolysaccharidosis (Morquio's syndrome, Hurler's syndrome)	Deficiencies of specific lysosomal acid hydrolases, with lysosomal storage of mucopolysaccharides
Hypertrophic zone — Degenerative zone		Ca²⁺ release begins	Ca²⁺ passes into matrix	Begin Ca²⁺ uptake		
Hypertrophic zone — Zone of provisional calcification	Disaggregated proteoglycans (acid mucopolysaccharides) permit calcification	Ca²⁺ released	Matrix calcified	Crystals in and on vesicles	Rickets, osteomalacia (also, defects in metaphysis)	Insufficiency of Ca²⁺ and/or Pᵢ for normal calcification of matrix
Ossification zone — Primary spongiosa					Metaphyseal chondro-dysplasia (Jansen and Schmid types)	Extension of hypertrophic cells into metaphysis
					Acute hematogenous osteomyelitis	Flourishing of bacteria due to sluggish circulation, low PO₂, reticuloendothelial deficiency
Ossification zone — Secondary spongiosa					Osteopetrosis	Abnormality of osteoclasts (internal remodeling)
					Osteogenesis imperfecta	Abnormality of osteoblasts and collagen synthesis
					Scurvy	Inadequate collagen formation
					Metaphyseal dysplasia (Pyle's disease)	Abnormality of funnelization (external remodeling)

8.17 PATHOPHYSIOLOGY OF THE GROWTH PLATE

Diseases that affect stature (either dwarfism or gigantism) are the result of nonnormal processes in the zone of proliferation, such as increased or decreased cartilage cell proliferation. Anomalies of bone tissue (e.g., rickets, osteomalacia, osteogenesis imperfecta, scurvy) originate in the metaphysis where bone forms in the epiphyseal plate.

CLINICAL POINT

Lines of arrested growth. Any disruption of growth results in a diminished production of cartilage cells in the epiphyseal plate, but ossification is less affected, and there is a resulting increase in bone density. These dense lines (Harris lines or lines of arrested growth) can be seen near the epiphyses in an X-ray of an adult bone as a record of acute trauma or insult during the growth period.

SKELETON OF FULL-TERM NEWBORN: TIME OF APPEARANCE OF OSSIFICATION CENTERS (PRIMARY UNLESS OTHERWISE INDICATED)

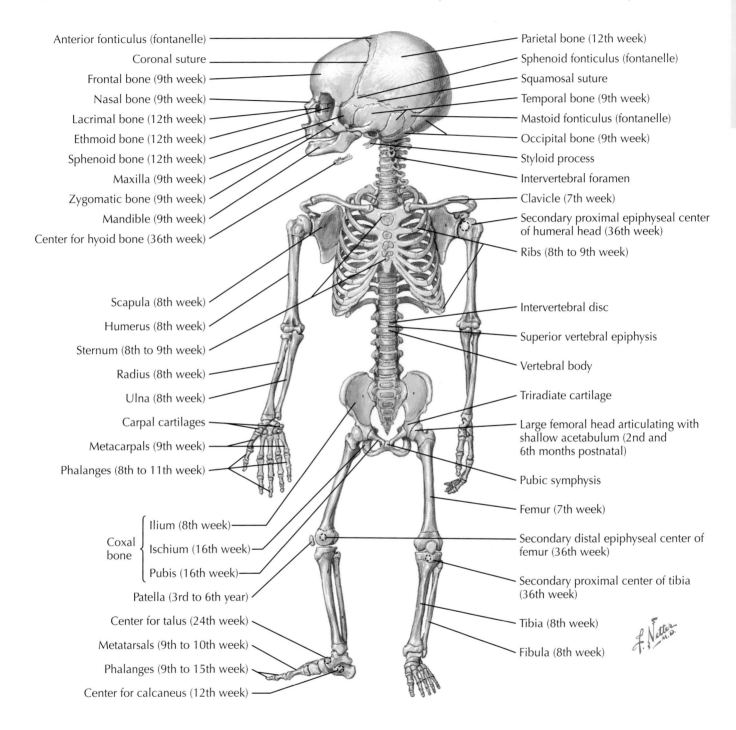

Anterior fonticulus (fontanelle)
Coronal suture
Frontal bone (9th week)
Nasal bone (9th week)
Lacrimal bone (12th week)
Ethmoid bone (12th week)
Sphenoid bone (12th week)
Maxilla (9th week)
Zygomatic bone (9th week)
Mandible (9th week)
Center for hyoid bone (36th week)

Scapula (8th week)
Humerus (8th week)
Sternum (8th to 9th week)
Radius (8th week)
Ulna (8th week)
Carpal cartilages
Metacarpals (9th week)
Phalanges (8th to 11th week)

Coxal bone {
Ilium (8th week)
Ischium (16th week)
Pubis (16th week)
}
Patella (3rd to 6th year)
Center for talus (24th week)
Metatarsals (9th to 10th week)
Phalanges (9th to 15th week)
Center for calcaneus (12th week)

Parietal bone (12th week)
Sphenoid fonticulus (fontanelle)
Squamosal suture
Temporal bone (9th week)
Mastoid fonticulus (fontanelle)
Occipital bone (9th week)
Styloid process
Intervertebral foramen
Clavicle (7th week)
Secondary proximal epiphyseal center of humeral head (36th week)
Ribs (8th to 9th week)

Intervertebral disc
Superior vertebral epiphysis
Vertebral body
Triradiate cartilage
Large femoral head articulating with shallow acetabulum (2nd and 6th months postnatal)
Pubic symphysis
Femur (7th week)
Secondary distal epiphyseal center of femur (36th week)
Secondary proximal center of tibia (36th week)
Tibia (8th week)
Fibula (8th week)

8.18 OSSIFICATION IN THE NEWBORN SKELETON

Most fetal bone is woven bone. Lamellae and osteons form with the postnatal increase in size of the skeleton. The diaphyses are mostly ossified at birth, and the secondary centers are just beginning to appear. The epiphyseal growth plates persist through the adolescent years. Once they have ossified, growth in the length of the bones (and the stature of an individual) can no longer occur.

CLINICAL POINT

Physiological measures of postnatal development. Stature and body weight have a large environmental component and are poor measures of physiological development in growing children. Measures with a large genetic component are times of tooth eruption. Close behind the status of dental eruption are the times of fusion of epiphyses to diaphysis as seen in X-rays of older children and the appearance of secondary centers of ossification in infants as indicated in the newborn skeleton in Fig. 8.18.

Development of three types of synovial joints

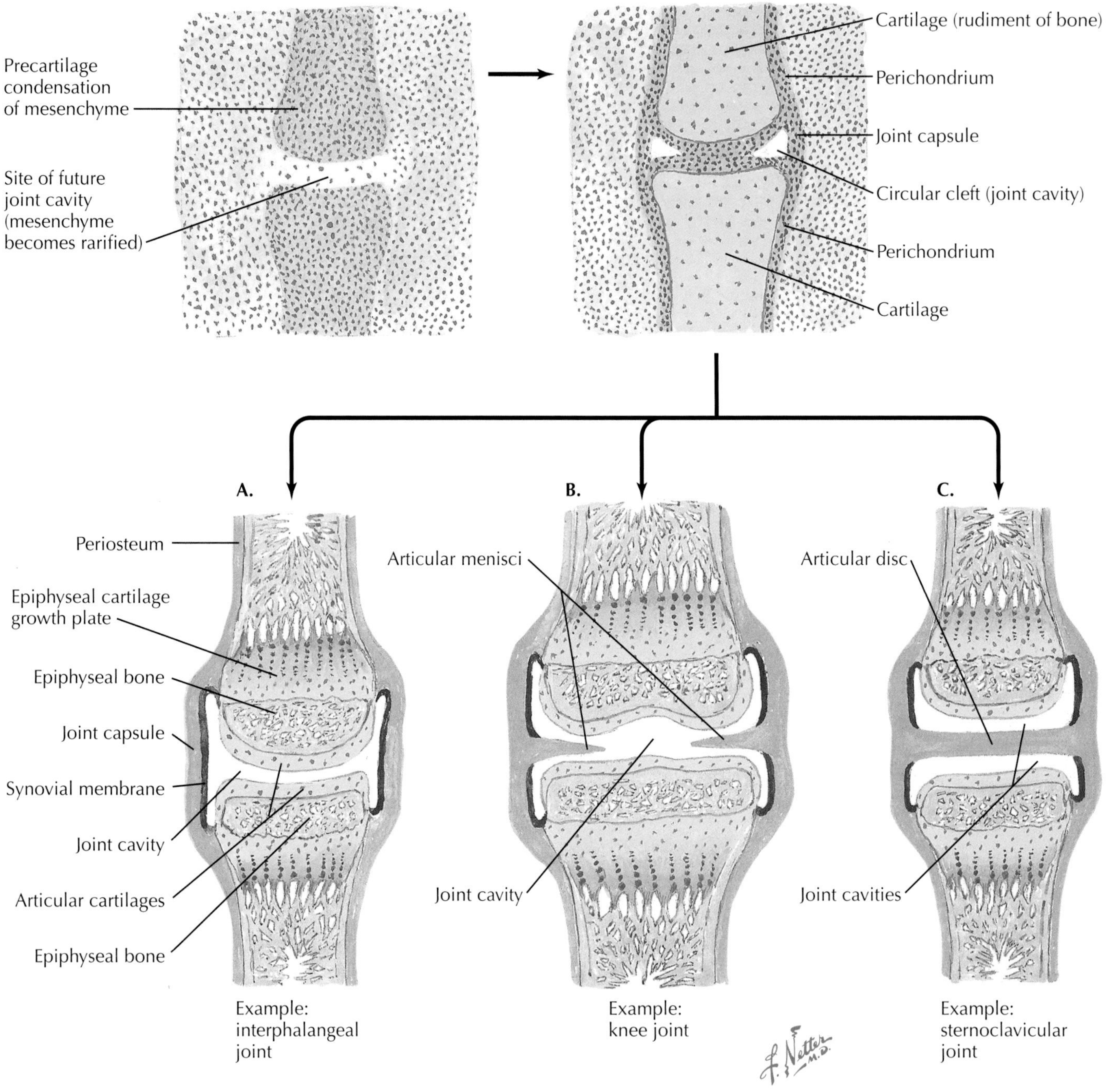

Precartilage condensation of mesenchyme

Site of future joint cavity (mesenchyme becomes rarified)

Cartilage (rudiment of bone)

Perichondrium

Joint capsule

Circular cleft (joint cavity)

Perichondrium

Cartilage

A.

Periosteum

Epiphyseal cartilage growth plate

Epiphyseal bone

Joint capsule

Synovial membrane

Joint cavity

Articular cartilages

Epiphyseal bone

Example: interphalangeal joint

B.

Articular menisci

Joint cavity

Example: knee joint

C.

Articular disc

Joint cavities

Example: sternoclavicular joint

8.19 JOINT DEVELOPMENT

The classification of joints is based on the fate of the mesenchyme between the early bony precursors. **Cartilaginous joints (synchondroses)** are designed to withstand compressive forces and have hyaline cartilage connecting the bony elements (e.g., spheno-occipital synchondrosis and epiphyseal plates). Dense connective tissue unites the bones in **fibrous joints**. The fibrous joints of the neurocranium resist tensile forces from the growing brain. **Synovial joints** have a joint cavity designed for movement and may have an articular disc. The mesenchyme disappears, and hyaline cartilage caps the articular ends of the bones. Synovial joints are the most common of the three types.

DIFFERENTIATION OF SOMITES INTO MYOTOMES, SCLEROTOMES, AND DERMATOMES: CROSS SECTION OF HUMAN EMBRYOS

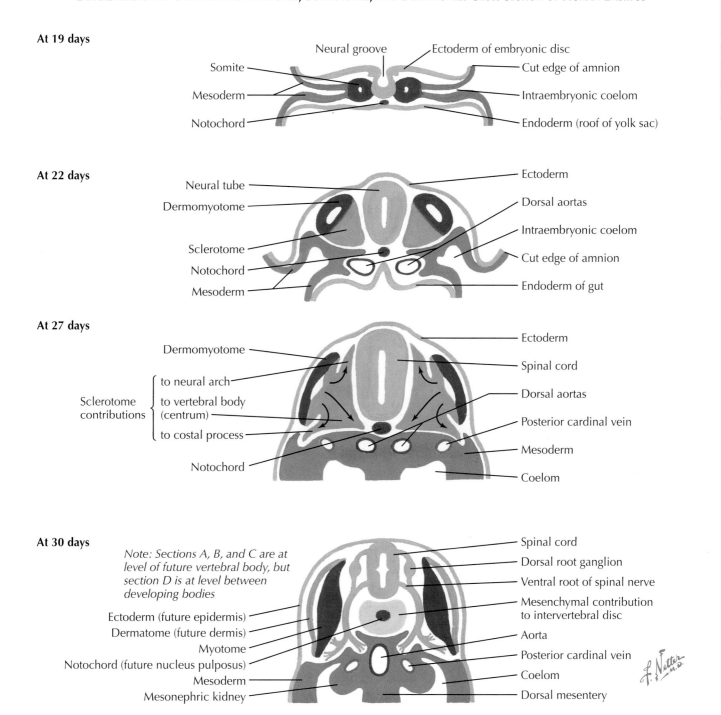

At 19 days

Neural groove — Ectoderm of embryonic disc
Somite — Cut edge of amnion
Mesoderm — Intraembryonic coelom
Notochord — Endoderm (roof of yolk sac)

At 22 days

Neural tube — Ectoderm
Dermomyotome — Dorsal aortas
— Intraembryonic coelom
Sclerotome — Cut edge of amnion
Notochord
Mesoderm — Endoderm of gut

At 27 days

Dermomyotome — Ectoderm
— Spinal cord
Sclerotome contributions { to neural arch
to vertebral body (centrum)
to costal process — Dorsal aortas
— Posterior cardinal vein
— Mesoderm
Notochord — Coelom

At 30 days

Note: Sections A, B, and C are at level of future vertebral body, but section D is at level between developing bodies

— Spinal cord
— Dorsal root ganglion
— Ventral root of spinal nerve
— Mesenchymal contribution to intervertebral disc
Ectoderm (future epidermis) — Aorta
Dermatome (future dermis) — Posterior cardinal vein
Myotome — Coelom
Notochord (future nucleus pulposus)
Mesoderm — Dorsal mesentery
Mesonephric kidney

8.20 MUSCULAR SYSTEM: PRIMORDIA

Skeletal (striated) muscles develop from the myotome of somites and somatopleure mesoderm. Myotomes give rise to the muscles of the trunk and some muscles in the head. Muscle cells of the limbs are derived from migrating myotome cells, whereas the connective tissue elements of muscle—tendons, endomysium, perimysium, and epimysium—come from somatopleure mesenchyme of the limbs. Mesoderm of somatopleure can also differentiate into muscle, as it appears to do in the ventral trunk region.

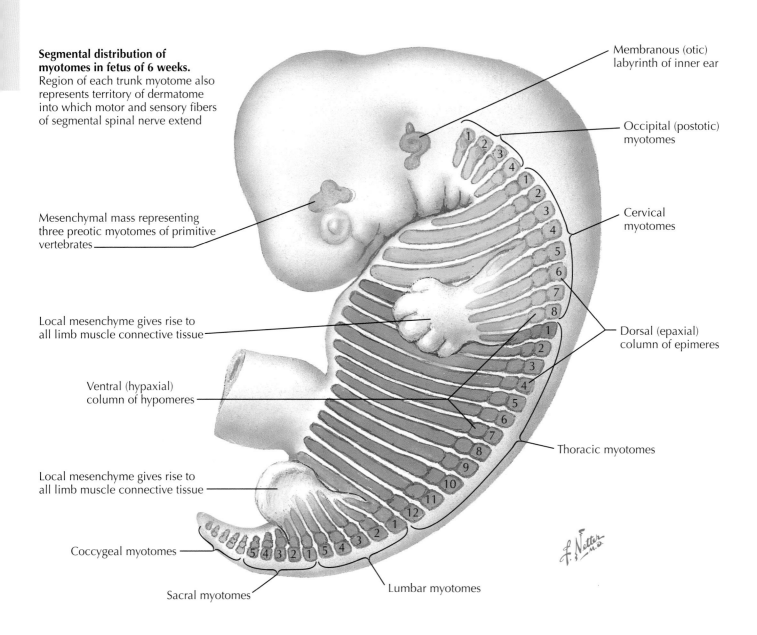

Segmental distribution of myotomes in fetus of 6 weeks.
Region of each trunk myotome also represents territory of dermatome into which motor and sensory fibers of segmental spinal nerve extend

Mesenchymal mass representing three preotic myotomes of primitive vertebrates

Local mesenchyme gives rise to all limb muscle connective tissue

Ventral (hypaxial) column of hypomeres

Local mesenchyme gives rise to all limb muscle connective tissue

Coccygeal myotomes

Sacral myotomes

Lumbar myotomes

Membranous (otic) labyrinth of inner ear

Occipital (postotic) myotomes

Cervical myotomes

Dorsal (epaxial) column of epimeres

Thoracic myotomes

8.21 SEGMENTATION AND DIVISION OF MYOTOMES

Like the somites from which they are derived, the myotomes have a segmental distribution in the embryo, and each segment is innervated by a spinal nerve (cervical, thoracic, lumbar, or sacral). The myotomes begin to divide into a small dorsal segment called an **epimere** and a larger ventral segment called the **hypomere**. Adjacent myotomes fuse to form individual skeletal muscles, so most muscles are innervated by more than one spinal segment (e.g., C3, C4, and C5). This occurs by innervation from multiple spinal nerves (back and abdominal muscles of the trunk) or the joining of multiple spinal segments into single nerves in the brachial and lumbosacral plexuses for limb muscle innervation.

A. Innervation of somatopleure (body wall) derivatives by the somatic nervous system (spinal nerves)

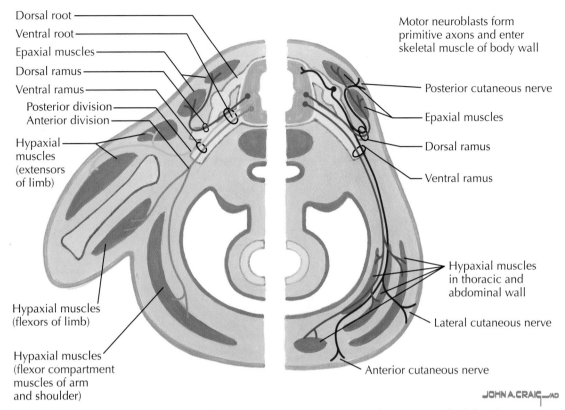

Dorsal root
Ventral root
Epaxial muscles
Dorsal ramus
Ventral ramus
Posterior division
Anterior division
Hypaxial muscles (extensors of limb)

Motor neuroblasts form primitive axons and enter skeletal muscle of body wall

Posterior cutaneous nerve
Epaxial muscles
Dorsal ramus
Ventral ramus

Hypaxial muscles in thoracic and abdominal wall

Lateral cutaneous nerve

Hypaxial muscles (flexors of limb)

Hypaxial muscles (flexor compartment muscles of arm and shoulder)

Anterior cutaneous nerve

JOHN A. CRAIG—AD

Innervation of somatopleure (body wall) derivatives by the somatic nervous system (spinal nerves). On the left is the organization of motor innervation to the back *(blue neurons)* and limbs *(yellow and green neurons)*. On the right is motor innervation to trunk muscles and sensory innervation in cutaneous nerves. Sensory nerve processes are found in all nerves to muscle in addition to cutaneous nerves. Sympathetic fibers supplying arterial smooth muscle are also in every spinal nerve branch.

B. Organizational summary of spinal nerve branches and the muscle group primordia they supply

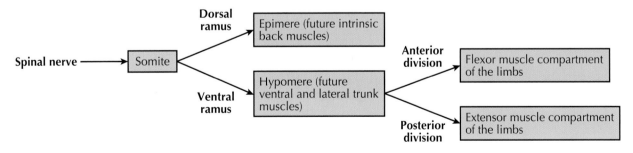

Spinal nerve → Somite

Dorsal ramus → Epimere (future intrinsic back muscles)

Ventral ramus → Hypomere (future ventral and lateral trunk muscles)

Anterior division → Flexor muscle compartment of the limbs

Posterior division → Extensor muscle compartment of the limbs

8.22 EPIMERE, HYPOMERE, AND MUSCLE GROUPS

The **epimere** of a myotome is innervated by the **dorsal primary ramus** of a spinal nerve (blue motor neurons on the left in Fig. 8.22A) and gives rise to the **intrinsic back muscles** (the spinotransverse [splenius] group, the erector spinae, and the transversospinalis group). The **hypomere** is supplied by the **ventral primary ramus** of a spinal nerve. The lateral and ventral muscles of the trunk and all of the muscle cells of the limbs come from hypomeres, which further divide in the limbs into ventral **flexor compartment muscle groups** and dorsal **extensor compartment muscle groups**. The flexors are innervated by **anterior division branches** of ventral rami (green motor neurons on the left in Fig. 8.22A) in the brachial plexus and lumbosacral plexus, the extensors by **posterior divisions** of ventral rami (yellow neurons). All nerves supplying muscles contain sensory (and sympathetic) neurons.

LIMB BUDS IN 6-WEEK EMBRYO

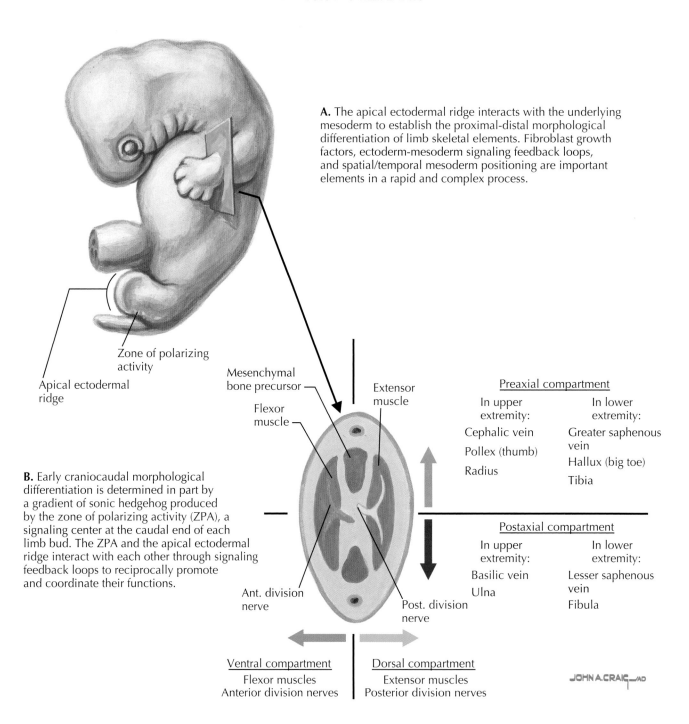

A. The apical ectodermal ridge interacts with the underlying mesoderm to establish the proximal-distal morphological differentiation of limb skeletal elements. Fibroblast growth factors, ectoderm-mesoderm signaling feedback loops, and spatial/temporal mesoderm positioning are important elements in a rapid and complex process.

Zone of polarizing activity

Apical ectodermal ridge

Mesenchymal bone precursor

Flexor muscle

Extensor muscle

Preaxial compartment

In upper extremity:
Cephalic vein
Pollex (thumb)
Radius

In lower extremity:
Greater saphenous vein
Hallux (big toe)
Tibia

B. Early craniocaudal morphological differentiation is determined in part by a gradient of sonic hedgehog produced by the zone of polarizing activity (ZPA), a signaling center at the caudal end of each limb bud. The ZPA and the apical ectodermal ridge interact with each other through signaling feedback loops to reciprocally promote and coordinate their functions.

Postaxial compartment

In upper extremity:
Basilic vein
Ulna

In lower extremity:
Lesser saphenous vein
Fibula

Ant. division nerve

Post. division nerve

Ventral compartment
Flexor muscles
Anterior division nerves

Dorsal compartment
Extensor muscles
Posterior division nerves

JOHN A. CRAIG—AD

8.23 DEVELOPMENT AND ORGANIZATION OF LIMB BUDS

Limb buds develop as paddlelike extensions of the ventrolateral body wall. They contain somatopleure mesenchyme capped by an **apical ectodermal ridge**. Hypomere cells from somite myotomes migrate into the buds to form muscle cells. The connective tissue of muscle comes from somatopleure mesenchyme. Limb bud organization is based on transverse and dorsoventral planes.

The cranial half of a limb bud is the **preaxial compartment**; the caudal half is the **postaxial compartment**. More functionally important, the buds are divided into a ventral **flexor compartment** and dorsal **extensor compartment**. Signals from somites trigger limb bud formation. See Fig. 1.14 for the roles of various growth factors in development of the limb. Although their actions seem straightforward, the control of their expression is complicated.

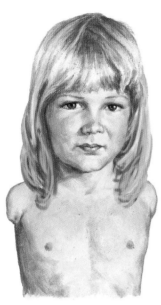
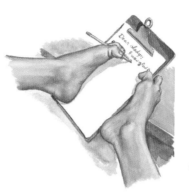
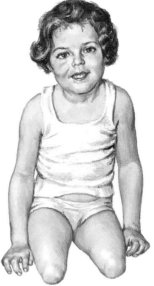
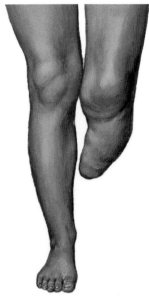

A. Amelia with complete absence of upper extremities

B. Amelia with compensation by prehensile use of the feet

C. Hemiamelia above the knee

D. Hemiamelia below the knee

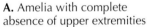
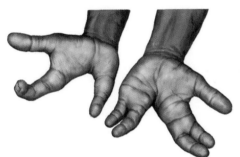
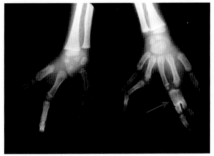
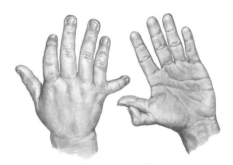

E. Deficiency of middle digital rays (lobster claw deformity, left). Partial syndactyly of digits 2 and 3 (right). See X-rays in **F.**

F. X-rays of hands seen in **E.** Complete absence of digits 3 and 4 on the left. partial fusion of proximal phalanges on the right (red arrow).

G. Polydactyly (extra digits). Postaxial type on the left; preaxial type on the right

8.24 LIMB ANOMALIES

Amelia, the absence of a limb, or **meromelia**, the partial absence of a limb, depends on the stage of development affected: suppression of limb bud development in the early embryo (Fig. 8.24A) versus inhibition of limb development later in time (Figs. 8.24C and 8.24D). Any component of a limb can be affected. Limb anomalies can be related to chromosomal abnormalities (e.g., trisomy 18), specific gene mutations (e.g., Hox genes, BMP, Shh, Wnt7), vascular disruption, environmental teratogens (e.g., thalidomide), uterine constriction of the fetus, or a combination of genetic and environmental factors, as in congenital dislocation of the hip. The digits begin to develop as digital rays of condensed mesenchyme in the hand and foot plates with notches in between. The tissue between the rays resorbs to form elongated fingers and toes. **Syndactyly** (fused digits) can be cutaneous syndactyly (webbed fingers or toes) or osseous syndactyly (bony digit fusion, Figs. 8.24E and 8.24F). Syndactyly can be inherited as a dominant or simple recessive trait. **Polydactyly** (supernumerary digits) is inherited as a dominant trait and is usually expressed as an extra digit or partial digit on the ulnar (postaxial) side of the hand, less often on the thumb (preaxial) side (Fig. 8.24G). It is 10 times more common in African and African American populations. Both syndactyly and polydactyly can result from mutations in pattern formation genes that will have them expressed as one feature in a syndrome of multiple anomalies. If a newborn has syndactyly or polydactyly, a search for more serious anomalies is in order.

CHANGES IN POSITION OF LIMBS BEFORE BIRTH

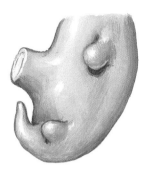
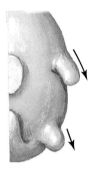

At 5 weeks. Upper and lower limbs have formed as finlike appendages pointing laterally and caudally

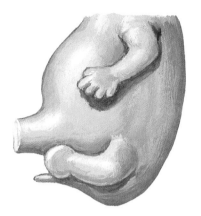
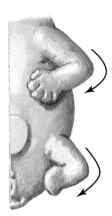

At 6 weeks. Limbs bend anteriorly, so elbows and knees point laterally, palms and soles face trunk

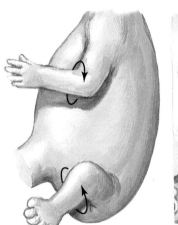
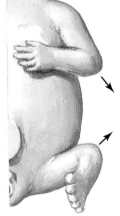

At 7 weeks. Upper and lower limbs have undergone 90-degree torsion about their long axes, but in opposite directions, so elbows point caudally and knees cranially

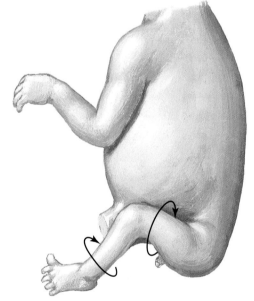
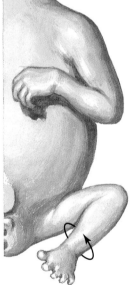

At 8 weeks. Torsion of lower limbs results in twisted or "barber pole" arrangement of their cutaneous innervation

8.25 ROTATION OF THE LIMBS

The limb buds are first oriented with their ventral surfaces facing medially and dorsal surfaces facing laterally. "Dorsal" and "ventral" in early limbs do not refer to adult anatomical directions but rather to continuity with the ventral and dorsal surfaces of the embryonic trunk. The upper extremity rotates 90 degrees laterally so that the ventral flexor compartment faces anteriorly. The lower extremity rotates 90 degrees medially so that the embryonic ventral flexor compartment is posterior in the lower limb and the extensors are anterior. The rotation occurs as a torsion in the femoral (and humeral) shaft. The flexors and extensors of the hip are mostly unaffected. Hip flexors are anterior; extensors are posterior.

Changes in ventral dermatome pattern (cutaneous sensory nerve distribution) during limb development

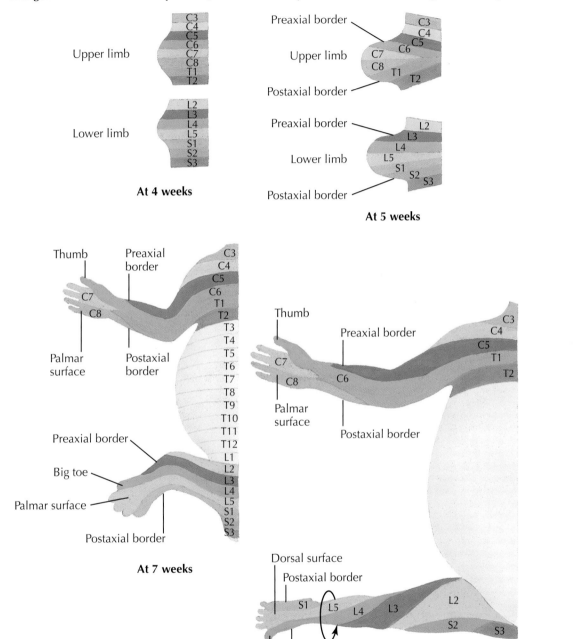

8.26 LIMB ROTATION AND DERMATOMES

Rotation of the lower limb results in a reversal of the preaxial and postaxial borders and a spiral, or "barber pole," arrangement of dermatomes. Spinal nerve segments on the anterior surface of the lower extremity extend medially and inferiorly, and the big toe (hallux) gets a higher dermatome (L4) than the little toe (S1). The lower extremity is an extension of the trunk, and the lowest dermatomes (sacral and coccygeal) are in the perineum, not the foot.

Comparison of embryonic limb organization to the plan of the brachial plexus

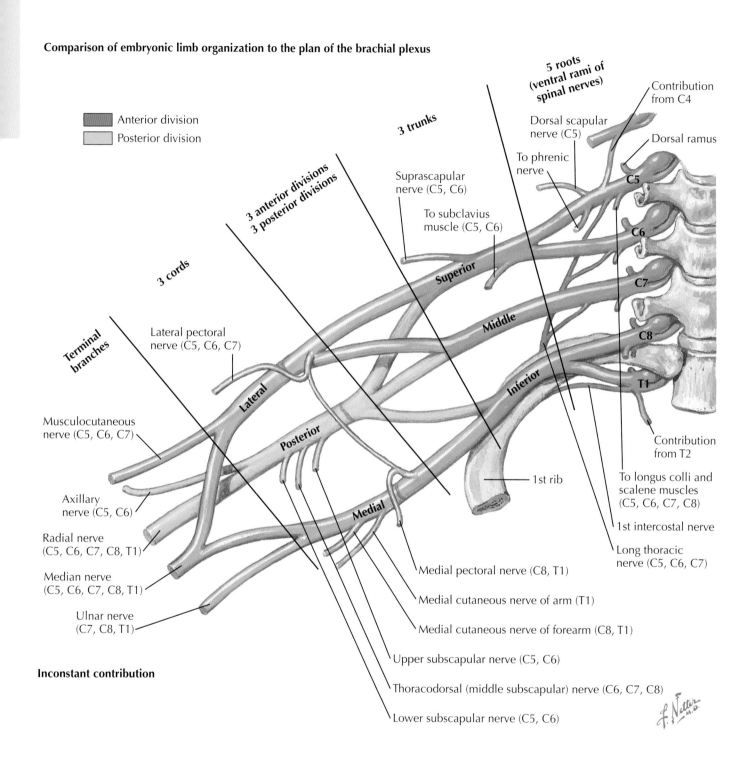

Anterior division
Posterior division

5 roots (ventral rami of spinal nerves)

3 trunks

3 anterior divisions
3 posterior divisions

3 cords

Terminal branches

Contribution from C4

Dorsal scapular nerve (C5)

Dorsal ramus

To phrenic nerve

Suprascapular nerve (C5, C6)

To subclavius muscle (C5, C6)

Superior

Middle

Inferior

C5

C6

C7

C8

T1

Lateral pectoral nerve (C5, C6, C7)

Lateral

Posterior

Musculocutaneous nerve (C5, C6, C7)

Axillary nerve (C5, C6)

Radial nerve (C5, C6, C7, C8, T1)

Median nerve (C5, C6, C7, C8, T1)

Ulnar nerve (C7, C8, T1)

Medial

1st rib

Contribution from T2

To longus colli and scalene muscles (C5, C6, C7, C8)

1st intercostal nerve

Long thoracic nerve (C5, C6, C7)

Medial pectoral nerve (C8, T1)

Medial cutaneous nerve of arm (T1)

Medial cutaneous nerve of forearm (C8, T1)

Upper subscapular nerve (C5, C6)

Thoracodorsal (middle subscapular) nerve (C6, C7, C8)

Lower subscapular nerve (C5, C6)

Inconstant contribution

8.27 EMBRYONIC PLAN OF THE BRACHIAL PLEXUS

The separation of the ventral rami and nerve trunks into anterior and posterior divisions is the most functionally important component of the brachial plexus. This relates to the embryonic separation of the myotome hypomeres into flexor and extensor compartment muscle groups. Nerve branches of anterior divisions (musculocutaneous, median, ulnar) go to flexor compartment muscles; branches of posterior divisions (axillary, radial, thoracodorsal, subscapular) supply extensor compartment muscles (see Fig. 8.22B).

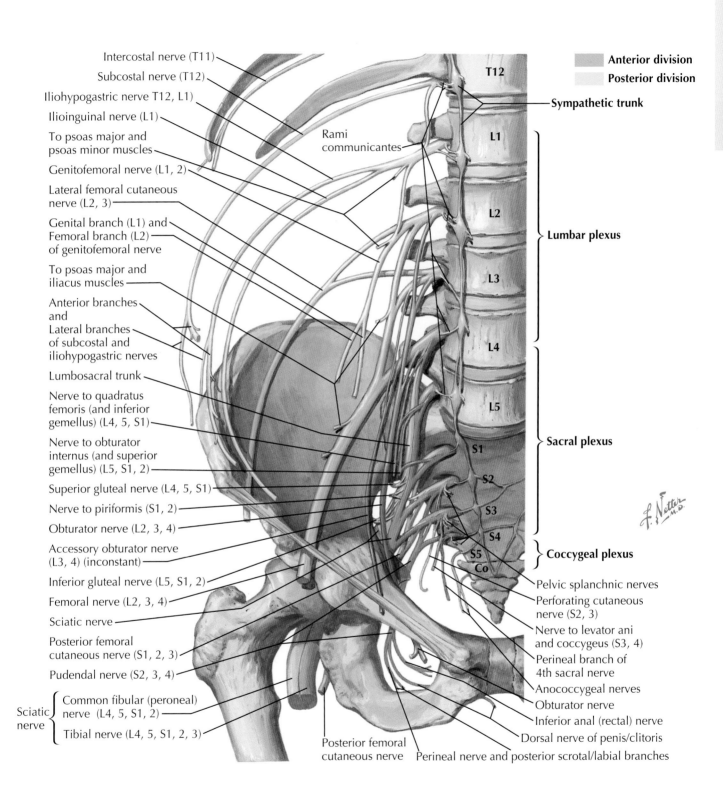

Intercostal nerve (T11)

Subcostal nerve (T12)

Iliohypogastric nerve T12, L1)

Ilioinguinal nerve (L1)

To psoas major and
psoas minor muscles

Genitofemoral nerve (L1, 2)

Lateral femoral cutaneous
nerve (L2, 3)

Genital branch (L1) and
Femoral branch (L2)
of genitofemoral nerve

To psoas major and
iliacus muscles

Anterior branches
and
Lateral branches
of subcostal and
iliohypogastric nerves

Lumbosacral trunk

Nerve to quadratus
femoris (and inferior
gemellus) (L4, 5, S1)

Nerve to obturator
internus (and superior
gemellus) (L5, S1, 2)

Superior gluteal nerve (L4, 5, S1)

Nerve to piriformis (S1, 2)

Obturator nerve (L2, 3, 4)

Accessory obturator nerve
(L3, 4) (inconstant)

Inferior gluteal nerve (L5, S1, 2)

Femoral nerve (L2, 3, 4)

Sciatic nerve

Posterior femoral
cutaneous nerve (S1, 2, 3)

Pudendal nerve (S2, 3, 4)

Sciatic nerve { Common fibular (peroneal) nerve (L4, 5, S1, 2)

Tibial nerve (L4, 5, S1, 2, 3)

Rami
communicantes

T12

L1

L2

L3

L4

L5

S1

S2

S3

S4

S5

Co

Anterior division
Posterior division

Sympathetic trunk

Lumbar plexus

Sacral plexus

Coccygeal plexus

Pelvic splanchnic nerves

Perforating cutaneous
nerve (S2, 3)

Nerve to levator ani
and coccygeus (S3, 4)

Perineal branch of
4th sacral nerve

Anococcygeal nerves

Obturator nerve

Inferior anal (rectal) nerve

Dorsal nerve of penis/clitoris

Posterior femoral
cutaneous nerve

Perineal nerve and posterior scrotal/labial branches

8.28 DIVISIONS OF THE LUMBOSACRAL PLEXUS

Anterior division nerves (tibial, obturator) to flexors are on the posterior aspect of the lower extremity, medial thigh, and sole of the foot. Posterior division nerves (femoral, common fibular) for extensors are mostly anterior in the adult.

Developing skeletal muscles at 8 weeks (superficial exposure)

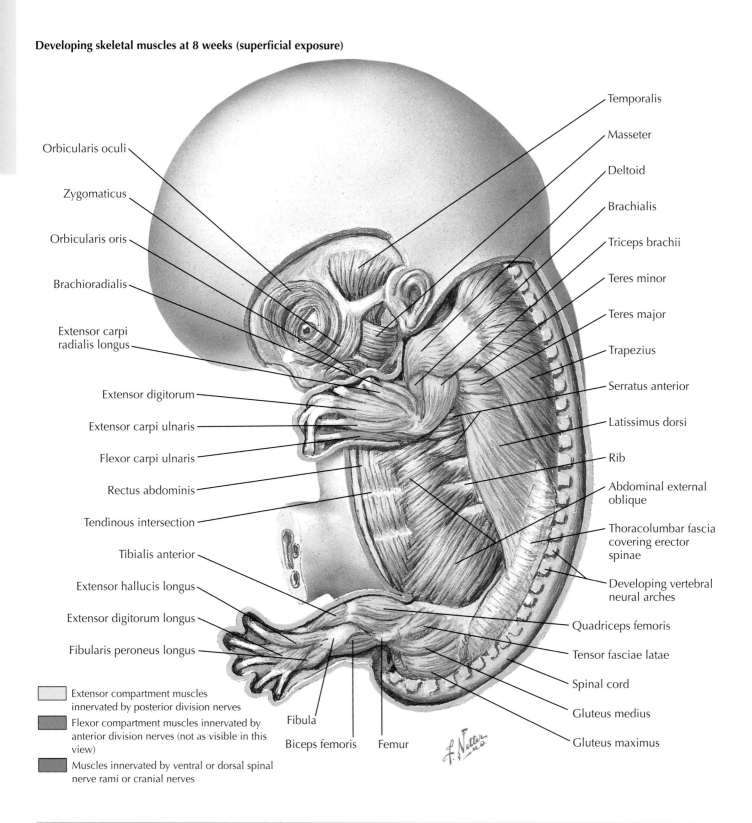

Orbicularis oculi

Zygomaticus

Orbicularis oris

Brachioradialis

Extensor carpi radialis longus

Extensor digitorum

Extensor carpi ulnaris

Flexor carpi ulnaris

Rectus abdominis

Tendinous intersection

Tibialis anterior

Extensor hallucis longus

Extensor digitorum longus

Fibularis peroneus longus

Temporalis

Masseter

Deltoid

Brachialis

Triceps brachii

Teres minor

Teres major

Trapezius

Serratus anterior

Latissimus dorsi

Rib

Abdominal external oblique

Thoracolumbar fascia covering erector spinae

Developing vertebral neural arches

Quadriceps femoris

Tensor fasciae latae

Spinal cord

Gluteus medius

Gluteus maximus

Fibula

Biceps femoris

Femur

Extensor compartment muscles innervated by posterior division nerves

Flexor compartment muscles innervated by anterior division nerves (not as visible in this view)

Muscles innervated by ventral or dorsal spinal nerve rami or cranial nerves

8.29 DEVELOPING SKELETAL MUSCLES

Muscles of the head and neck are derived from somitomeres—some (extraocular eye muscles and tongue muscles) directly and the rest (muscles of mastication and facial expression, and neck and larynx muscles) via somitic cell migration into the pharyngeal arches. Intercostal and abdominal muscles are innervated by the ventral rami of spinal nerves, and the limbs are innervated by the separation of the ventral rami into anterior and posterior division nerves of the brachial plexus and lumbosacral plexus. Most of the flexor muscles (green) are not visible in Fig. 8.29 because the flexor compartments are in the medial, ventral half of the limb buds. The ventral surface of the limb buds is continuous with the ventral surface of the trunk.

Terminology

Amelia
(G., "absence of (a) limb") The absence of an entire upper or lower extremity. Subcategories (meromelia) can be the absence of any component of a limb.

Apical ectodermal ridge
A ridge of ectoderm at the distal margin of the limb buds that plays an important signaling role in the determination of proximal-distal morphological differentiation of the limb bones.

Appendicular skeleton
(L., appendix—"appendage") Limb bones, including anchoring girdle bones—the clavicle, scapula, and pelvis.

Axial skeleton
The skeleton along the vertical axis of the body: the skull, vertebral column, and ribs.

Cancellous bone
Spongy or trabecular bone that forms the interior of most bones.

Cement line
Thin line surrounding osteons consisting of highly mineralized bone lacking collagen fibers.

Cranium
Skull, except the mandible.

Diaphysis
Shaft of a long bone formed by a primary center of ossification.

Diploë
Cancellous bone between inner and outer layers of compact bone in the flat neurocranial bones.

Endochondral bone
Bones that begin with a hyaline cartilaginous model. Includes most of the postcranial bones and the cranial base at the interface between the neurocranium (braincase) and viscerocranium (facial skeleton).

Endomysium
Thin, connective tissue layer surrounding each skeletal muscle cell.

Endosteum
Equivalent of periosteum on the inside of the wall of compact bone.

Epimere
Dorsal part of a somite myotome that forms the intrinsic back muscles and is innervated by the dorsal rami of spinal nerves.

Epimysium
Dense connective tissue enveloping a muscle.

Epiphysis
The ends of long bones formed from secondary centers of ossification.

Fiber
A muscle cell or a nerve cell.

Filaments
Threads of actin and myosin molecules within muscle cells.

Hyaline cartilage
Most common type of cartilage; it has a homogeneous matrix and is found in ribs, most of the larynx, rings of the airway, articular cartilage, and epiphyseal plates. The other two types of cartilage, elastic cartilage and fibrocartilage, are classified by the type of fibers embedded in the cartilage matrix.

Hypomere
Ventral part of a somite myotome that forms all muscles other than intrinsic back muscles (intercostal and abdominal muscles, and all muscle cells in the limbs). Hypomeres are innervated by the ventral rami of spinal nerves.

Interstitial growth
Addition of new cells and connective tissue matrix from within the matrix. Cartilage grows interstitially; bone does not.

Lacunae
(L., "little lakes") Spaces in bone matrix where osteocytes reside. Bone cells in lacunae are osteocytes. Cells on bone surface are osteoblasts.

Lamellae
Layers of bone in mature, compact bone. Organized as circumferential lamellae, concentric lamellae of osteons, and interstitial lamellae between osteons. Separated by thin layers of collagen fibers that are parallel within layers and perpendicular between layers.

Metaphysis
Flaring ends of a long bone under the epiphyseal growth plates where new bone is deposited with the growth in length of the bone.

Neurocranium
Bones surrounding the brain. The bottom of the neurocranium is the cranial base at the interface between neurocranium and viscerocranium.

Terminology—cont'd

Osteoid	Organic component of bone matrix that is deposited by osteoblasts before it becomes mineralized by membrane-bound packets of hydroxyapatite crystals.
Osteon	A haversian system, the structural unit of mature, compact bone consisting of a series of concentric lamellae surrounding a central (haversian) canal containing an arteriole, nerve, and other cells.
Perimysium	Connective tissue surrounding groups of skeletal muscle cells or larger units within a muscle. It has epithelial, contractile, and connective tissue properties.
Periosteum	Outer fibrous covering of bones with an outer, dense connective tissue layer and inner osteogenic layer.
Plexus	(L., "braid") Interconnecting nerves or vessels.
Polydactyly	(G., "many fingers") Supernumerary fingers or toes.
Postcranial	Beneath the cranium. Postcranial skeleton consists of all bones except the skull.
Sclerotome	(G., "hard cutting") Ventromedial part of a somite that forms the endochondral bone of the vertebral column, ribs, and cranial base.
Scoliosis	Lateral curvature of the vertebral column.
Skull	Cranium plus the mandible.
Spina bifida	(L., "split spine") Defective development of a vertebral arch consisting of pedicles, laminae, and vertebral spine. It is usually accompanied by herniation of meninges and or the spinal cord through the defect onto the surface of the back.
Syndactyly	(G., "together – finger") Fusion of digits during development. It can be cutaneous (webbed fingers or toes) or fusion of phalangeal bone.
Trabeculae	(L., "little beams") Interconnecting bony spicules of spongy (or cancellous or trabecular) bone.
Viscerocranium	Facial skeleton consisting of the upper and lower jaws, nasal bones, and bony eye sockets.
Woven bone	Immature, nonlamellar bone where the collagen fibers are in a random "woven" orientation in the matrix. Bone is always deposited as woven bone; most of the embryonic and fetal skeleton is woven bone.
Zone of polarizing activity	A signaling center at the caudal end of each limb bud that plays important roles in determining cranio-caudal differentiation of the limbs and interaction with the apical ectodermal ridge.

9

HEAD AND NECK

PRENATAL TIME SCALE (MONTHS)

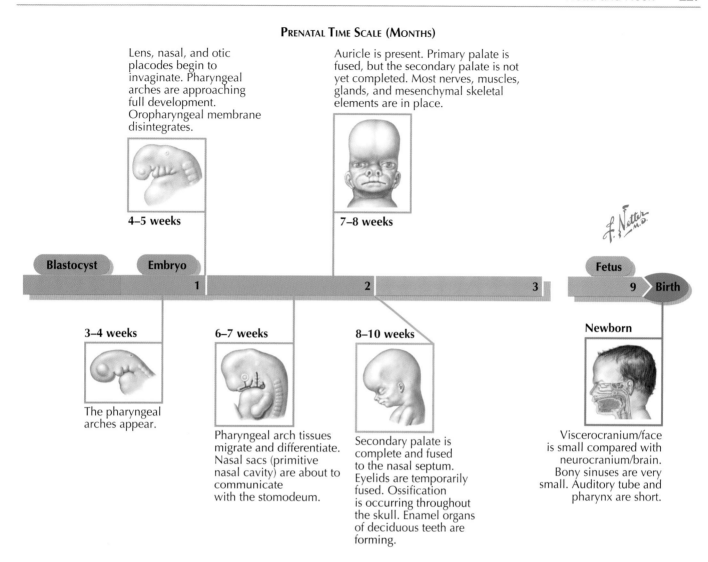

Lens, nasal, and otic placodes begin to invaginate. Pharyngeal arches are approaching full development. Oropharyngeal membrane disintegrates.

4–5 weeks

Auricle is present. Primary palate is fused, but the secondary palate is not yet completed. Most nerves, muscles, glands, and mesenchymal skeletal elements are in place.

7–8 weeks

Blastocyst   Embryo   Fetus   Birth

1   2   3   9

3–4 weeks

The pharyngeal arches appear.

6–7 weeks

Pharyngeal arch tissues migrate and differentiate. Nasal sacs (primitive nasal cavity) are about to communicate with the stomodeum.

8–10 weeks

Secondary palate is complete and fused to the nasal septum. Eyelids are temporarily fused. Ossification is occurring throughout the skull. Enamel organs of deciduous teeth are forming.

Newborn

Viscerocranium/face is small compared with neurocranium/brain. Bony sinuses are very small. Auditory tube and pharynx are short.

9.1 TIMELINE

MESODERMAL PRIMORDIA
Postotic somites, preotic somitomeres, head mesenchyme from neural crest, pharyngeal arch mesenchyme (from neural crest and somitomeres).

ECTODERMAL PRIMORDIA
Surface ectoderm, lining of the stomodeum (primitive oral and nasal cavities), pharyngeal grooves between the pharyngeal arches, and surface placodes.

ENDODERMAL PRIMORDIA
Foregut, pharyngeal pouches between the pharyngeal arches.

PLAN
The head and neck have segmental motor and sensory innervation like the rest of the body, but there are several new features. The head region is underdeveloped at the time of gastrulation, and little primitive streak mesoderm other than somitomeres extends into the head. The neural crest is the origin of most head mesenchyme, and much of it is organized into a series of horizontal bars flanking the foregut. These pharyngeal arches evolved as the gill apparatus in fish but form most of the structures in the head and neck of higher animals. Some alternative and clinical resources refer to these structures as the "branchial arches," linked to the gill appearance, although "pharyngeal" is now regarded as the

more accurate term for human anatomy. The head also has special sensory organs and related neurons that derive from ectodermal surface placodes. Even the predominant type of ossification in the head—intramembranous—is different than the endochondral bone formation in the postcranial skeleton.

INCLUSION AND BIAS CONSIDERATION: SPECIAL SENSORY DEVELOPMENT
Like the considerations presented in Chapter 3, understanding the development of structures of the head and neck region is critical in understanding the structure of special sensory organs. Such organs can be important in informing individuals' interactions with the world, in addition to expression of behaviors. It is important to recognize the role of respecting "neurodiversity" and emphasis on supporting individual autonomy. For example, this chapter details ear development, which relates to the diversity of the deaf and hearing community. Lowercase "deaf" is frequently used when referring to an audiological condition, whereas uppercase "Deaf" is the preferred term of individuals who identify with the Deaf community and ascribe to Deaf culture. Deaf culture has unique shared values and behaviors, including use of sign language as their primary language. Individuals should be comfortable discussing such terms and having clinical and educational spaces representative of these. This is just one example of how understanding language of sensory organs is essential to inclusive practices.

EMBRYO AT 3 TO 5 WEEKS

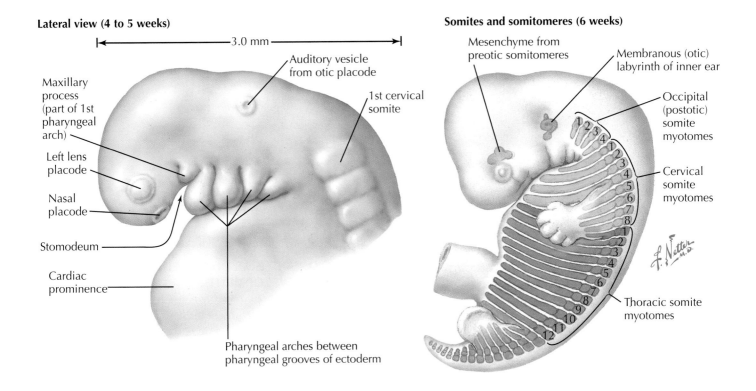

Lateral view (3 to 4 weeks)

1.0 mm

Forebrain
Left optic vesicle
Otic placode
1st cervical somite
Stomodeum
Cardiac prominence
2nd pharyngeal elevation (future hyoid arch)
1st pharyngeal elevation (future mandibular arch)

Sagittal section (3 to 4 weeks)

Future brain ventricle
Neural crest mesenchyme (surrounds brain)
Rathke's pouch
Oropharyngeal membrane
Ectoderm
Foregut
Forebrain (neural tube)
Future thyroid gland
Anterior neuropore
Future lung bud
Stomodeum
Future thoracic wall
Midgut
Heart
Future liver
Pericardial coelom
Yolk sac wall
Amnion
Extraembryonic coelom

Lateral view (4 to 5 weeks)

3.0 mm

Maxillary process (part of 1st pharyngeal arch)
Auditory vesicle from otic placode
1st cervical somite
Left lens placode
Nasal placode
Stomodeum
Cardiac prominence
Pharyngeal arches between pharyngeal grooves of ectoderm

Somites and somitomeres (6 weeks)

Mesenchyme from preotic somitomeres
Membranous (otic) labyrinth of inner ear
Occipital (postotic) somite myotomes
Cervical somite myotomes
Thoracic somite myotomes

9.2 ECTODERM, ENDODERM, AND MESODERM

The surface ectoderm invaginates to form the **stomodeum**, the lining of the future oral and nasal cavities. The ectoderm thickens in three locations to form olfactory, lens, and otic **placodes** that relate to the special sensory cranial nerves I, II, and VIII, respectively. The endoderm of the foregut extends to the stomodeum and will line the pharynx, larynx, trachea, esophagus, and related structures. Mesoderm in the head is in the form of **somites** and **head mesenchyme** from the **neural crest**. The latter surrounds the developing brain and forms the **pharyngeal arches** innervated by nerves V, VII, IX, and X. Postotic somites become tongue muscles (nerve XII), and preotic somitomeres form eye muscles (nerves III, IV, and VI).

Embryo at 4 to 5 weeks: lateral view

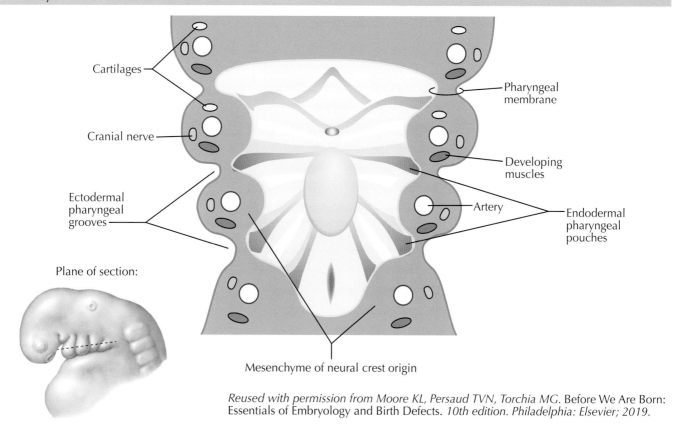

Cartilages

Cranial nerve

Ectodermal
pharyngeal
grooves

Pharyngeal
membrane

Developing
muscles

Artery

Endodermal
pharyngeal
pouches

Plane of section:

Mesenchyme of neural crest origin

Reused with permission from Moore KL, Persaud TVN, Torchia MG. Before We Are Born:
Essentials of Embryology and Birth Defects. *10th edition. Philadelphia: Elsevier; 2019.*

Pharyngeal pouches and aortic arch arteries: lateral view

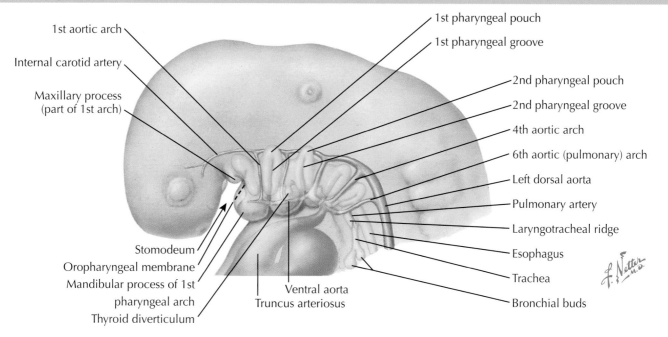

1st aortic arch

Internal carotid artery

Maxillary process
(part of 1st arch)

Stomodeum
Oropharyngeal membrane
Mandibular process of 1st
pharyngeal arch
Thyroid diverticulum

Ventral aorta
Truncus arteriosus

1st pharyngeal pouch

1st pharyngeal groove

2nd pharyngeal pouch

2nd pharyngeal groove

4th aortic arch

6th aortic (pulmonary) arch

Left dorsal aorta

Pulmonary artery

Laryngotracheal ridge

Esophagus

Trachea

Bronchial buds

9.3 PHARYNGEAL (BRANCHIAL) ARCHES

The pharyngeal (branchial) arches are transverse swellings of mesenchyme that flank the foregut. They are covered with surface ectoderm on the outside and endoderm of the foregut on the inside. **Pharyngeal grooves** of ectoderm separate each pharyngeal arch on the surface, and **pharyngeal pouches** of foregut endoderm are their equivalent on the inside. Six arches originally evolved in fish as the primordia of the gill apparatus and viscerocranium. There are five arches in mammals, designated 1, 2, 3, 4, and 6 (arch 5 does not develop); they form most of the structures in the face and neck. Each mesodermal arch has a cranial nerve, a piece of cartilage, and an aortic arch artery.

Ventral view

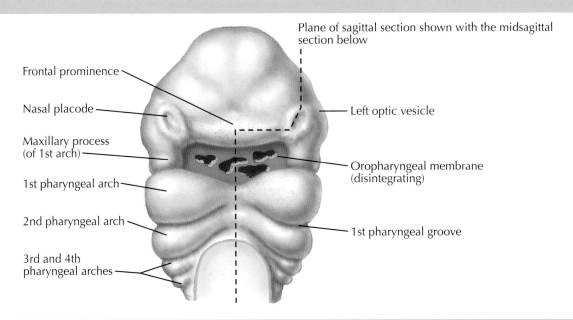

Plane of sagittal section shown with the midsagittal section below

Frontal prominence

Nasal placode

Maxillary process (of 1st arch)

1st pharyngeal arch

2nd pharyngeal arch

3rd and 4th pharyngeal arches

Left optic vesicle

Oropharyngeal membrane (disintegrating)

1st pharyngeal groove

Midsagittal section

Infundibulum (posterior lobe)
Rathke's pouch (anterior lobe) } Pituitary gland

Hypothalamus of brain

Frontal prominence

Nasal placode

Stomodeum

1st pharyngeal arch

Thyroid diverticulum

1st pharyngeal pouch

Oropharyngeal membrane (disintegrating)

Pharynx

Laryngotracheal ridge or groove

Esophagus

Bronchial bud

9.4 VENTRAL AND MIDSAGITTAL VIEWS

The first pharyngeal arch has maxillary and mandibular parts that form the lateral and inferior boundaries of the stomodeum, respectively. The maxillary (V2) and mandibular (V3) divisions of the trigeminal nerve supply the two primordia. Because of its relationship to the stomodeum, the first pharyngeal arch has ectoderm on the outside and inside, with more intense general sensory (somatic) innervation than the visceral sensory nerves that supply the endoderm on the inside of the other arches and the gut in general. The maxillary part of the first arch gives rise to the maxilla and structures of the midface, apart from the nose. The mandibular arch develops into the mandible and related structures.

CLINICAL POINT

Pierre Robin sequence, typically from a de novo mutation, is a group of facial anomalies caused by insufficient migration of mesenchyme into the first branchial arch. Major features include a small mandible (micrognathia), a resultant displaced tongue that compresses the upper airway, and often a cleft palate. Incidence is about 1 in 10,000.

CLINICAL POINT

Treacher Collins syndrome (from an autosomal dominant mutation) only affects zygomatic bone development in the upper jaw with a characteristic flattening of that facial region. Anomalies in the lower eyelids and the external ear may also be present.

EMBRYO AT **4** TO **5** WEEKS

Pharynx (ventral view)

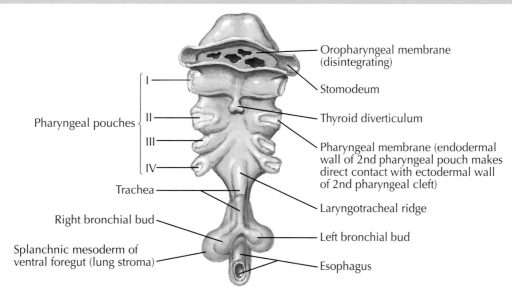

Oropharyngeal membrane (disintegrating)

Stomodeum

Thyroid diverticulum

Pharyngeal membrane (endodermal wall of 2nd pharyngeal pouch makes direct contact with ectodermal wall of 2nd pharyngeal cleft)

Laryngotracheal ridge

Left bronchial bud

Esophagus

Pharyngeal pouches { I, II, III, IV

Trachea

Right bronchial bud

Splanchnic mesoderm of ventral foregut (lung stroma)

Pharynx (anterior view of left side)

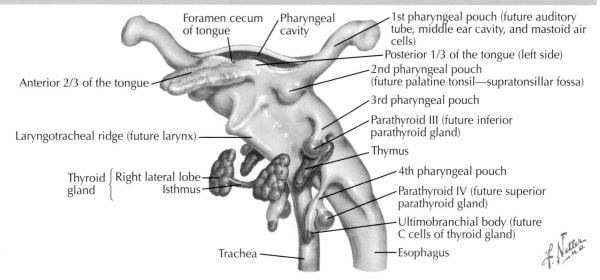

Foramen cecum of tongue

Pharyngeal cavity

1st pharyngeal pouch (future auditory tube, middle ear cavity, and mastoid air cells)

Posterior 1/3 of the tongue (left side)

2nd pharyngeal pouch (future palatine tonsil—supratonsillar fossa)

3rd pharyngeal pouch

Parathyroid III (future inferior parathyroid gland)

Thymus

4th pharyngeal pouch

Parathyroid IV (future superior parathyroid gland)

Ultimobranchial body (future C cells of thyroid gland)

Esophagus

Anterior 2/3 of the tongue

Laryngotracheal ridge (future larynx)

Thyroid gland { Right lateral lobe, Isthmus

Trachea

9.5 FATE OF THE PHARYNGEAL POUCHES

Pouch 1 forms the auditory tube, middle ear cavity, and mastoid air cells. Pouch 2 forms the epithelial crypts of the palatine tonsil. Epithelial cells from the rest of the pouches migrate to form the thymus gland (pouch 3), parathyroid glands (pouches 3 and 4), and parafollicular cells (C cells) of the thyroid gland (pouch 4). Parathyroid glands from pouch 3 become the inferior parathyroid glands as they descend with the thymus gland to a lower position than the superior parathyroid glands from pouch 4. The thyroid gland has its own diverticulum off the back of the tongue. It descends as a thyroglossal duct to its position anterior to the trachea.

CLINICAL POINT

DiGeorge syndrome. Improper development of pouch 3 (and sometimes 4) is a component of **DiGeorge syndrome**, an autosomal dominant mutation in chromosome 22 that affects many organs and facial morphology. The pouch 3 effect is the absence or underdevelopment of the thymus gland and subsequent absent or severely depressed T-cell–mediated immunity. The inferior parathyroid glands are also affected, causing hypocalcemia.

CLINICAL POINT

Otitis media (middle ear inflammation) is the most common illness pediatricians encounter and is reported to occur in 90% of preschool children. Not only does the auditory tube of the first pharyngeal pouch connect the middle ear to the nasopharynx, but it is shorter and more horizontal in children, predisposing to infection from the pharynx.

CLINICAL POINT

Thyroid anomalies. The most common **thyroid anomalies** are anterior midline **thyroid cysts** or **ectopic thyroid tissue** that may persist anywhere from the foramen cecum to the trachea. There also may be an undescended lingual thyroid gland.

Midsagittal section at 5 to 6 weeks

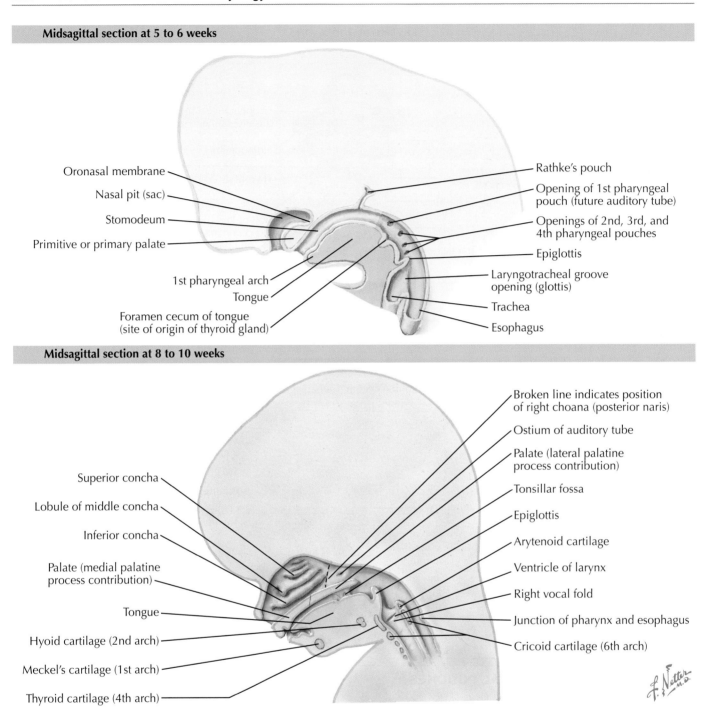

Oronasal membrane

Nasal pit (sac)

Stomodeum

Primitive or primary palate

1st pharyngeal arch

Tongue

Foramen cecum of tongue
(site of origin of thyroid gland)

Rathke's pouch

Opening of 1st pharyngeal
pouch (future auditory tube)

Openings of 2nd, 3rd, and
4th pharyngeal pouches

Epiglottis

Laryngotracheal groove
opening (glottis)

Trachea

Esophagus

Midsagittal section at 8 to 10 weeks

Superior concha

Lobule of middle concha

Inferior concha

Palate (medial palatine
process contribution)

Tongue

Hyoid cartilage (2nd arch)

Meckel's cartilage (1st arch)

Thyroid cartilage (4th arch)

Broken line indicates position
of right choana (posterior naris)

Ostium of auditory tube

Palate (lateral palatine
process contribution)

Tonsillar fossa

Epiglottis

Arytenoid cartilage

Ventricle of larynx

Right vocal fold

Junction of pharynx and esophagus

Cricoid cartilage (6th arch)

9.6 MIDSAGITTAL VIEW OF THE PHARYNX

Only the first and second pharyngeal pouches have derivatives visible in the pharynx after 10 weeks. The yellow portion of Fig. 9.6B (8–10 weeks) shows the superior extent of the foregut where it joins the ectoderm of the nasal and oral cavities at the site of the former oropharyngeal membrane. The opening of the **auditory tube** (pouch 1) is clearly seen above the soft palate in the **nasopharynx**. Below the soft palate is the **oropharynx** with the **palatine tonsils** and their epithelial crypts derived from the second pharyngeal pouch. The laryngopharynx surrounds the epiglottis and entrance to the larynx. Epithelial cells from pouches 3 and 4 migrate to form glands, and the lateral walls of the pharynx behind and below the palatine tonsils are smooth.

CLINICAL POINT

Developmental implications of head proportions for the pediatric airway. Compared with an adult, the infant has a relatively large occiput and neurocranium in general, predisposing the neck to flexion when supine that can cause airway obstruction. Also contributing to obstruction is the hyperextension that can result from the flexibility of the relatively large head. Exacerbating the risk of obstruction is a large infant tongue in a small viscerocranium. On the positive side, the infant pharynx is relatively short, facilitating alignment of the oral, pharyngeal, and tracheal axes in airway management.

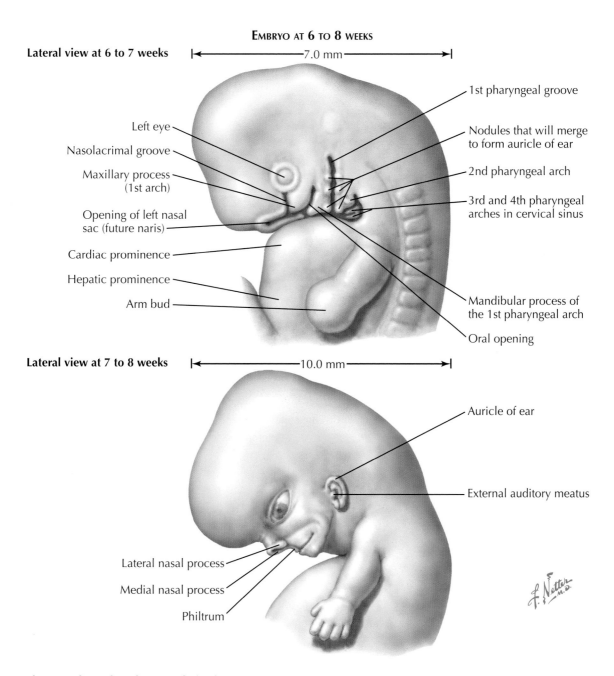

EMBRYO AT 6 TO 8 WEEKS

Lateral view at 6 to 7 weeks |← 7.0 mm →|

- 1st pharyngeal groove
- Nodules that will merge to form auricle of ear
- 2nd pharyngeal arch
- 3rd and 4th pharyngeal arches in cervical sinus
- Left eye
- Nasolacrimal groove
- Maxillary process (1st arch)
- Opening of left nasal sac (future naris)
- Cardiac prominence
- Hepatic prominence
- Arm bud
- Mandibular process of the 1st pharyngeal arch
- Oral opening

Lateral view at 7 to 8 weeks |← 10.0 mm →|

- Auricle of ear
- External auditory meatus
- Lateral nasal process
- Medial nasal process
- Philtrum

Pharyngeal pouch and groove derivatives

No.	From Pouches	From Grooves
1	Auditory tube, middle ear cavity, mastoid air cells	External auditory meatus
2	Palatine tonsil crypts	Cervical sinus (disappears)
3	Inferior parathyroids, thymus	Cervical sinus (disappears)
4	Superior parathyroids, parafollicular cells (C cells) of thyroid	Cervical sinus (disappears)

9.7 FATE OF THE PHARYNGEAL GROOVES

The ectoderm overlying arches 2 through 6 does not grow much and contributes little to the skin in adults. Pharyngeal grooves 2, 3, and 4 merge to form a **cervical sinus** that sinks beneath the surface as a cervical cyst that disappears. The external auditory meatus, the remnant of the first pharyngeal groove, is the only invagination on the side of the adult head and the only derivative of the pharyngeal grooves.

A. Adult fistulas

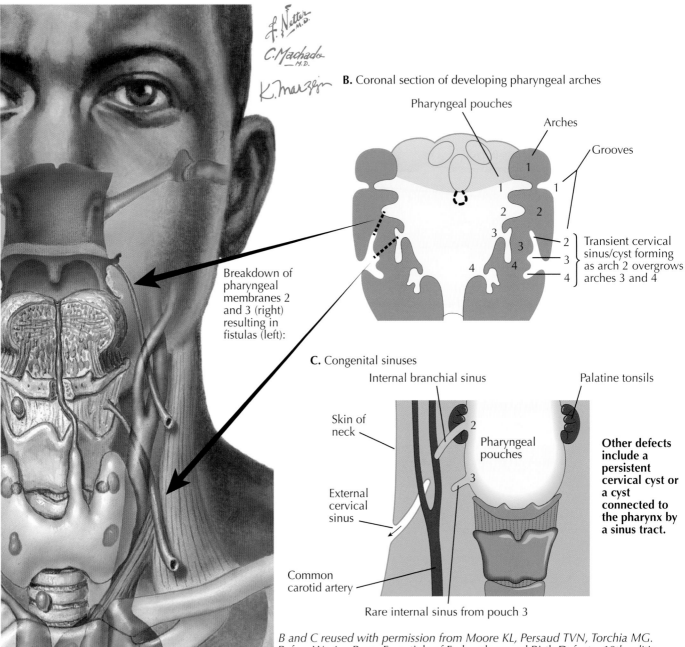

Breakdown of pharyngeal membranes 2 and 3 (right) resulting in fistulas (left):

B. Coronal section of developing pharyngeal arches

Pharyngeal pouches

Arches

Grooves

1
1
2   2
3   3   2
4   4   3
4

Transient cervical sinus/cyst forming as arch 2 overgrows arches 3 and 4

C. Congenital sinuses

Internal branchial sinus

Palatine tonsils

Skin of neck

External cervical sinus

Common carotid artery

Pharyngeal pouches

2

3

Rare internal sinus from pouch 3

Other defects include a persistent cervical cyst or a cyst connected to the pharynx by a sinus tract.

B and C reused with permission from Moore KL, Persaud TVN, Torchia MG. Before We Are Born: Essentials of Embryology and Birth Defects. 10th edition. Philadelphia: Elsevier; 2019.

9.8 PHARYNGEAL CYST, SINUS, AND FISTULA FORMATION

Pharyngeal cysts, sinuses, and fistulas in the neck result from disruptions in the process of the disappearance of branchial grooves 2, 3, and 4, and their relationship to pharyngeal pouches 2, 3, and 4. Fig. 9.8A shows examples of adult fistulas, and Fig. 9.8B shows the embryonic mechanism for their creation. Branchial grooves 2, 3, and 4 merge with each other as arch 2 overgrows the lower arches. They form a sinus and then a cervical cyst that typically disappears. Early in this process, they still abut against their corresponding pharyngeal pouches via the developing cyst. The dashed lines in Fig. 9.8B show where the breakdown of the pharyngeal membranes occurs (at an earlier date). Fig. 9.8C shows congenital sinuses that may be external or internal, with a summary description of congenital cysts.

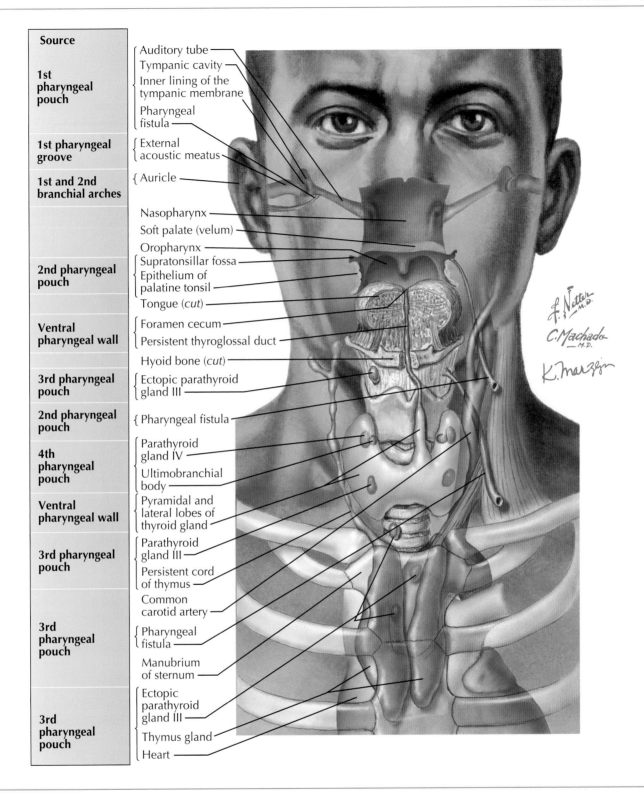

Source	
1st pharyngeal pouch	Auditory tube
	Tympanic cavity
	Inner lining of the tympanic membrane
	Pharyngeal fistula
1st pharyngeal groove	External acoustic meatus
1st and 2nd branchial arches	Auricle
	Nasopharynx
	Soft palate (velum)
	Oropharynx
2nd pharyngeal pouch	Supratonsillar fossa
	Epithelium of palatine tonsil
	Tongue (*cut*)
Ventral pharyngeal wall	Foramen cecum
	Persistent thyroglossal duct
	Hyoid bone (*cut*)
3rd pharyngeal pouch	Ectopic parathyroid gland III
2nd pharyngeal pouch	Pharyngeal fistula
4th pharyngeal pouch	Parathyroid gland IV
	Ultimobranchial body
Ventral pharyngeal wall	Pyramidal and lateral lobes of thyroid gland
3rd pharyngeal pouch	Parathyroid gland III
	Persistent cord of thymus
	Common carotid artery
3rd pharyngeal pouch	Pharyngeal fistula
	Manubrium of sternum
3rd pharyngeal pouch	Ectopic parathyroid gland III
	Thymus gland
	Heart

9.9 SUMMARY OF PHARYNGEAL GROOVE AND POUCH ANOMALIES

The only visible derivate of the branchial grooves of ectoderm is the lining of the external auditory meatus and external surface of the tympanic membrane. The only visible derivatives of the endodermal pharyngeal pouches are the opening of the auditory tube (pouch 1) and lining of the palatine tonsil (pouch 2). Pouch 3 is the most common source of ectopic tissue because its thymus gland derivate must migrate a long distance into the mediastinum.

There is more opportunity for an undescended thymus gland or the trailing of thymic tissue along the path of descent. Parathyroid glands from pouch 3 may be carried with the thymus into the thorax or also be located anywhere along the path of descent. The thyroid gland has its own dedicated midline bud off the back of the tongue. Also note the path of a persistent **thyroglossal duct** from the tongue to the gland's location anterior to the trachea. It may present as midline cysts, ectopic thyroid tissue, or an undescended thyroid gland imbedded in the tongue.

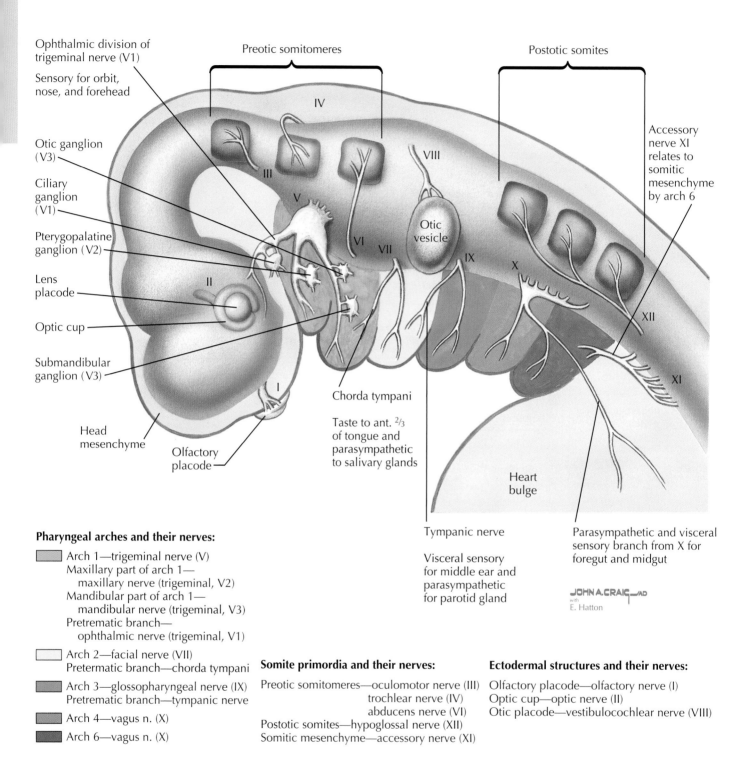

Ophthalmic division of
trigeminal nerve (V1)

Sensory for orbit,
nose, and forehead

Otic ganglion
(V3)

Ciliary
ganglion
(V1)

Pterygopalatine
ganglion (V2)

Lens
placode

Optic cup

Submandibular
ganglion (V3)

Head
mesenchyme

Olfactory
placode

Preotic somitomeres

Postotic somites

Accessory
nerve XI
relates to
somitic
mesenchyme
by arch 6

Otic
vesicle

Chorda tympani

Taste to ant. $^2/_3$
of tongue and
parasympathetic
to salivary glands

Heart
bulge

Tympanic nerve

Visceral sensory
for middle ear and
parasympathetic
for parotid gland

Parasympathetic and visceral
sensory branch from X for
foregut and midgut

JOHN A. CRAIG
with
E. Hatton

Pharyngeal arches and their nerves:

Arch 1—trigeminal nerve (V)
  Maxillary part of arch 1—
    maxillary nerve (trigeminal, V2)
  Mandibular part of arch 1—
    mandibular nerve (trigeminal, V3)
  Pretrematic branch—
    ophthalmic nerve (trigeminal, V1)

Arch 2—facial nerve (VII)
  Pretrematic branch—chorda tympani

Arch 3—glossopharyngeal nerve (IX)
  Pretrematic branch—tympanic nerve

Arch 4—vagus n. (X)

Arch 6—vagus n. (X)

Somite primordia and their nerves:

Preotic somitomeres—oculomotor nerve (III)
            trochlear nerve (IV)
            abducens nerve (VI)
Postotic somites—hypoglossal nerve (XII)
Somitic mesenchyme—accessory nerve (XI)

Ectodermal structures and their nerves:

Olfactory placode—olfactory nerve (I)
Optic cup—optic nerve (II)
Otic placode—vestibulocochlear nerve (VIII)

9.10 CRANIAL NERVE PRIMORDIA

The 12 pairs of cranial nerves exit the developing brain in
sequence, except for the accessory nerve (XI). The nerves relate to
surface placodes, the optic cup, head somites, or the pharyngeal
arches and innervate all of the structures and tissues that derive

from them. The vagus nerve supplies both arches 4 and 6 (the latter branch was formerly considered the "cranial root" of XI). The
mesoderm of the accessory nerve (formerly the "spinal root" of
XI) is somitic mesenchyme in the vicinity of pharyngeal arch 6.

SPECIAL SENSORY AND SOMATOMOTOR CRANIAL NERVE NEURON COMPONENTS

Nerve	Primordium Innervated	Neuron Components
Olfactory (I) Optic (II) Vestibulocochlear (VIII)	Olfactory placode Optic cup Otic placode	Special sensory (olfaction) Special sensory (vision) Special sensory (hearing and balance)
Oculomotor (III)	Preotic somitomere	Somatomotor to extraocular eye muscles Parasympathetics to ciliary ganglion (for pupil constrictor and ciliary muscle)
Trochlear (IV) Abducens (VI) Hypoglossal (XII) Accessory (XI)	Preotic somitomere Preotic somitomere Postotic somites Somitic mesenchyme by arch 6	Somatomotor to superior oblique muscle Somatomotor to lateral rectus muscle Somatomotor to tongue muscles Somatomotor to sternocleidomastoid and trapezius

PHARYNGEAL ARCH CRANIAL NERVE NEURON COMPONENTS

Nerve	Arch	Neuron Components
Trigeminal (V)	1	General sensory (face, orbit, nasal, and oral cavities) Branchiomotor (muscles of mastication; tensor tympani; tensor veli palatini)

Facial (VII)	2	Branchiomotor (muscles of facial expression; stylohyoid; posterior
		    digastric; stapedius)
		Special sensory (taste to anterior two-thirds of tongue)
		Parasympathetic to pterygopalatine and submandibular ganglia
		    (for lacrimal gland, nasal mucosa, and salivary glands)

Glossopharyngeal (IX)	3	Visceral sensory to pharynx Branchiomotor to stylopharyngeus Parasympathetic to otic ganglion (for the parotid gland) Special sensory (taste to posterior tongue; carotid body and sinus)
Vagus (X)	4 and 6	Branchiomotor (pharynx and larynx) Visceral sensory (larynx; foregut below pharynx and midgut) General sensory to external acoustic meatus Parasympathetics (enteric ganglia of foregut and midgut) Special sensory (taste in laryngopharynx; carotid body and sinus)

9.11 CRANIAL NERVE NEURON COMPONENTS

The pharyngeal arch nerves are the territorial nerves of the head and neck with more than one neuron type. Most have branchiomotor neurons for skeletal muscles derived from arch mesenchyme, visceral sensory neurons for the inner endodermal linings of the arches (pharynx and larynx), and general sensory neurons for surface ectoderm or lining of the stomodeum. The somites give rise to extraocular eye and tongue muscles, and the placodes and optic cup relate to the special sensory organs of the head. Cranial nerves III, VII, IX, and X also exit the brain with presynaptic parasympathetic neurons that are mostly destined for structures in territories distant from their nerve of origin.

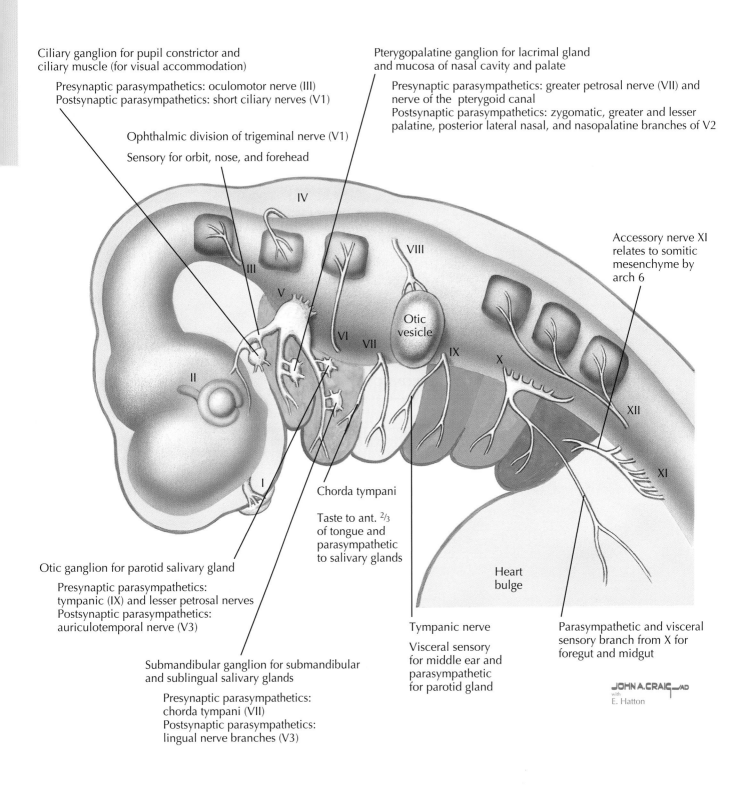

Ciliary ganglion for pupil constrictor and
ciliary muscle (for visual accommodation)

Presynaptic parasympathetics: oculomotor nerve (III)
Postsynaptic parasympathetics: short ciliary nerves (V1)

Ophthalmic division of trigeminal nerve (V1)

Sensory for orbit, nose, and forehead

Pterygopalatine ganglion for lacrimal gland
and mucosa of nasal cavity and palate

Presynaptic parasympathetics: greater petrosal nerve (VII) and
nerve of the pterygoid canal
Postsynaptic parasympathetics: zygomatic, greater and lesser
palatine, posterior lateral nasal, and nasopalatine branches of V2

Accessory nerve XI
relates to somitic
mesenchyme by
arch 6

Otic
vesicle

Otic ganglion for parotid salivary gland

Presynaptic parasympathetics:
tympanic (IX) and lesser petrosal nerves
Postsynaptic parasympathetics:
auriculotemporal nerve (V3)

Submandibular ganglion for submandibular
and sublingual salivary glands

Presynaptic parasympathetics:
chorda tympani (VII)
Postsynaptic parasympathetics:
lingual nerve branches (V3)

Chorda tympani

Taste to ant. $^2/_3$
of tongue and
parasympathetic
to salivary glands

Heart
bulge

Tympanic nerve

Visceral sensory
for middle ear and
parasympathetic
for parotid gland

Parasympathetic and visceral
sensory branch from X for
foregut and midgut

JOHN A.CRAIG __/AD
with
E. Hatton

9.12 PARASYMPATHETIC INNERVATION AND UNIQUE NERVES

Presynaptic parasympathetic neurons exit the brain with the cranial nerves III, VII, IX, and X, but all structures in the head that need parasympathetic innervation are in the territory of the trigeminal nerve. Parasympathetics from cranial nerves III, VII, and IX synapse in one of four ganglia, then travel with trigeminal branches to their targets. The **accessory nerve** (XI) is unique. It exits the spinal cord in line with branchiomotor roots of cranial nerves, enters the skull through the foramen magnum, and then exits the skull via the jugular canal to innervate neck muscles. In the **pretrematic nerve concept,** the first three pharyngeal arch nerves have branches that leave their arch of origin to provide sensory innervation to the territory immediately preceding its arch.

What the sensory nerve territories would be if the embryonic pattern of the pharyngeal arches was retained

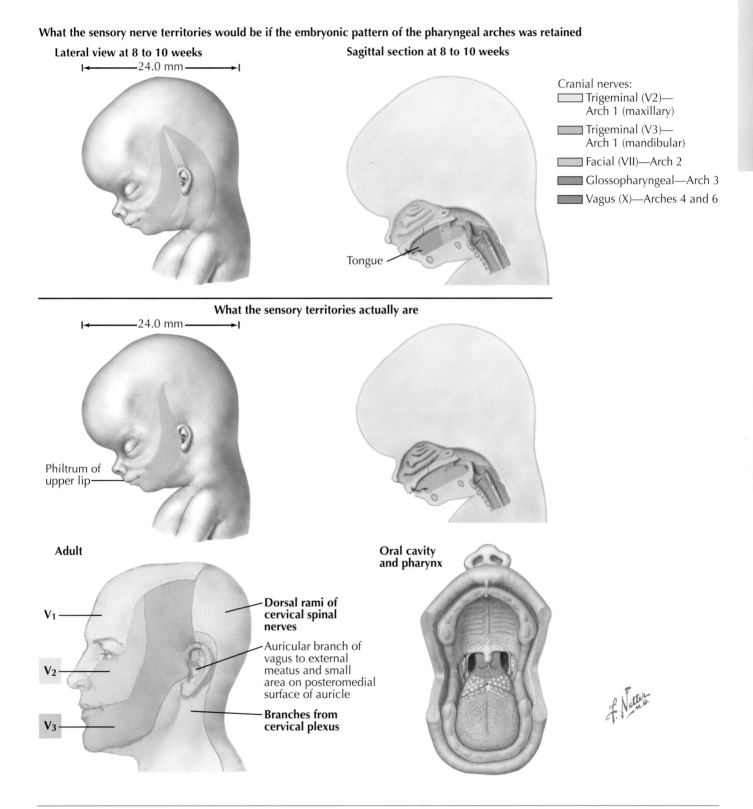

Lateral view at 8 to 10 weeks

|←——24.0 mm——→|

Sagittal section at 8 to 10 weeks

Cranial nerves:
- ▢ Trigeminal (V2)—Arch 1 (maxillary)
- ▢ Trigeminal (V3)—Arch 1 (mandibular)
- ▢ Facial (VII)—Arch 2
- ▢ Glossopharyngeal—Arch 3
- ▢ Vagus (X)—Arches 4 and 6

Tongue

What the sensory territories actually are

|←——24.0 mm——→|

Philtrum of upper lip

Adult

Oral cavity and pharynx

V_1

V_2

V_3

Dorsal rami of cervical spinal nerves

Auricular branch of vagus to external meatus and small area on posteromedial surface of auricle

Branches from cervical plexus

f. Netter

9.13 SENSORY INNERVATION TERRITORIES

The adult segmental pattern of cranial nerve innervation differs from the embryonic pattern because of two events:

1. The ectodermal linings on the surface of arches 2 through 6 do not grow. They merge into the cervical sinus and disappear. The result is that cervical spinal nerve territory is immediately below trigeminal nerve territory of the first pharyngeal arch.

2. The inside lining of arch 2 mostly disappears except, perhaps, for a little sensation on the soft palate. The back of the tongue behind arch 1 territory should be innervated by the facial nerve, but it is supplied by the glossopharyngeal nerve from arch 3.

ORIGINS AND INNERVATION OF SOMITE MYOTOME MUSCLES (BROWN) AND PHARYNGEAL ARCH MUSCLES (OTHER COLORS)

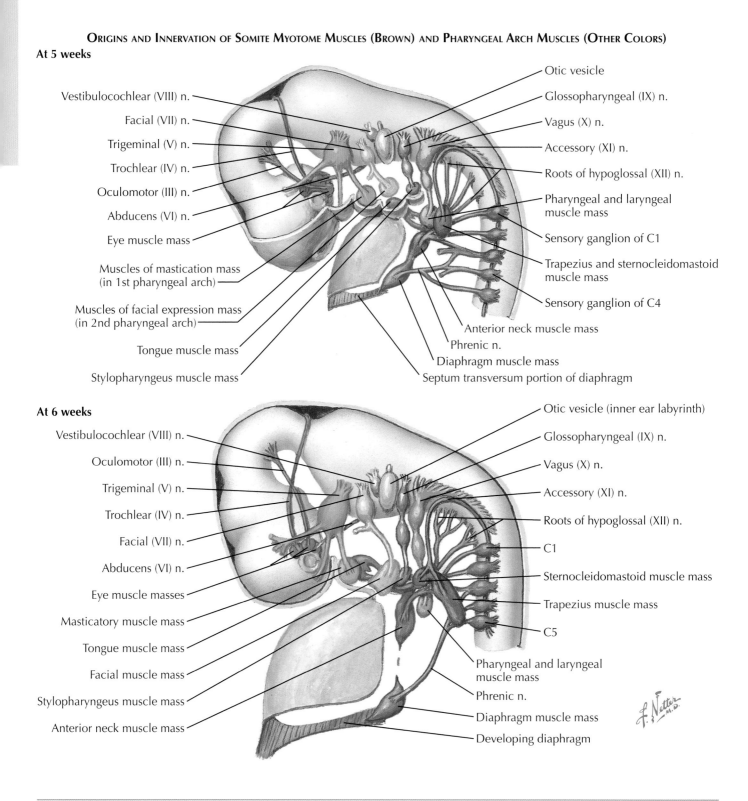

At 5 weeks

Vestibulocochlear (VIII) n.
Facial (VII) n.
Trigeminal (V) n.
Trochlear (IV) n.
Oculomotor (III) n.
Abducens (VI) n.
Eye muscle mass
Muscles of mastication mass (in 1st pharyngeal arch)
Muscles of facial expression mass (in 2nd pharyngeal arch)
Tongue muscle mass
Stylopharyngeus muscle mass

Otic vesicle
Glossopharyngeal (IX) n.
Vagus (X) n.
Accessory (XI) n.
Roots of hypoglossal (XII) n.
Pharyngeal and laryngeal muscle mass
Sensory ganglion of C1
Trapezius and sternocleidomastoid muscle mass
Sensory ganglion of C4
Anterior neck muscle mass
Phrenic n.
Diaphragm muscle mass
Septum transversum portion of diaphragm

At 6 weeks

Vestibulocochlear (VIII) n.
Oculomotor (III) n.
Trigeminal (V) n.
Trochlear (IV) n.
Facial (VII) n.
Abducens (VI) n.
Eye muscle masses
Masticatory muscle mass
Tongue muscle mass
Facial muscle mass
Stylopharyngeus muscle mass
Anterior neck muscle mass

Otic vesicle (inner ear labyrinth)
Glossopharyngeal (IX) n.
Vagus (X) n.
Accessory (XI) n.
Roots of hypoglossal (XII) n.
C1
Sternocleidomastoid muscle mass
Trapezius muscle mass
C5
Pharyngeal and laryngeal muscle mass
Phrenic n.
Diaphragm muscle mass
Developing diaphragm

9.14 EARLY DEVELOPMENT OF PHARYNGEAL ARCH MUSCLES

The neural crest mesenchyme in the pharyngeal arches gives rise to the connective tissue component of muscles (tendons, epimysium, perimysium, and endomysium). Cells from somite myotomes migrate into the arches to differentiate into muscle cells. The pattern is the same as for muscle development in the limb buds: The muscle cells are somitic in origin, and the connective tissue comes from local mesenchyme (somatopleure in the limbs and neural crest in the pharyngeal arches). The first arch gives rise to the muscles of mastication, the second arch to the muscles of facial expression, the third to the stylopharyngeus muscle, and the fourth to the laryngeal muscles and constrictors of the pharynx.

Superficial muscles

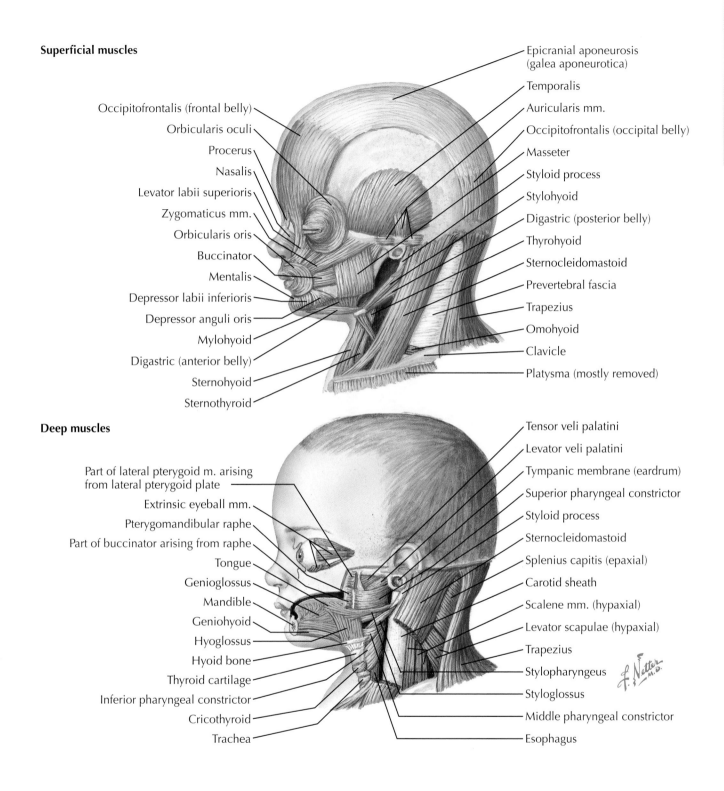

Occipitofrontalis (frontal belly)

Orbicularis oculi

Procerus

Nasalis

Levator labii superioris

Zygomaticus mm.

Orbicularis oris

Buccinator

Mentalis

Depressor labii inferioris

Depressor anguli oris

Mylohyoid

Digastric (anterior belly)

Sternohyoid

Sternothyroid

Epicranial aponeurosis (galea aponeurotica)

Temporalis

Auricularis mm.

Occipitofrontalis (occipital belly)

Masseter

Styloid process

Stylohyoid

Digastric (posterior belly)

Thyrohyoid

Sternocleidomastoid

Prevertebral fascia

Trapezius

Omohyoid

Clavicle

Platysma (mostly removed)

Deep muscles

Part of lateral pterygoid m. arising from lateral pterygoid plate

Extrinsic eyeball mm.

Pterygomandibular raphe

Part of buccinator arising from raphe

Tongue

Genioglossus

Mandible

Geniohyoid

Hyoglossus

Hyoid bone

Thyroid cartilage

Inferior pharyngeal constrictor

Cricothyroid

Trachea

Tensor veli palatini

Levator veli palatini

Tympanic membrane (eardrum)

Superior pharyngeal constrictor

Styloid process

Sternocleidomastoid

Splenius capitis (epaxial)

Carotid sheath

Scalene mm. (hypaxial)

Levator scapulae (hypaxial)

Trapezius

Stylopharyngeus

Styloglossus

Middle pharyngeal constrictor

Esophagus

9.15 LATER DEVELOPMENT OF PHARYNGEAL ARCH MUSCLES

The extraocular eye muscles originate from preotic somitomeres and are supplied by cranial nerves III (oculomotor), IV (trochlear), and VI (abducens). The tongue muscles develop from postotic somites innervated by the hypoglossal nerve (XII). Somitic muscles innervated by cervical spinal nerves are the infrahyoid "strap" muscles of the neck and the diaphragm. The trapezius and sternocleidomastoid muscles originate from an early migration of somitic cells in the vicinity of the sixth pharyngeal arch. They are innervated by the accessory nerve, a "cranial" nerve (XI) that arises from the cervical spinal cord. The former spinal root of the accessory nerve is now the accessory nerve proper, and the former cranial root of XI is part of the vagus nerve.

Embryo at 7 to 8 weeks: Cartilage primordia

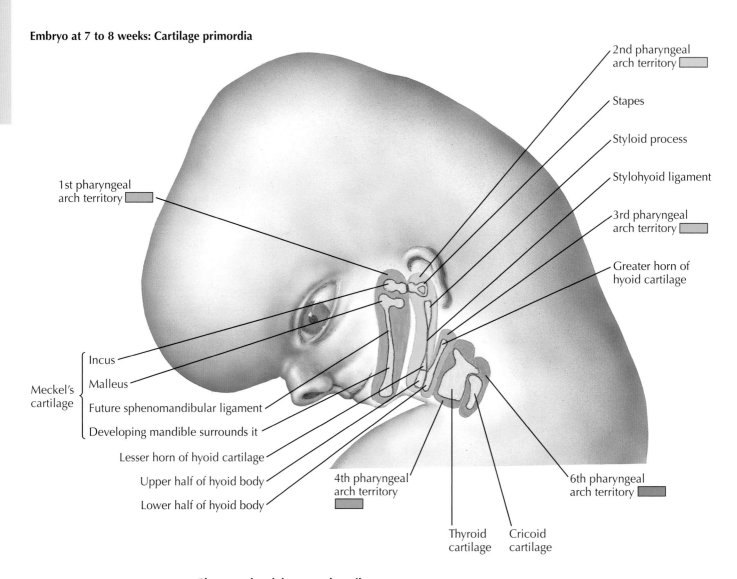

2nd pharyngeal arch territory

Stapes

Styloid process

Stylohyoid ligament

3rd pharyngeal arch territory

Greater horn of hyoid cartilage

1st pharyngeal arch territory

Meckel's cartilage
- Incus
- Malleus
- Future sphenomandibular ligament
- Developing mandible surrounds it

Lesser horn of hyoid cartilage

Upper half of hyoid body

Lower half of hyoid body

4th pharyngeal arch territory

6th pharyngeal arch territory

Thyroid cartilage

Cricoid cartilage

Pharyngeal arch bones and cartilage

Arch #	Derivatives of Arch Cartilages
1	Malleus, incus, sphenomandibular ligament
2	Stapes, styloid process, stylohyoid ligament, upper half of hyoid
3	Lower half and greater horns of hyoid
4	Thyroid and epiglottic cartilages of larynx
6	Cricoid, arytenoid, and corniculate cartilages of larynx

9.16 PHARYNGEAL ARCH CARTILAGES

The mandible primarily develops from intramembranous ossification of the first branchial arch mesenchyme that condenses around Meckel's cartilage. Secondary cartilages appear in arch 1 mesenchyme to form endochondral bone of the mandibular condyle, symphysis, and coronoid process.

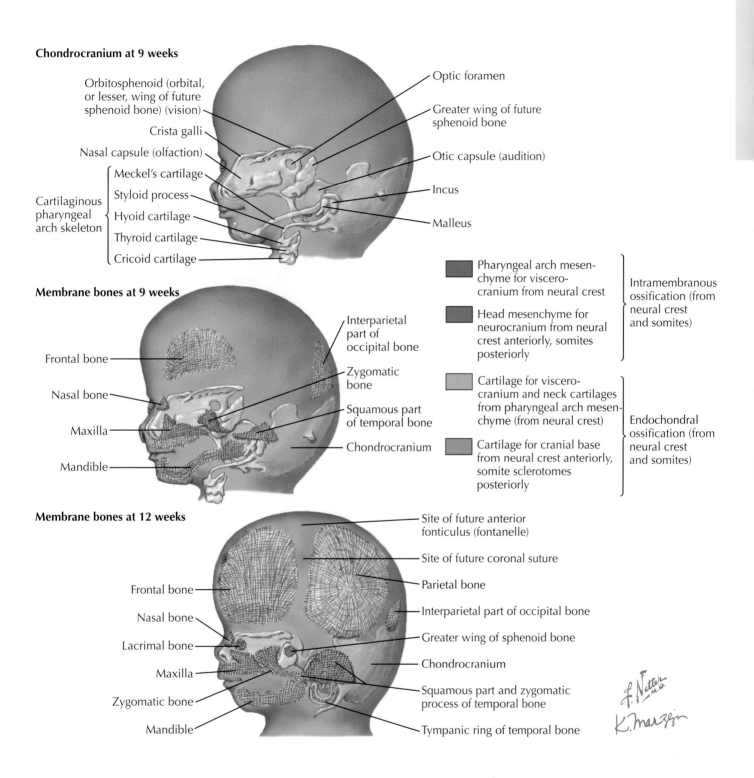

Chondrocranium at 9 weeks

Orbitosphenoid (orbital, or lesser, wing of future sphenoid bone) (vision)

Crista galli

Nasal capsule (olfaction)

Cartilaginous pharyngeal arch skeleton {
Meckel's cartilage
Styloid process
Hyoid cartilage
Thyroid cartilage
Cricoid cartilage
}

Optic foramen

Greater wing of future sphenoid bone

Otic capsule (audition)

Incus

Malleus

Membrane bones at 9 weeks

Frontal bone

Nasal bone

Maxilla

Mandible

Interparietal part of occipital bone

Zygomatic bone

Squamous part of temporal bone

Chondrocranium

Pharyngeal arch mesenchyme for viscerocranium from neural crest

Head mesenchyme for neurocranium from neural crest anteriorly, somites posteriorly
} Intramembranous ossification (from neural crest and somites)

Cartilage for viscerocranium and neck cartilages from pharyngeal arch mesenchyme (from neural crest)

Cartilage for cranial base from neural crest anteriorly, somite sclerotomes posteriorly
} Endochondral ossification (from neural crest and somites)

Membrane bones at 12 weeks

Frontal bone

Nasal bone

Lacrimal bone

Maxilla

Zygomatic bone

Mandible

Site of future anterior fonticulus (fontanelle)

Site of future coronal suture

Parietal bone

Interparietal part of occipital bone

Greater wing of sphenoid bone

Chondrocranium

Squamous part and zygomatic process of temporal bone

Tympanic ring of temporal bone

9.17 OSSIFICATION OF THE SKULL

The skull develops from both intramembranous and endochondral ossification, and the source of mesenchyme or cartilage depends on whether a bone is anterior or posterior in the skull, regardless of the type of ossification. Bones anterior to the coronal suture and middle of the sphenoid bone develop from neural crest mesenchyme. Bones posterior to these boundaries develop from paraxial mesoderm (somites). The frontal bone develops via intramembranous ossification from mesenchyme from the neural crest. The parietal bones and the upper, interparietal part of the occipital bone are also from intramembranous ossification, but the source of mesenchyme is paraxial mesoderm, not neural crest. (*Topic continued in 9.18.*)

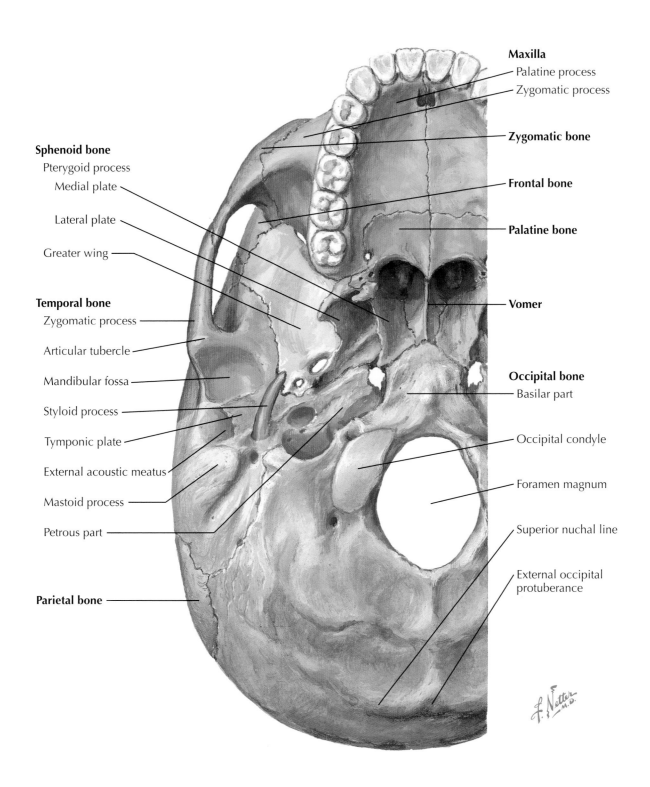

Maxilla
- Palatine process
- Zygomatic process

Sphenoid bone
- Pterygoid process
  - Medial plate
  - Lateral plate
  - Greater wing

Zygomatic bone

Frontal bone

Palatine bone

Temporal bone
- Zygomatic process
- Articular tubercle
- Mandibular fossa
- Styloid process
- Tymponic plate
- External acoustic meatus
- Mastoid process
- Petrous part

Vomer

Occipital bone
- Basilar part

Occipital condyle

Foramen magnum

Superior nuchal line

External occipital protuberance

Parietal bone

9.18 OSSIFICATION OF THE SKULL (CONTINUED)

Endochondral bone of the cranial base comes from neural crest mesenchyme anteriorly (ethmoid bone, anterior half of the sphenoid) and somite sclerotomes posteriorly (posterior half of the sphenoid, petrous and mastoid parts of the temporal bone, and basilar, condylar, and lower squamous part of the occipital bone).

All of the endochondral and intramembranous bones that develop from the pharyngeal (branchial) arches come from neural crest cells that invade the arches to form most of their mesenchyme. Some bones, such as the temporal and sphenoid bones, develop from both types of ossification.

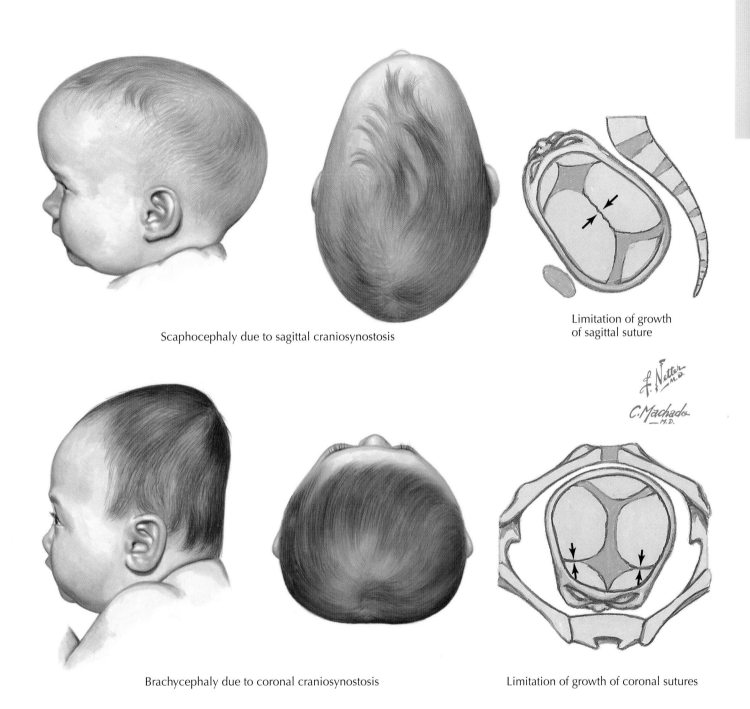

Scaphocephaly due to sagittal craniosynostosis

Limitation of growth
of sagittal suture

Brachycephaly due to coronal craniosynostosis

Limitation of growth of coronal sutures

9.19 PREMATURE SUTURE CLOSURE

Enlargement of the neurocranium occurs from bony deposition at the sutures. If the process is interrupted at one suture, growth in the direction of deposition is impeded, and compensation occurs by more rapid deposition in the other sutures. Premature closure of the sagittal suture prevents growth in width and results in a long, narrow neurocranium. The viscerocranium is largely unaffected. Growth compensation for early closure of the coronal or lambdoidal suture produces a short, wide neurocranium. Premature closure can be caused by a difficult birth (Fig. 9.19) or genetic factors and can involve only one side of the skull. Normal fusion begins in the 20s at the top of the skull and proceeds throughout life toward the ear region.

A. Fate of body, costal process, and neural arch components of cervical and thoracic vertebra, with sites and time of appearance of ossification centers

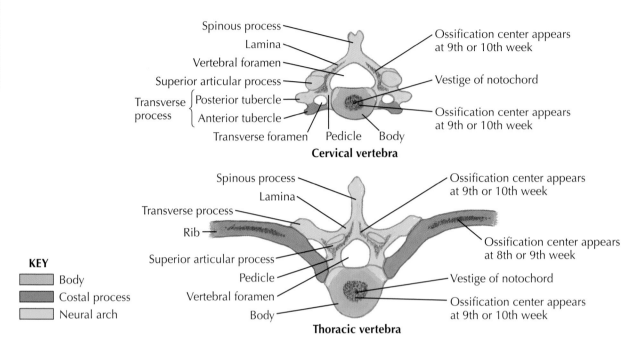

Spinous process
Lamina
Vertebral foramen
Superior articular process
Transverse { Posterior tubercle
process { Anterior tubercle
Transverse foramen   Pedicle   Body
Ossification center appears at 9th or 10th week
Vestige of notochord
Ossification center appears at 9th or 10th week
Cervical vertebra

Spinous process
Lamina
Transverse process
Rib
Superior articular process
Pedicle
Vertebral foramen
Body
Ossification center appears at 9th or 10th week
Ossification center appears at 8th or 9th week
Vestige of notochord
Ossification center appears at 9th or 10th week
Thoracic vertebra

KEY
- Body
- Costal process
- Neural arch

B. First and second cervical vertebrae at birth

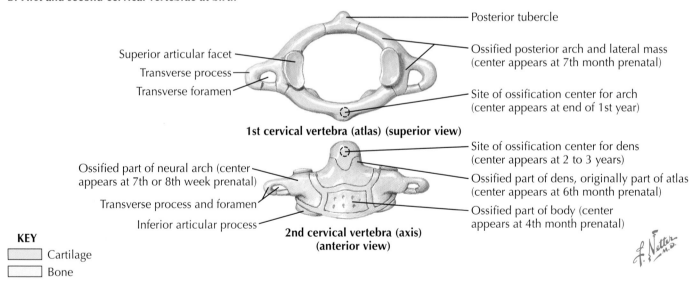

Superior articular facet
Transverse process
Transverse foramen
Posterior tubercle
Ossified posterior arch and lateral mass (center appears at 7th month prenatal)
Site of ossification center for arch (center appears at end of 1st year)
1st cervical vertebra (atlas) (superior view)

Ossified part of neural arch (center appears at 7th or 8th week prenatal)
Transverse process and foramen
Inferior articular process
Site of ossification center for dens (center appears at 2 to 3 years)
Ossified part of dens, originally part of atlas (center appears at 6th month prenatal)
Ossified part of body (center appears at 4th month prenatal)
2nd cervical vertebra (axis) (anterior view)

KEY
- Cartilage
- Bone

9.20 CERVICAL OSSIFICATION

Cervical vertebrae develop from the endochondral ossification of somite sclerotome mesoderm that condenses around the neural tube. The anterior tubercle of the transverse process is homologous to the rib ossification center related to a thoracic vertebra. The body of the atlas (C1) fuses to the axis (C2) to form the **odontoid process** or **dens** (Fig. 9.20A). Most cervical ossification anomalies produce the fusion of adjacent vertebrae. This can involve most of the cervical spine (Klippel-Feil syndrome), C2 to C3, the atlas to the occipital bone, or the dens to the atlas (os odontoideum). Intervertebral joint instability between the atlas and axis can result in narrowing the vertebral canal upon flexion and extension with possible spinal cord damage.

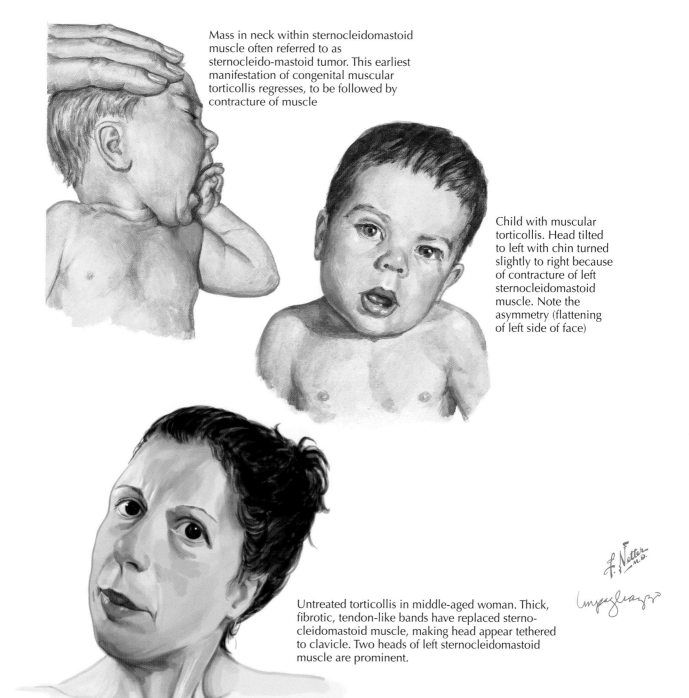

Mass in neck within sternocleidomastoid muscle often referred to as sternocleido-mastoid tumor. This earliest manifestation of congenital muscular torticollis regresses, to be followed by contracture of muscle

Child with muscular torticollis. Head tilted to left with chin turned slightly to right because of contracture of left sternocleidomastoid muscle. Note the asymmetry (flattening of left side of face)

Untreated torticollis in middle-aged woman. Thick, fibrotic, tendon-like bands have replaced sterno-cleidomastoid muscle, making head appear tethered to clavicle. Two heads of left sternocleidomastoid muscle are prominent.

9.21 TORTICOLLIS

"Torticollis" literally means a twisting of the neck and can be caused by partial disarticulation (subluxation) and fixation of the atlas and axis, or more commonly by damage to or dysfunction of one sternocleidomastoid muscle. The result is a shortening or contracture of one sternocleidomastoid muscle that puts the head and neck in a configuration that is a sum of all the actions of the muscle on the affected side:

- Flexion of the neck at the lower cervical intervertebral joints
- Extension at the atlanto-occipital joint
- Lateral bending of the neck at cervical intervertebral joints
- Rotation of the head and neck (at all cervical intervertebral joints) to the opposite side of the contracting muscle

THE CERVICAL PLEXUS AND HYPOGLOSSAL NERVE IN A 5- TO 6-WEEK EMBRYO

Innervation of muscle masses of tongue, neck, and diaphragm (lateral view)

Myelencephalon (future medulla oblongata)

Spinal cord

Myotome of 1st cervical somite

Sensory ganglion of 1st cervical nerve

Superior root of ansa cervicalis

Inferior root of ansa cervicalis

Ansa cervicalis

Hypoglossal (XII) nerve

Lingual muscle mass (future tongue)

Infrahyoid muscle mass (future so-called strap muscles)

Diaphragmatic muscle mass

Septum transversum (future anterior portion of diaphragm)

Phrenic nerve

4th cervical nerve

Cervical plexus: schema

Hypoglossal nerve (XII)

Accessory nerve (XI)

Great auricular nerve

Lesser occipital nerve

To geniohyoid muscle

To thyrohyoid muscle

Communication to vagus nerve

To rectus capitis lateralis, longus capitis and rectus capitis anterior muscles

Transverse cervical nerves

To omohyoid muscle (superior belly)

To longus capitis and longus coli muscles

Ansa cervicalis { Superior root / Inferior root

To sternothyroid muscle

To sternohyoid muscle

To omohyoid muscle (inferior belly)

To scalene and levator scapulae muscles

Supraclavicular nerves

Phrenic nerve

Note: S = Gray ramus from superior cervical sympathetic ganglion

9.22 CERVICAL PLEXUS

The cervical plexus of spinal nerves supplies the infrahyoid strap muscles, diaphragm, and other neck muscles. It is closely related to cranial nerve XII, the hypoglossal nerve. Both innervate muscles derived from sequential somites that continue from the neck into the head. This explains why some C1 fibers end up in the sheath of the hypoglossal nerve. The **ansa cervicalis**, the **phrenic nerve**, and direct branches to the scalene muscles, levator scapulae, and the longus capitis and colli muscles are the main motor components of the cervical plexus. Cutaneous branches are the greater auricular, lesser occipital, transverse cervical, and suprascapular nerves.

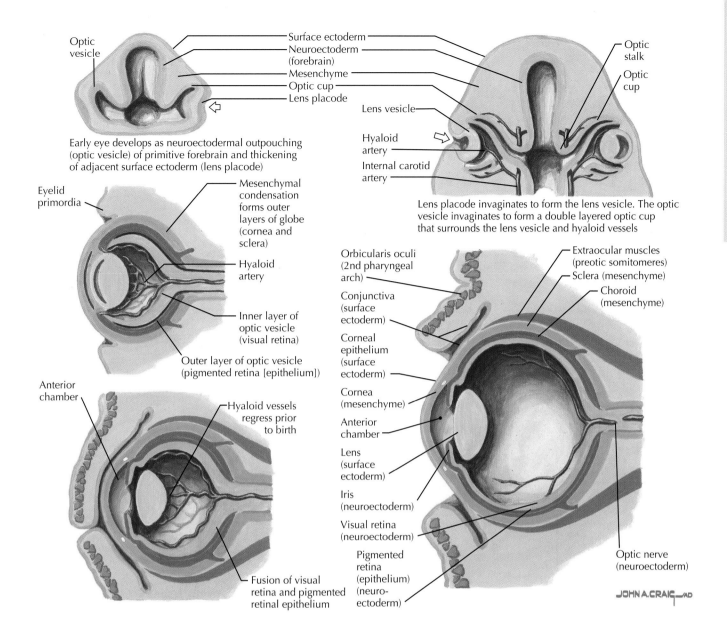

Optic vesicle

Surface ectoderm
Neuroectoderm (forebrain)
Mesenchyme
Optic cup
Lens placode

Optic stalk
Optic cup

Early eye develops as neuroectodermal outpouching (optic vesicle) of primitive forebrain and thickening of adjacent surface ectoderm (lens placode)

Lens vesicle
Hyaloid artery
Internal carotid artery

Lens placode invaginates to form the lens vesicle. The optic vesicle invaginates to form a double layered optic cup that surrounds the lens vesicle and hyaloid vessels

Eyelid primordia

Mesenchymal condensation forms outer layers of globe (cornea and sclera)
Hyaloid artery
Inner layer of optic vesicle (visual retina)
Outer layer of optic vesicle (pigmented retina [epithelium])

Anterior chamber

Hyaloid vessels regress prior to birth

Fusion of visual retina and pigmented retinal epithelium

Orbicularis oculi (2nd pharyngeal arch)
Conjunctiva (surface ectoderm)
Corneal epithelium (surface ectoderm)
Cornea (mesenchyme)
Anterior chamber
Lens (surface ectoderm)
Iris (neuroectoderm)
Visual retina (neuroectoderm)
Pigmented retina (epithelium) (neuro-ectoderm)

Extraocular muscles (preotic somitomeres)
Sclera (mesenchyme)
Choroid (mesenchyme)

Optic nerve (neuroectoderm)

JOHN A. CRAIG—AD

Primordia and derivatives

Primordium	Derivative	Related Nerve
Optic cup	Retina, optic nerve, ciliary and iris epithelium, and pupil constrictor and dilator muscles	Optic nerve (II)
Head mesenchyme	Cornea, sclera, meninges, choroid, ciliary muscle and connective tissue, and iris connective tissue	Ophthalmic nerve (V1)
Somites	Extraocular eye muscles	III, IV, and VI
Surface ectoderm	Eyelid epidermis, conjunctiva, lacrimal gland	Ophthalmic nerve (V1)
2nd pharyngeal arch	Orbicularis oculi muscle	Facial nerve (VII)
Lens placode	Lens	

9.23 ORBIT

The retina and optic nerve develop as a double-layered extension of the neural tube that surrounds the lens vesicle of surface origin. The optic cup has a ventral cleft for blood vessels to reach the developing lens. The iris is at the reflection of the two layers, and both the iris and ciliary body are formed in part from optic cup epithelium.

Connective tissue elements of the eye—sclera, cornea, and the vascular choroid layer—develop from a condensation of head mesenchyme around the optic cup. Extraocular muscles come from somitomeres. The epidermis of the eyelids develops from surface ectoderm and is continuous with the conjunctiva and corneal epithelium.

CLINICAL POINT

The two layers of the optic cup never become firmly attached. This is the embryonic basis of a **detached retina**. A blow to the orbit can cause the visual retina to separate from the pigmented retina. If not treated early, loss of vision can result that progresses like a black curtain being drawn over the visual field.

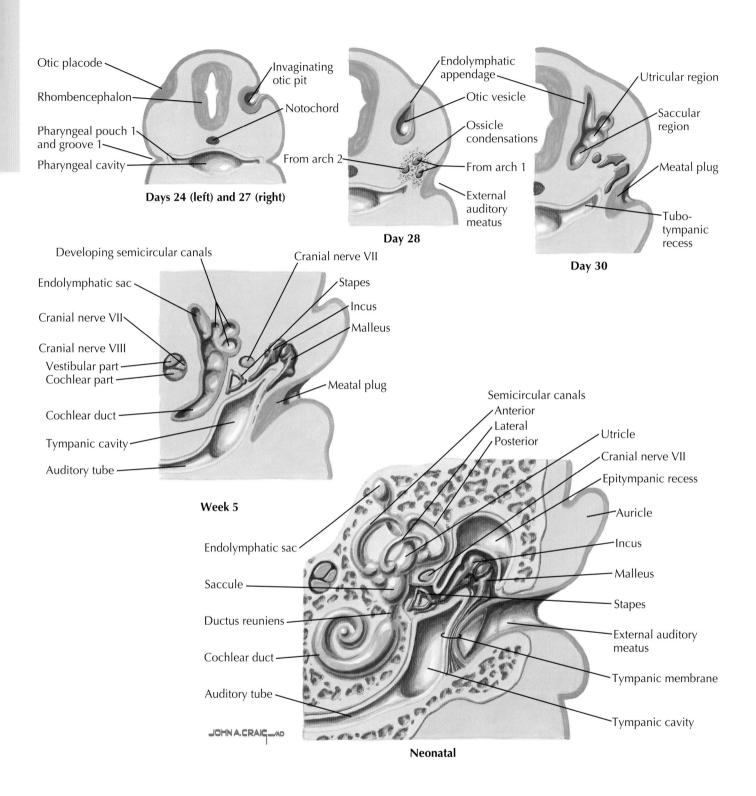

Otic placode
Rhombencephalon
Pharyngeal pouch 1 and groove 1
Pharyngeal cavity
Invaginating otic pit
Notochord

Days 24 (left) and 27 (right)

Endolymphatic appendage
Otic vesicle
Ossicle condensations
From arch 2
From arch 1
External auditory meatus

Day 28

Utricular region
Saccular region
Meatal plug
Tubo-tympanic recess

Day 30

Developing semicircular canals
Endolymphatic sac
Cranial nerve VII
Cranial nerve VIII
Vestibular part
Cochlear part
Cochlear duct
Tympanic cavity
Auditory tube
Cranial nerve VII
Stapes
Incus
Malleus
Meatal plug

Week 5

Semicircular canals
Anterior
Lateral
Posterior
Endolymphatic sac
Saccule
Ductus reuniens
Cochlear duct
Auditory tube
Utricle
Cranial nerve VII
Epitympanic recess
Auricle
Incus
Malleus
Stapes
External auditory meatus
Tympanic membrane
Tympanic cavity

JOHN A. CRAIG—AD

Neonatal

9.24 EAR DEVELOPMENT

The ear is organized into external, middle, and inner parts that differ from each other in structure and embryonic origins. The external ear consists of the auricle and external auditory meatus extending to the tympanic membrane (eardrum). The middle ear cavity, an extension of the nasopharynx housing the three ear ossicles, is deep to the tympanic membrane. The external auditory meatus and middle ear develop from the first pharyngeal groove and pouch, respectively. The otic placode gives rise to the inner ear, which consists of the organs of hearing and balance: the cochlea and vestibular apparatus (saccule, utricle, and semicircular canals). These are imbedded in the petrous part of the temporal bone.

Bony and membranous labyrinths: schema

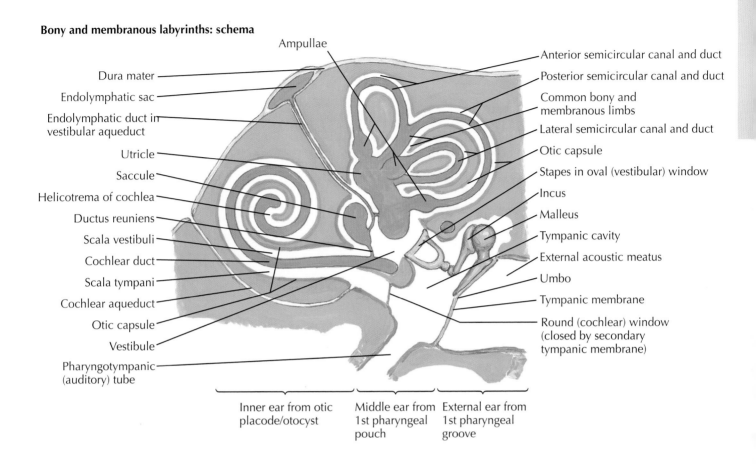

Ampullae

Dura mater

Endolymphatic sac

Endolymphatic duct in vestibular aqueduct

Utricle

Saccule

Helicotrema of cochlea

Ductus reuniens

Scala vestibuli

Cochlear duct

Scala tympani

Cochlear aqueduct

Otic capsule

Vestibule

Pharyngotympanic (auditory) tube

Anterior semicircular canal and duct

Posterior semicircular canal and duct

Common bony and membranous limbs

Lateral semicircular canal and duct

Otic capsule

Stapes in oval (vestibular) window

Incus

Malleus

Tympanic cavity

External acoustic meatus

Umbo

Tympanic membrane

Round (cochlear) window (closed by secondary tympanic membrane)

Inner ear from otic placode/otocyst

Middle ear from 1st pharyngeal pouch

External ear from 1st pharyngeal groove

Section through turn of cochlea

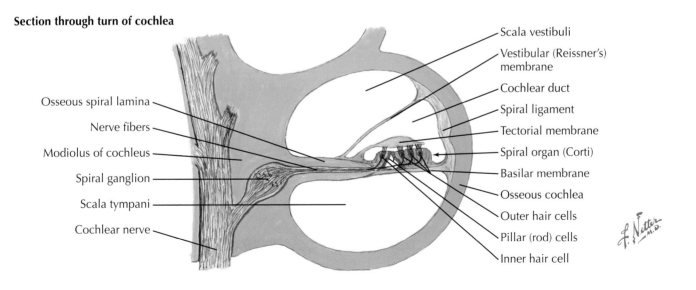

Osseous spiral lamina

Nerve fibers

Modiolus of cochleus

Spiral ganglion

Scala tympani

Cochlear nerve

Scala vestibuli

Vestibular (Reissner's) membrane

Cochlear duct

Spiral ligament

Tectorial membrane

Spiral organ (Corti)

Basilar membrane

Osseous cochlea

Outer hair cells

Pillar (rod) cells

Inner hair cell

9.25 ADULT EAR ORGANIZATION

The inner ear is a **membranous labyrinth** of sacs (utricle and saccule) and ducts (cochlea and semicircular ducts) housed within a **bony labyrinth**, which is the space in the petrous part of the temporal bone consisting of the cochlear and semicircular canals and vestibule. The membranous labyrinth contains a fluid called **endolymph** and is surrounded by **perilymph** in the **scala vestibuli** and **scala tympani** on either side of the cochlear duct within the cochlear canal. Sound waves in the external auditory meatus are transferred as vibrations in the following sequence of structures: tympanic membrane → middle ear ossicles → perilymph in scala tympani → endolymph in cochlear duct → tectorial membrane hair cells → impulses in cochlear part of nerve VIII that the brain interprets as sounds.

Primordia of the outer, middle, and inner ear

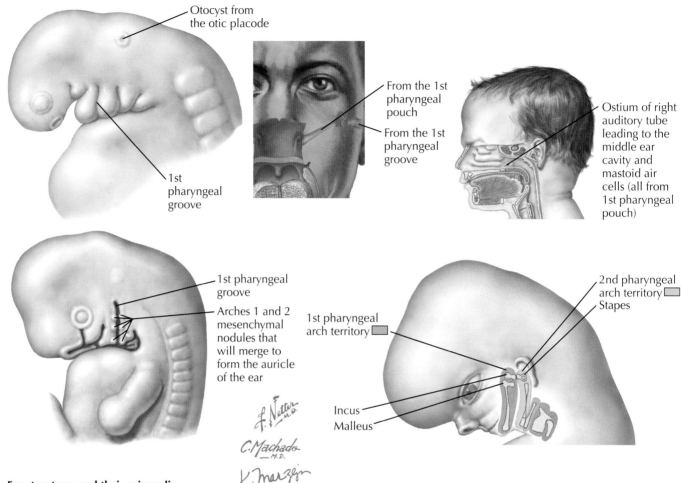

Otocyst from the otic placode

1st pharyngeal groove

From the 1st pharyngeal pouch

From the 1st pharyngeal groove

Ostium of right auditory tube leading to the middle ear cavity and mastoid air cells (all from 1st pharyngeal pouch)

1st pharyngeal groove

Arches 1 and 2 mesenchymal nodules that will merge to form the auricle of the ear

1st pharyngeal arch territory

2nd pharyngeal arch territory

Stapes

Incus

Malleus

Ear structures and their primordia

Structures	Primordia
Auricle	Mesenchyme of the 1st and 2nd pharyngeal arches
External auditory meatus	1st pharyngeal groove (ectoderm)
Middle ear cavity; auditory tube, mastoid air cells	1st pharyngeal pouch (endoderm)
Cochlea and vestibular apparatus	Otic placode/otocyst (ectoderm)
Tympanic membrane	1st pharyngeal membrane (ectoderm/endoderm) with intervening mesenchyme
Ear ossicles	1st pharyngeal arch cartilage (incus and malleus)
	2nd pharyngeal arch cartilage (stapes)
Temporal bone	Occipital sclerotomes (mastoid and petrous parts)
	2nd pharyngeal arch cartilage (styloid process)
	1st pharyngeal arch mesenchyme (squamous and tympanic parts)

9.26 SUMMARY OF EAR DEVELOPMENT

Structures of the external, middle, and inner ear develop from the first and second pharyngeal arches and the groove and pouch between them. Cranial nerve VIII (vestibulocochlear) relates to the otic placode and vesicle and provides the special sensations of hearing and balance. The mandibular nerve (V3 from arch 1) supplies the tensor tympani muscle that dampens the malleus, and the facial nerve (arch 2) supplies the stapedius muscle. Not so obvious is the innervation of the external acoustic meatus and the middle ear. General sensation for the former is by the vagus nerve, its only cutaneous branch. Visceral sensation for the middle ear is by the tympanic branch of the glossopharyngeal nerve, the pretrematic branch of IX that is out of its territory (arch 3).

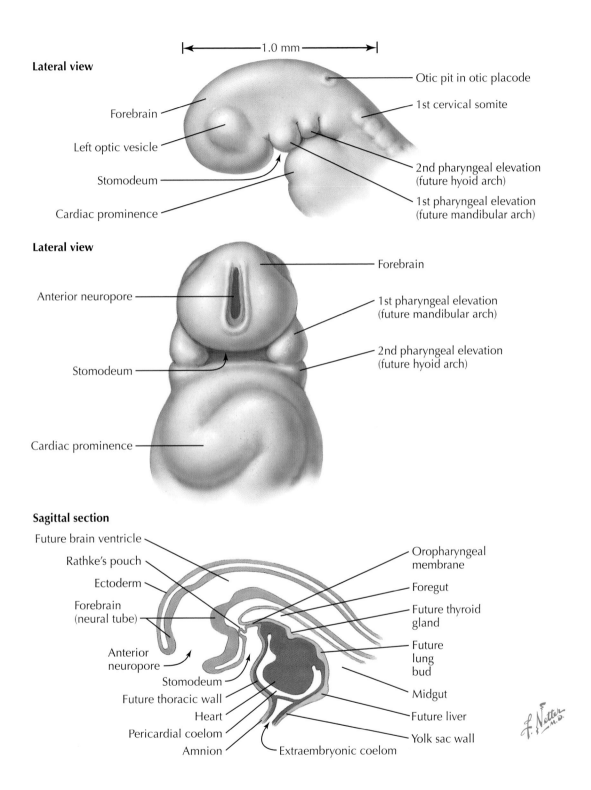

Lateral view

1.0 mm

Forebrain

Left optic vesicle

Stomodeum

Cardiac prominence

Otic pit in otic placode

1st cervical somite

2nd pharyngeal elevation
(future hyoid arch)

1st pharyngeal elevation
(future mandibular arch)

Lateral view

Anterior neuropore

Stomodeum

Cardiac prominence

Forebrain

1st pharyngeal elevation
(future mandibular arch)

2nd pharyngeal elevation
(future hyoid arch)

Sagittal section

Future brain ventricle

Rathke's pouch

Ectoderm

Forebrain
(neural tube)

Anterior
neuropore

Stomodeum

Future thoracic wall

Heart

Pericardial coelom

Amnion

Oropharyngeal
membrane

Foregut

Future thyroid
gland

Future
lung
bud

Midgut

Future liver

Yolk sac wall

Extraembryonic coelom

9.27 DEVELOPMENT OF THE FACE: 3 TO 4 WEEKS

The face and head at weeks 3 to 4 are dominated by the appearance of the pharyngeal arches and the invagination of surface ectoderm between relatively huge forebrain and cardiac prominence. This ectodermal recess is the stomodeum, the primitive oral cavity. The otic placode of surface ectoderm is beginning to invaginate to form the otocyst. The lens and nasal placodes are soon to appear. The bulging optic vesicle is the beginning of the formation of the optic cup of neural ectoderm.

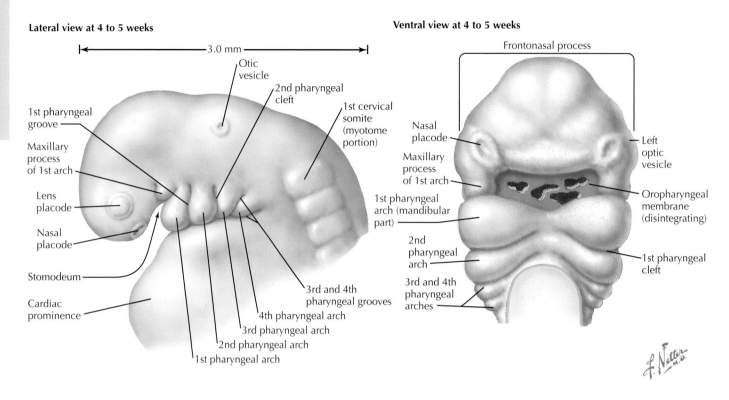

Lateral view at 4 to 5 weeks

Ventral view at 4 to 5 weeks

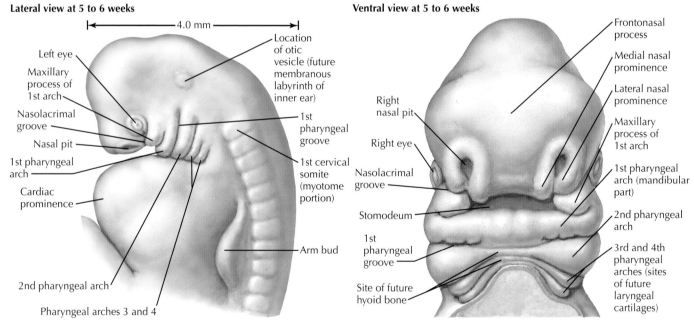

Lateral view at 5 to 6 weeks

Ventral view at 5 to 6 weeks

9.28 DEVELOPMENT OF THE FACE: 4 TO 6 WEEKS

By week 4, the mesenchyme around the swelling of the forebrain cranial to the first pharyngeal arch forms a **frontonasal process** that includes the nasal placodes. As the nasal placodes invaginate, **medial and lateral nasal swellings** of mesenchyme form on either side of what are now **nasal pits** or **sacs** in the frontonasal process.

The cleft between the lateral nasal prominence of the frontonasal process and the maxillary part of the first pharyngeal arch is the **nasolacrimal groove**. It extends from the medial corner of the developing eye to part of the future nasal cavity and pinches off beneath the surface to form the **nasolacrimal duct** that drains lacrimal gland secretions (tears) into the inferior meatus of the nasal cavity.

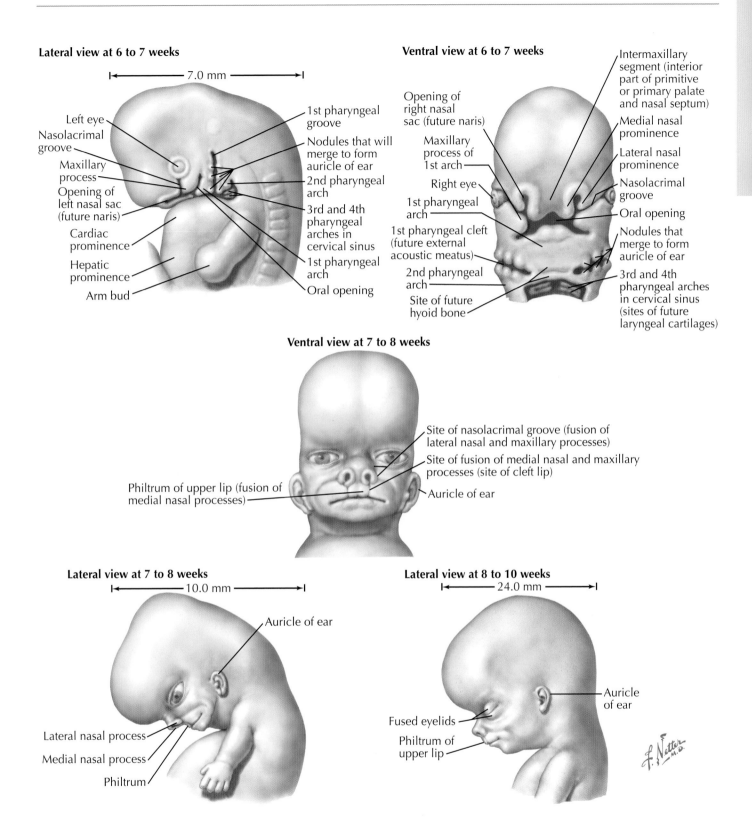

Lateral view at 6 to 7 weeks

|← 7.0 mm →|

Left eye
Nasolacrimal groove
Maxillary process
Opening of left nasal sac (future naris)
Cardiac prominence
Hepatic prominence
Arm bud

1st pharyngeal groove
Nodules that will merge to form auricle of ear
2nd pharyngeal arch
3rd and 4th pharyngeal arches in cervical sinus
1st pharyngeal arch
Oral opening

Ventral view at 6 to 7 weeks

Opening of right nasal sac (future naris)
Maxillary process of 1st arch
Right eye
1st pharyngeal arch
1st pharyngeal cleft (future external acoustic meatus)
2nd pharyngeal arch
Site of future hyoid bone

Intermaxillary segment (interior part of primitive or primary palate and nasal septum)
Medial nasal prominence
Lateral nasal prominence
Nasolacrimal groove
Oral opening
Nodules that merge to form auricle of ear
3rd and 4th pharyngeal arches in cervical sinus (sites of future laryngeal cartilages)

Ventral view at 7 to 8 weeks

Philtrum of upper lip (fusion of medial nasal processes)

Site of nasolacrimal groove (fusion of lateral nasal and maxillary processes)
Site of fusion of medial nasal and maxillary processes (site of cleft lip)
Auricle of ear

Lateral view at 7 to 8 weeks

|← 10.0 mm →|

Auricle of ear
Lateral nasal process
Medial nasal process
Philtrum

Lateral view at 8 to 10 weeks

|← 24.0 mm →|

Auricle of ear
Fused eyelids
Philtrum of upper lip

9.29 DEVELOPMENT OF THE FACE: 6 TO 10 WEEKS

The **intermaxillary segment** formed by fusion of the **medial nasal processes** is named for its position between the maxillary processes of the first pharyngeal arch (with which it fuses). It gives rise to most of the external nose, the **philtrum** of the upper lip, and the **primary palate**. The ophthalmic division of the trigeminal nerve (V1), the nerve of the frontonasal process, provides general sensory innervation for all of these midline structures, as well as the forehead and orbit. The maxillary nerve (V2) supplies the midface, including most of the maxilla, nasal cavity, and roof of the oral cavity. The mandibular nerve (V3) innervates the mandible and overlying skin in addition to the floor of the oral cavity proper and vestibule.

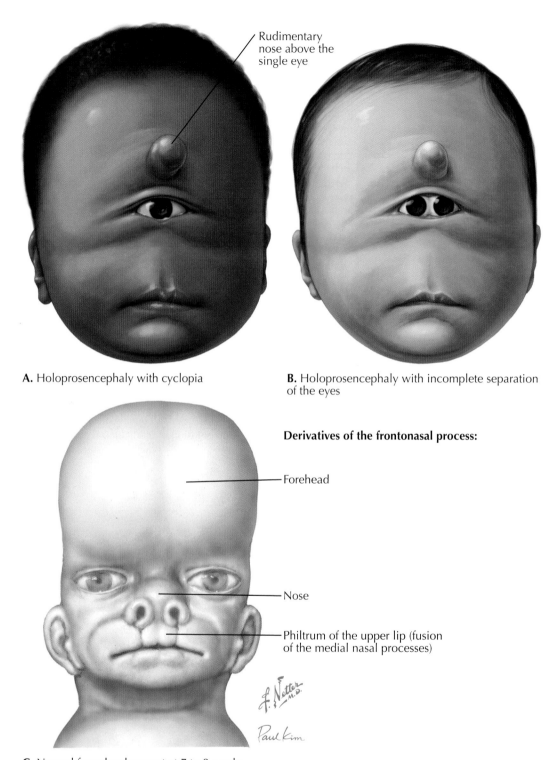

A. Holoprosencephaly with cyclopia

B. Holoprosencephaly with incomplete separation of the eyes

Derivatives of the frontonasal process:

Forehead

Nose

Philtrum of the upper lip (fusion of the medial nasal processes)

C. Normal face development at 7 to 8 weeks

9.30 HOLOPROSENCEPHALY

Holoprosencephaly results from incomplete division of the forebrain hemispheres caused by cell death near the midline of the embryonic disc in week 3. At the more extreme end of a range of phenotypes in the newborn, the eyes are fused (cyclopia, Fig. 9.30A) or nearly fused (Fig. 9.30B), and a primitive nose is above them. The nose develops with the forehead from the embryonic frontonasal process (Fig. 9.30C), and if the eyes are not separate, the nose cannot extend down between them. Holoprosencephaly is related to a variety of genetic anomalies, such as trisomy 13 or sonic hedgehog gene mutations, maternal diabetes, and severe fetal alcohol syndrome. The incidence is 1.3 in 10,000 live births and twice as common in males. Because most cases result in miscarriage, the frequency of holoprosencephaly in all pregnancies is 10–20 times higher, and that is for the more severely affected, more easily detectable individuals.

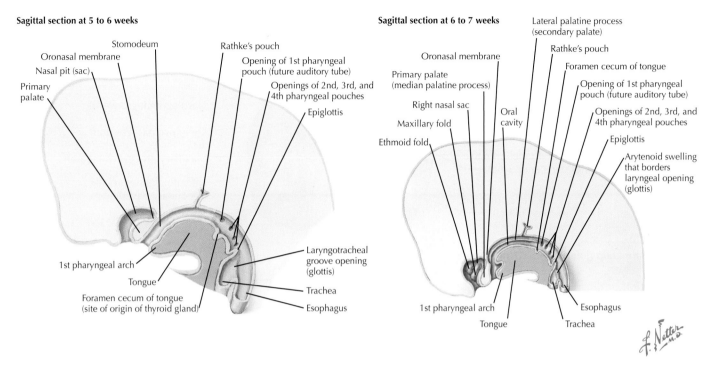

Sagittal section at 5 to 6 weeks

Stomodeum
Oronasal membrane
Nasal pit (sac)
Primary palate
Rathke's pouch
Opening of 1st pharyngeal pouch (future auditory tube)
Openings of 2nd, 3rd, and 4th pharyngeal pouches
Epiglottis
1st pharyngeal arch
Tongue
Foramen cecum of tongue (site of origin of thyroid gland)
Laryngotracheal groove opening (glottis)
Trachea
Esophagus

Sagittal section at 6 to 7 weeks

Lateral palatine process (secondary palate)
Rathke's pouch
Foramen cecum of tongue
Opening of 1st pharyngeal pouch (future auditory tube)
Openings of 2nd, 3rd, and 4th pharyngeal pouches
Epiglottis
Arytenoid swelling that borders laryngeal opening (glottis)
Oronasal membrane
Primary palate (median palatine process)
Right nasal sac
Maxillary fold
Ethmoid fold
Oral cavity
1st pharyngeal arch
Tongue
Esophagus
Trachea

Sagittal section at 7 to 8 weeks

Olfactory bulb
Axons of nerve cells passing from olfactory epithelium of nasal cavity to olfactory bulb
Ethmoid fold
Maxillary fold
Ostium of auditory tube
Right lateral palatine process of secondary palate
Cut surface of tongue
Epiglottis
Pharynx
Larynx
Cricoid cartilage
Right cerebral hemisphere
Primary palate
Hyoid cartilage
Meckel's cartilage
Thyroid cartilage
Tracheal cartilage
Trachea
Esophagus

Sagittal section at 8 to 10 weeks

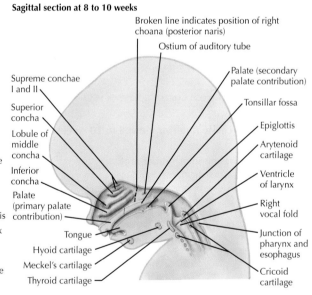

Broken line indicates position of right choana (posterior naris)
Ostium of auditory tube
Palate (secondary palate contribution)
Tonsillar fossa
Epiglottis
Arytenoid cartilage
Ventricle of larynx
Right vocal fold
Junction of pharynx and esophagus
Cricoid cartilage
Supreme conchae I and II
Superior concha
Lobule of middle concha
Inferior concha
Palate (primary palate contribution)
Tongue
Hyoid cartilage
Meckel's cartilage
Thyroid cartilage

9.31 PALATE FORMATION

At weeks 5 to 6, the nasal sacs are separated from the stomodeum by a thin **oronasal membrane**. The block of tissue between the nasal sacs and stomodeum is the **primary palate**. **Lateral palatine processes** begin to grow from the maxillary part of the first pharyngeal arch to form the future **secondary palate** posterior to the primary palate. The nasal cavity is derived from the nasal sacs and the posterior portion of the stomodeum above the lateral palatine processes. The **nasal septum** grows inferiorly in the midline. The lateral palatine processes fuse with the nasal septum, and the primary palate fuses with the secondary palate to complete palate formation.

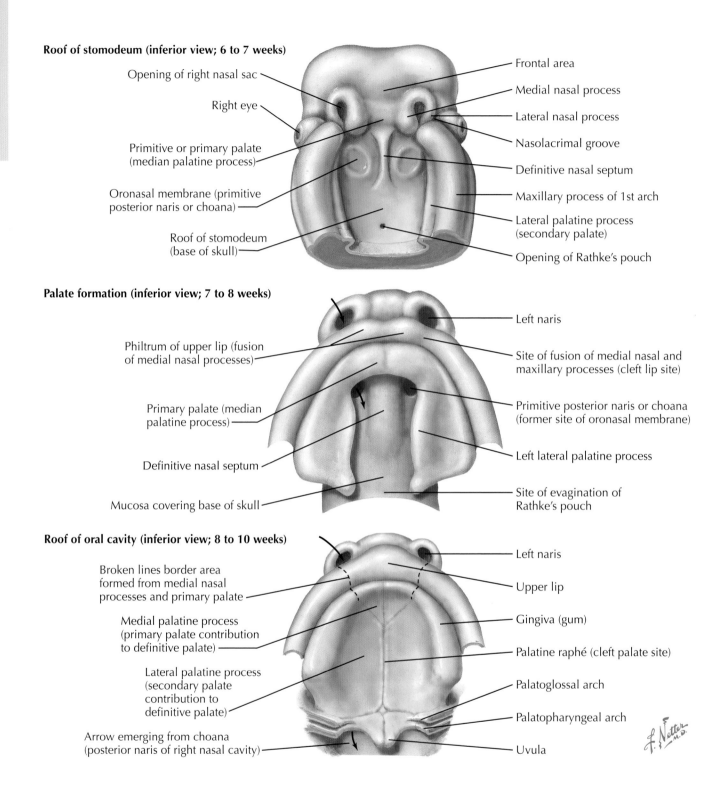

Roof of stomodeum (inferior view; 6 to 7 weeks)

- Opening of right nasal sac
- Right eye
- Primitive or primary palate (median palatine process)
- Oronasal membrane (primitive posterior naris or choana)
- Roof of stomodeum (base of skull)
- Frontal area
- Medial nasal process
- Lateral nasal process
- Nasolacrimal groove
- Definitive nasal septum
- Maxillary process of 1st arch
- Lateral palatine process (secondary palate)
- Opening of Rathke's pouch

Palate formation (inferior view; 7 to 8 weeks)

- Philtrum of upper lip (fusion of medial nasal processes)
- Primary palate (median palatine process)
- Definitive nasal septum
- Mucosa covering base of skull
- Left naris
- Site of fusion of medial nasal and maxillary processes (cleft lip site)
- Primitive posterior naris or choana (former site of oronasal membrane)
- Left lateral palatine process
- Site of evagination of Rathke's pouch

Roof of oral cavity (inferior view; 8 to 10 weeks)

- Broken lines border area formed from medial nasal processes and primary palate
- Medial palatine process (primary palate contribution to definitive palate)
- Lateral palatine process (secondary palate contribution to definitive palate)
- Arrow emerging from choana (posterior naris of right nasal cavity)
- Left naris
- Upper lip
- Gingiva (gum)
- Palatine raphé (cleft palate site)
- Palatoglossal arch
- Palatopharyngeal arch
- Uvula

9.32 INFERIOR VIEW OF PALATE FORMATION, ROOF OF THE ORAL CAVITY

The oronasal membranes break down, and the nasal sacs communicate with the stomodeum. The medial nasal processes of the frontonasal process fuse to form an intermaxillary segment that develops into the philtrum (middle portion) of the upper lip and primary palate. The primary palate gives rise to the **premaxillary ossification center** of the maxilla containing the maxillary incisor teeth. The latter palatine processes form the secondary palate that gives rise to the palatine bones, soft palate, and the rest of the rest of the maxilla.

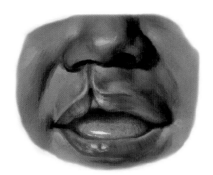

Unilateral cleft lip—partial

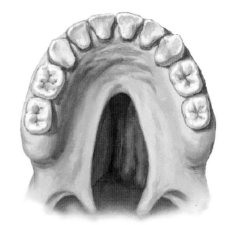

Partial cleft of palate

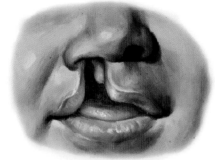

Unilateral cleft of primary palate—
complete, involving lip and complete,
involving lip, mucosa, and bone

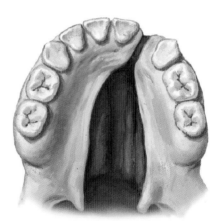

Complete cleft of secondary palate
and unilateral cleft of primary palate

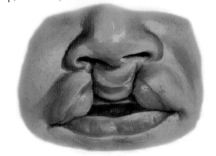

Bilateral cleft lip

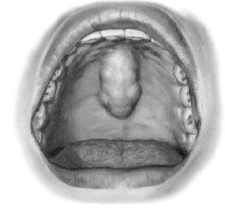

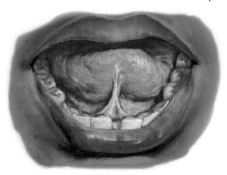

Ankyloglossia—restricted tongue movement
from a short lingual frenulum

Torus palatinus—bone deposition on palate

9.33 CONGENITAL ANOMALIES OF THE ORAL CAVITY

Clefts can occur at any point along the site of fusion of the inter-maxillary segment of the frontonasal process and the lateral palatine processes. They are classified as anterior or posterior according to their relationships to the incisive foramen located between the primary and secondary palates. Anterior clefts can involve the lip, the alveolar process of the maxilla, or the entire primary palate, and they can be unilateral or bilateral. Posterior clefts may affect just the soft palate or the soft and posterior bony palate (secondary palate). These are midline clefts, and the nasal septum may be fused to the hard palate on one side or not at all. Anterior and posterior clefts are unrelated; they have different frequencies and population occurrences.

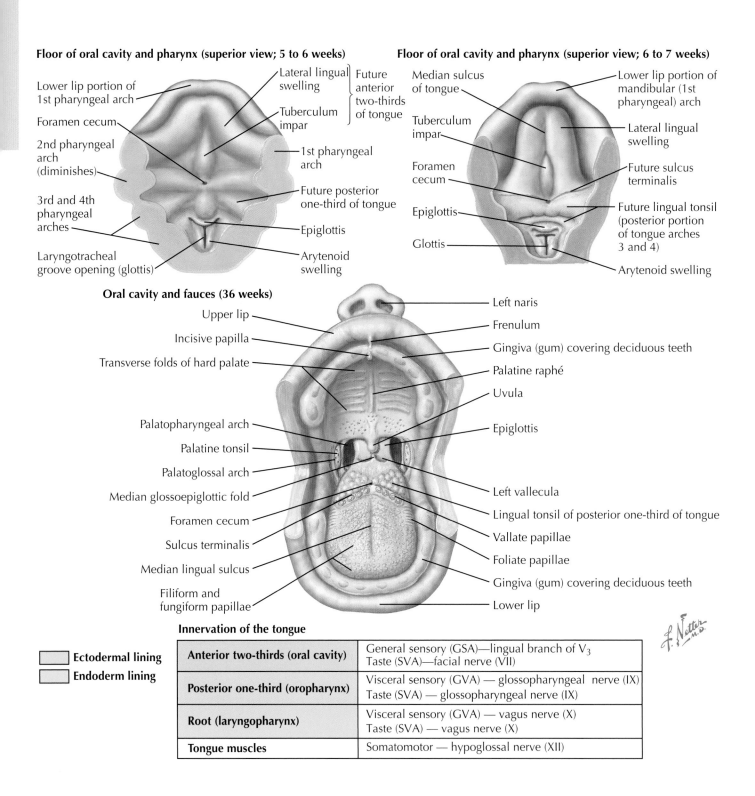

Floor of oral cavity and pharynx (superior view; 5 to 6 weeks)

- Lower lip portion of 1st pharyngeal arch
- Foramen cecum
- 2nd pharyngeal arch (diminishes)
- 3rd and 4th pharyngeal arches
- Laryngotracheal groove opening (glottis)
- Lateral lingual swelling
- Tuberculum impar
- Future anterior two-thirds of tongue
- 1st pharyngeal arch
- Future posterior one-third of tongue
- Epiglottis
- Arytenoid swelling

Floor of oral cavity and pharynx (superior view; 6 to 7 weeks)

- Median sulcus of tongue
- Tuberculum impar
- Foramen cecum
- Epiglottis
- Glottis
- Lower lip portion of mandibular (1st pharyngeal) arch
- Lateral lingual swelling
- Future sulcus terminalis
- Future lingual tonsil (posterior portion of tongue arches 3 and 4)
- Arytenoid swelling

Oral cavity and fauces (36 weeks)

- Upper lip
- Incisive papilla
- Transverse folds of hard palate
- Palatopharyngeal arch
- Palatine tonsil
- Palatoglossal arch
- Median glossoepiglottic fold
- Foramen cecum
- Sulcus terminalis
- Median lingual sulcus
- Filiform and fungiform papillae
- Left naris
- Frenulum
- Gingiva (gum) covering deciduous teeth
- Palatine raphé
- Uvula
- Epiglottis
- Left vallecula
- Lingual tonsil of posterior one-third of tongue
- Vallate papillae
- Foliate papillae
- Gingiva (gum) covering deciduous teeth
- Lower lip

Ectodermal lining
Endoderm lining

Innervation of the tongue

Anterior two-thirds (oral cavity)	General sensory (GSA)—lingual branch of V₃ Taste (SVA)—facial nerve (VII)
Posterior one-third (oropharynx)	Visceral sensory (GVA) — glossopharyngeal nerve (IX) Taste (SVA) — glossopharyngeal nerve (IX)
Root (laryngopharynx)	Visceral sensory (GVA) — vagus nerve (X) Taste (SVA) — vagus nerve (X)
Tongue muscles	Somatomotor — hypoglossal nerve (XII)

9.34 FLOOR OF THE ORAL CAVITY

The ectoderm of the oral cavity receives a very rich general sensation; the foregut is supplied with less intense visceral sensation, with the degree of sensation diminishing from the pharynx to the esophagus. Because the lining of arch 2 does not grow much, the facial nerve does not contribute to the general or visceral sensation of the tongue.

Frontal (coronal) section at 7 to 8 weeks

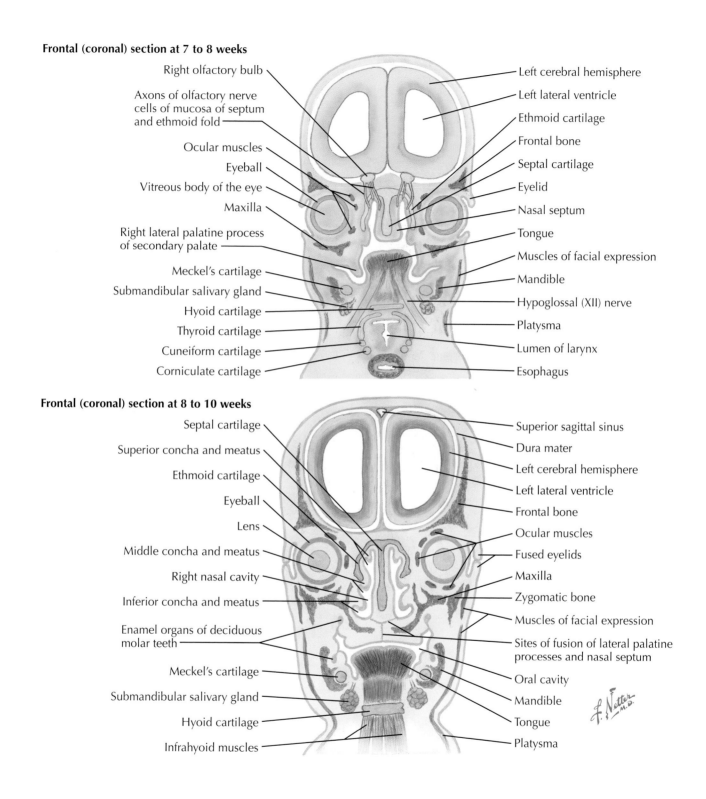

Right olfactory bulb

Axons of olfactory nerve cells of mucosa of septum and ethmoid fold

Ocular muscles

Eyeball

Vitreous body of the eye

Maxilla

Right lateral palatine process of secondary palate

Meckel's cartilage

Submandibular salivary gland

Hyoid cartilage

Thyroid cartilage

Cuneiform cartilage

Corniculate cartilage

Left cerebral hemisphere

Left lateral ventricle

Ethmoid cartilage

Frontal bone

Septal cartilage

Eyelid

Nasal septum

Tongue

Muscles of facial expression

Mandible

Hypoglossal (XII) nerve

Platysma

Lumen of larynx

Esophagus

Frontal (coronal) section at 8 to 10 weeks

Septal cartilage

Superior concha and meatus

Ethmoid cartilage

Eyeball

Lens

Middle concha and meatus

Right nasal cavity

Inferior concha and meatus

Enamel organs of deciduous molar teeth

Meckel's cartilage

Submandibular salivary gland

Hyoid cartilage

Infrahyoid muscles

Superior sagittal sinus

Dura mater

Left cerebral hemisphere

Left lateral ventricle

Frontal bone

Ocular muscles

Fused eyelids

Maxilla

Zygomatic bone

Muscles of facial expression

Sites of fusion of lateral palatine processes and nasal septum

Oral cavity

Mandible

Tongue

Platysma

9.35 DEVELOPMENTAL CORONAL SECTIONS

Although thin in adults, the nasal septum in the embryo is thick and is a driving force in the vertical growth of the head. The lateral palatine processes (secondary palate) are angled inferiorly when they first develop. The tongue must drop down before they can swing up toward the nasal septum. The eyes face laterally on the embryonic head. The eyelids fuse in the early fetus (8–10 weeks) and reopen by week 26.

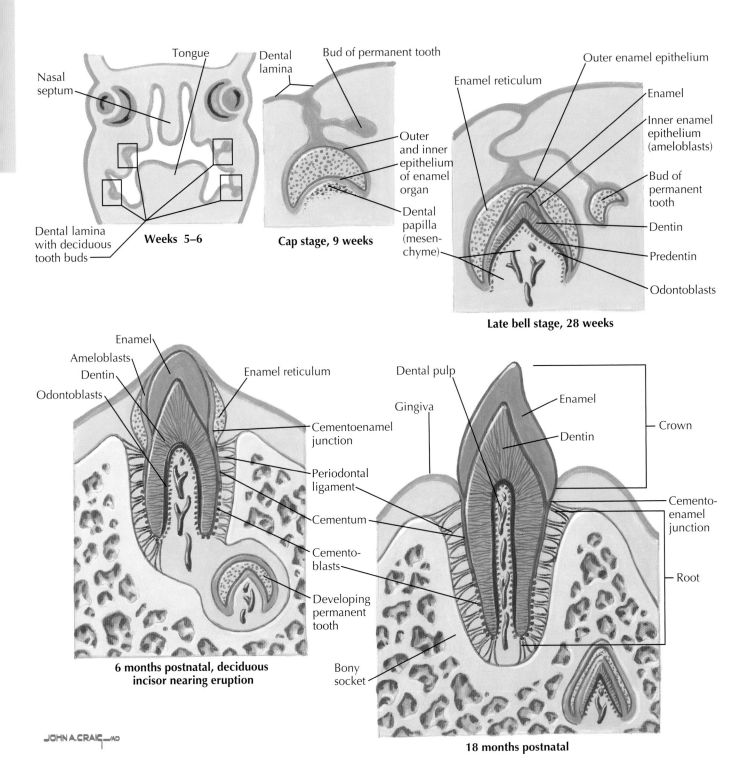

Nasal septum

Tongue

Dental lamina

Bud of permanent tooth

Dental lamina with deciduous tooth buds

Weeks 5–6

Outer and inner epithelium of enamel organ

Dental papilla (mesen-chyme)

Cap stage, 9 weeks

Outer enamel epithelium

Enamel reticulum

Enamel

Inner enamel epithelium (ameloblasts)

Bud of permanent tooth

Dentin

Predentin

Odontoblasts

Late bell stage, 28 weeks

Enamel

Ameloblasts

Dentin

Odontoblasts

Enamel reticulum

Cementoenamel junction

Periodontal ligament

Cementum

Cemento-blasts

Developing permanent tooth

6 months postnatal, deciduous incisor nearing eruption

Dental pulp

Gingiva

Enamel

Dentin

Crown

Cemento-enamel junction

Root

Bony socket

18 months postnatal

JOHN A.CRAIG—AD

9.36 TOOTH STRUCTURE AND DEVELOPMENT

In week 6, the oral ectoderm thickens to form U-shaped **dental laminae** in the upper and lower jaws. Extensions of the dental lamina give rise to epithelial **enamel organs** that surround mesenchymal **dental papillae** to form tooth buds by week 9. Enamel and dentin are secreted at the interface of the two primordia. The enamel-forming **ameloblasts** are on the inner layer of an enamel organ, and the outer mesenchymal cells of a dental papilla form an epithelial layer of **odontoblasts** that secrete dentin. Tooth formation involves a complicated series of inductive events between epithelium and mesenchyme (in both directions), with at least eight signaling molecules. The ectodermal epithelium initiates the cascade, and the mesenchyme determines whether a tooth becomes an incisor or molar.

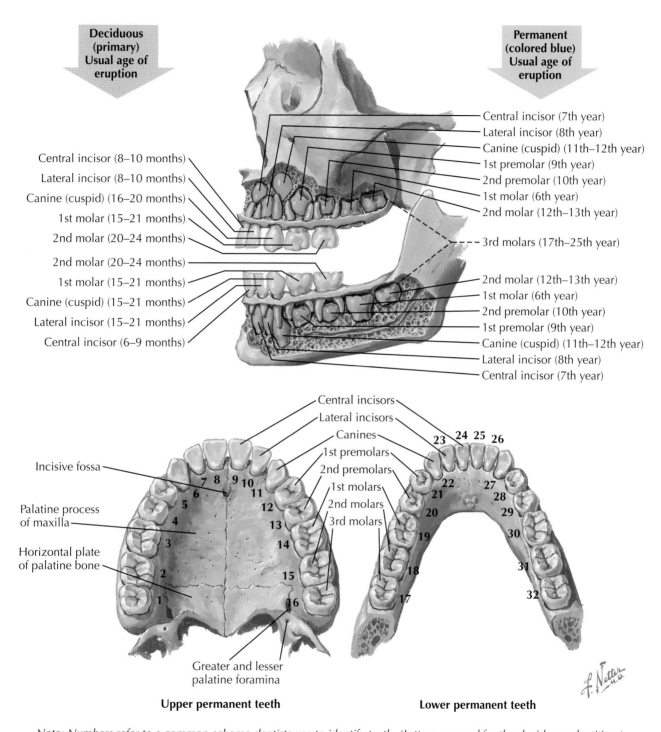

Deciduous (primary) Usual age of eruption

Central incisor (8–10 months)
Lateral incisor (8–10 months)
Canine (cuspid) (16–20 months)
1st molar (15–21 months)
2nd molar (20–24 months)

2nd molar (20–24 months)
1st molar (15–21 months)
Canine (cuspid) (15–21 months)
Lateral incisor (15–21 months)
Central incisor (6–9 months)

Permanent (colored blue) Usual age of eruption

Central incisor (7th year)
Lateral incisor (8th year)
Canine (cuspid) (11th–12th year)
1st premolar (9th year)
2nd premolar (10th year)
1st molar (6th year)
2nd molar (12th–13th year)

3rd molars (17th–25th year)

2nd molar (12th–13th year)
1st molar (6th year)
2nd premolar (10th year)
1st premolar (9th year)
Canine (cuspid) (11th–12th year)
Lateral incisor (8th year)
Central incisor (7th year)

Central incisors
Lateral incisors
Canines
1st premolars
2nd premolars
1st molars
2nd molars
3rd molars

Incisive fossa

Palatine process of maxilla

Horizontal plate of palatine bone

Greater and lesser palatine foramina

Upper permanent teeth   **Lower permanent teeth**

Note: Numbers refer to a common scheme dentists use to identify teeth. (Letters are used for the deciduous dentition.)

9.37 DENTAL ERUPTION

The crowns of the teeth are completely formed in the jaws before they erupt. Space constraints inhibit root development, which is completed during eruption of the tooth. Because enamel is acellular, no growth of a crown is possible after eruption. The deciduous (primary or "baby") teeth must be replaced by larger permanent teeth. The deciduous teeth fall out when their roots are resorbed as a result of development and eruption of the permanent crowns.

Terminology

Ankyloglossia	(G., "crooked tongue") Restricted mobility of the tongue caused by a short lingual frenulum, a frenulum attached too close to the tip of the tongue, or fusion of the tongue to the floor of the oral cavity.
Ansa cervicalis	(ansa, L., "handle") Nerve loop of the cervical plexus lying on the carotid sheath. It is motor to the infrahyoid strap muscles.
Branchial	(G., referring to "gills") Pharyngeal arches used to be called branchial arches in reference to the phylogenetic origin of the arches as the gill apparatus in fish. In higher animals, they flank the pharynx and become a variety of structures.
Branchiomotor	Classification of motor neurons to striated muscle derived from the pharyngeal arches. They differ from somatomotor neurons according to muscle primordia only.
Cervical sinus	Ectodermal invagination formed by the merging of pharyngeal grooves 2, 3, and 4. It disappears, and the ectoderm of arches 2 through 6 contributes to little in the adult.
Foramen cecum	Blind pit on the back of the tongue that is the site of the endodermal thyroid diverticulum that descends to its final location anterior to the trachea.
Hyoid arch	The second pharyngeal arch.
Hyomandibular cleft	The first pharyngeal groove between the mandibular part of the first pharyngeal arch and the second (hyoid) pharyngeal arch. It develops into the external auditory meatus.
Hypobranchial eminence	Mesenchymal swelling in the third and fourth pharyngeal arches that contributes to the posterior, pharyngeal part of the tongue and the epiglottis.
Meckel's cartilage	The cartilage of the first pharyngeal arch that becomes the malleus, incus, and sphenomandibular ligament. It does not contribute to the mandible, which is mostly membrane bone that condenses around the cartilage.
Nervus intermedius	The sensory (taste) and parasympathetic root of the facial nerve (cranial nerve VII). "Intermedius" refers to its location between the large branchiomotor root of VII and nerve VIII.
Neurocranium	The bones surrounding the brain. The bottom of the neurocranium is the cranial base at the interface between neurocranium and viscerocranium.
Oropharyngeal membrane	Membrane of ectoderm and endoderm in the gastrula that separates the stomodeum (primitive oral cavity) from the foregut (primitive pharynx). It breaks down in the fourth week.
Pharyngeal grooves	Ectodermal clefts between the pharyngeal arches on the surface. They persist as the external auditory meatus only.
Pharyngeal membranes	A membrane of ectoderm, mesoderm, and endoderm where a pharyngeal groove abuts a pharyngeal pouch between the pharyngeal arches. The first persists as the tympanic membrane (eardrum).
Pharyngeal pouches	Endodermal extensions of the foregut between the pharyngeal arches on the inside. They give rise to the auditory tube, middle ear cavity, mastoid air cells, thymus, parathyroid glands, and C cells of the thyroid.
Placode	Thickening of surface ectoderm that relates to special sensory nerves I, II, and VIII. They form olfactory epithelium and nerves, the lens of the eye, and the vestibulocochlear apparatus for balance and hearing.
Premaxilla	The part of the maxilla with the incisor teeth that is derived from the primary palate, the inferior part of the frontonasal process. Its ossification center fuses with the rest of the maxilla (from the lateral palatine processes) in humans.
Pretrematic	(trema, L., "slit") In front of the gill slit. Pretrematic nerves provide sensory innervation to the arch or area in front of their arches of origin. They are the ophthalmic division of the trigeminal nerve (V1), the chorda tympani (VII), and the tympanic nerve (IX).
Preotic	Refers to somitomeres in front of (cranial to) the otic placode that give rise to extraocular eye muscles. Postotic somites (or somitomeres) for tongue muscles are behind (caudal to) the otic placode.

Terminology—cont'd

Spinal accessory nerve	Traditionally considered the 11th cranial nerve with a cranial root accessory to the vagus nerve and a spinal root for the trapezius and sternocleidomastoid muscles. More recently thought that the cranial root has no connection to the spinal root and is part of the vagus nerve. The spinal root is the entire accessory nerve and is unique; it is not a cranial nerve and exits the spinal cord in a different location than cervical spinal nerves.
Stomodeum	Invagination of surface ectoderm that forms the primitive oral cavity and posterior part of the primitive nasal cavity.
Synostosis	The closure or ossification of sutures by the replacement of the fibrous connective tissue with bone.
Thyroglossal duct	An elongation of the thyroid diverticulum formed as the thyroid primordium descends from the back of the tongue to the front of the trachea. Initially, it has a lumen that may persist as a sinus or cyst in the tongue.
Tuberculum impar	A mesenchymal swelling on the floor of the stomodeum that, together with lateral lingual swellings of the first pharyngeal arch, forms the basis of the anterior two-thirds of the tongue.
Ultimobranchial body	An antiquated, cryptic term for the ultimate or last extension off the fourth pharyngeal pouch that develops into the calcitonin-producing parafollicular cells (C cells) of the thyroid gland. Also called the postbranchial body.

Neuron Terminology

Traditional Neuron Terminology	Terms Used in This Book
General somatic afferent (GSA)	General sensory
General somatic efferent (GSE)	Somatomotor
General visceral afferent (GVA)	Visceral sensory
General visceral efferent (GVE)	Parasympathetic
Special visceral efferent (SVE)	Branchiomotor
Special somatic afferent (SSA) (vision, hearing)	Special sensory
Special visceral afferent (SVA) (taste, smell)	Special sensory

APPENDIX

SUMMARY OF COMMON CONGENITAL ANOMALIES THROUGHOUT THE BODY AND THEIR EMBRYONIC CAUSES

Condition	Embryological Basis
Anencephaly	Absence of part of the brain from a neurulation defect where the neural tube does not close and the overlying skull is not able to form. It is the head equivalent of spina bifida with myelocele.
Anular pancreas	A pancreatic head that encircles the duodenum when the ventral pancreatic bud improperly migrates around both sides of the abdominal foregut tube to fuse with the dorsal pancreatic bud and trails pancreatic tissue along its bifid path.
Bladder-rectum fistula	Improper division of the hindgut cloaca into the rectum and urogenital sinus (bladder, urethra, and related glands).
Bicornuate uterus	Bifid uterus ("two horns") that develops from the left and right paramesonephric (Müllerian) ducts in addition to the fused uterovaginal primordium. Other abnormalities of the uterus and vagina result from improper development of the uterovaginal primordium and/or one or both of the ducts.
Cleft lip/primary palate	Failure of the lower part of the frontonasal process (intermaxillary segment with its median palatine process) to fuse with the maxillary part of the first pharyngeal arch. It can be unilateral or bilateral.
Cleft secondary palate	Failure of the lateral palatine processes of the maxillary part of the first pharyngeal arch to fuse with each other and/or the nasal septum.
Coloboma of the eye	Failure of closure of the ventral cleft in the optic cup. Can result in anything from a small defect in the iris to large gaps in the iris, ciliary body, and/or retina.
Cryptorchidism	Undescended testes in the abdominal cavity or inguinal canal. Sterility results if both testes are undescended.
Detached retina	The two layers of the optic cup never tightly fuse, and the inner layer (visual retina) can fall away from the outer layer (pigmented retina).
Diaphragmatic hernia	Most often a failure of the pleuroperitoneal membranes to close off the central tendon of the diaphragm to complete the separation of the pleural and peritoneal coelomic cavities.
DiGeorge syndrome	Absence of the thymus and parathyroid gland from defective development of the third and fourth pharyngeal pouches. Results in immune deficiency from defective T-cell function. Often accompanied by first arch defects of the face and ears.
Double aortic arch	Persistence of the proximal part of the right dorsal aorta to form a vascular sling around the trachea and esophagus. The aorta and the superior and inferior vena cavae are initially paired vessels that may persist.
Ectopia cordis	A gastroschisis-type defect of the thorax where the heart extends outside the thoracic wall.
Ectopic parathyroids	Typically, these are the inferior parathyroid glands from pharyngeal pouch 3. They descend with the thymus gland, sometimes all the way into the mediastinum. The superior parathyroid glands are from pouch 4 and do not migrate very far to their adult location behind the thyroid gland.
Ectopic thyroid tissue	Located anywhere along the path of the thyroglossal duct—from the tongue to the trachea anterior to the hyoid bone and larynx. There can also be cysts in a patent duct. The foramen cecum on the tongue is the site of the thyroid diverticulum.
Ectopic ureters	The metanephric ducts (ureters) can open in many locations in the bladder and other organs. They originate from the caudal end of the mesonephric duct and are often "carried" with it to a lower position than normal (e.g., urethra), particularly in the male infant.

Condition	Embryological Basis
Epispadius	A penile urethra that opens on the dorsal surface of the penis because of improper location of the phallic tubercle relative to the urogenital sinus.
Exstrophy of the bladder	A gastroschisis-type defect of the lower abdominal wall where a deficiency of ventral mesoderm results in a lower abdominal wall defect and absence of the anterior bladder wall. The posterior bladder wall protrudes through the abdominal wall defect. It is usually accompanied by external genital organ defects and pubic bone malformation.
External auditory meatus atresia	Failure of the cellular plug in the meatus (developing in the vicinity of the first pharyngeal groove) to canalize. Often related to first pharyngeal arch syndrome, in which neural crest cells fail to migrate into the arch in sufficient numbers.
Gartner's duct cyst	A remnant of the male duct primordium (the mesonephric or Wolffian duct) in the broad ligament of the uterus.
Gastroschisis	An abdominal hernia through a body wall defect resulting from incomplete folding of the gastrula or ventral muscle migration. It can look like an omphalocele, but the intestines do not extend into the umbilical cord (they are usually to the right of the umbilical ring), and the viscera are directly bathed in amniotic fluid. The "split stomach" term is a misnomer.
Hepatic segment of inferior vena cava absent	The vitelline veins fail to form the hepatic segment of the inferior vena cava. Blood from the lower inferior vena cava reaches the heart via the azygous vein.
Holoprosencephaly	The most severe consequence of fetal alcohol syndrome (or other causes), it is the failure of midline cleavage of the embryonic forebrain. Numerous abnormalities may include a small forebrain, a single forebrain ventricle, absence of olfactory bulbs and tracts (arrhinencephaly), and facial deformities (e.g., a single eye [cyclopia] or eyes close together beneath a rudimentary nose).
Horseshoe kidney	The left and right metanephric kidneys, with their ureteric buds, fuse in the midline of the pelvis and hook around the inferior mesenteric artery as they ascend.
Hydrocephaly	Excess cerebrospinal fluid (CSF) that dilates the ventricles within the brain or accumulates in the subarachnoid space around the brain. It results from blockage within the ventricular system (e.g., obstructive hydrocephaly, aqueductal stenosis, or atresia of the foramina of Luschka and Magendie) or in the flow of CSF within the subarachnoid space (communicating hydrocephaly).
Hypospadias	A penile urethra that opens on the ventral surface of the penis. The urogenital (UG) folds fail to enclose the distal part of the UG sinus on the ventral surface of the phallic tubercle (developing penis). The UG endoderm normally connects to an invagination of ectoderm from the tip of the glans penis to complete penile urethra development.
Indirect (congenital) hernia	A patent processus vaginalis (a fingerlike extension of parietal peritoneum through the inguinal canal that typically closes) is a ready-made hernial sac. Its partial closure can result in cysts.
Interatrial septal defect	The embryonic single atrium is divided into left and right chambers by a septum primum with a foramen secundum and a septum secundum with a foramen ovale. A septal defect usually results when one or both foramina are too large and they overlap too much.
Interventricular septal defect	The embryonic interventricular septum (which becomes the muscular interventricular [IV] septum) fails to fuse properly with the endocardial cushions and the spiral (aorticopulmonary) septum. This fusion defect is in the upper membranous part of the IV septum. Holes can also develop within the muscular IV septum.
Meckel's diverticulum	Remnant of the yolk sac stalk extending from the midgut (ileum). Its inflammation can mimic the pain of appendicitis. The stalk can also be a cyst or fistula.
Megacolon	Lack of peristalsis caused by the failure of neural crest cells to migrate into the colon and differentiate into neurons of the enteric nervous system in the smooth muscle wall of the colon.
Multiple renal vessels	A by-product of the unusual mechanism of kidney blood vessel development. Most organs (e.g., gonads, muscles) trail their blood supply as they migrate. As the kidneys ascend from the pelvis, new vessels develop and connect to them at successively higher levels. The lower ones usually disappear but may persist as multiple renal vessels from the aorta and/or inferior vena cava.
Nasolacrimal duct defect	A "tear duct" that opens on the surface at the side of the nose. Results from failure of the middle part of the frontonasal process alongside the developing nose to fuse with the maxillary part of the first pharyngeal (branchial) arch. The ectodermal cleft between these swellings normally invaginates to form the duct.

Condition	Embryological Basis
Oligohydramnios	Low amount of amniotic fluid that results in fetal compression and associated deformities (e.g., Potter's syndrome). May be caused by low fluid (urine) production from renal agenesis.
Omphalocele	Congenital umbilical hernia. The rapidly growing intestines of the midgut leave the fetal abdominal cavity and enter the umbilical cord as a normal part of development. Sometimes, they fail to return to the abdominal cavity.
Pelvic kidney	Failure of the kidneys to ascend from the pelvis, where the metanephric diverticulum originates from the caudal end of the mesonephric duct.
Pharyngeal (branchial) cysts and sinuses	A persistence of the typically transient cervical cyst, which is a fusion of pharyngeal grooves II, III, and IV below the surface. Communication of the cyst with the branchial grooves and/or their corresponding pharyngeal pouches results in internal or external sinuses or fistulas connecting the pharynx with the surface.
Pharyngeal (branchial) fistulas	Communication between the surface of the neck and the lumen of the pharynx (usually at the palatine tonsil) or larynx when a pharyngeal membrane breaks down between an external pharyngeal groove and internal pharyngeal pouch.
Polyhydramnios	Excess amniotic fluid that may result from anencephaly, esophageal atresia, or other anomalies that impair the drinking, swallowing, and/or absorption of amniotic fluid in the fetus.
Respiratory distress syndrome	The absence or reduction of surfactant, a detergent produced by type II alveolar cells (pneumocytes) that reduces the surface tension required to maintain alveolar patency. It results from premature birth (before 6 months) or damage to type II cells.
Scoliosis	Absence of a somite or sclerotome on one side of the embryo. Only half of a vertebra develops, and a congenital lateral bending of the vertebral column (scoliosis) is the result. Postnatal scoliosis is caused by an imbalance in the tone of the intrinsic back muscles on one side compared with the other.
Spina bifida	Neural tube defect. It can remain on the surface (spinal cord exposed) or sink below, but not enough for sclerotome cells to envelop it. All cases have an absent or incomplete vertebral arch over the spinal cord, hence the "bifid spine."
Tethered cord syndrome	A low positioning of the termination of the spinal cord below L1 by the filum terminale that may result from abnormal secondary neurulation. May be associated with sensory and motor symptoms in pelvic organs (e.g., incontinence) and the lower extremities.
Tetralogy of Fallot	An unequal division of the truncus arteriosus by the spiral septum, which leads to four major defects: (1) pulmonary trunk stenosis (narrowing), (2) interventricular (IV) septal defect, (3) large aorta overriding the IV defect and draining both ventricles, and (4) hypertrophy of the right ventricular wall.
Transposition of the great vessels	Failure of the spiral (aorticopulmonary) septum to take a spiral path in dividing the truncus arteriosus into the ascending aorta and pulmonary trunk. The aorta drains the right ventricle, and the pulmonary trunk the left ventricle. Pulmonary and systemic circulation are parallel systems, and oxygenated blood does not get to the body tissues. Death at birth results unless there is communication between the systems (e.g., septal defects).
Trisomy 21 (Down syndrome)	The trisomy of chromosome 21 occurs most often in children born later in the reproductive years of their mothers. Meiotic division of the chromatids normally stops in the fetus, then continues just before ovulation. This may be decades in older mothers, and the length of time in arrested meiosis presents more opportunity for errors in disjunction. There are no known behavioral or environmental causes.
Urachal cyst/sinus/fistula	The urachus is a remnant of the allantois, the fourth extraembryonic membrane that extends from the bladder into the umbilical cord. A cyst will be inferior to the level of umbilicus. Urine will pass to the surface of the abdomen through a urachal fistula.

INDEX

Page numbers followed by "*f*" indicate figures, "*t*" indicate tables, and "*b*" indicate boxes.